Health Care Consumers, Professionals, and Organizations

The Milbank Readers
John B. McKinlay, general editor

Health Care Consumers, Professionals, and Organizations

Milbank Reader 2

edited by John B. McKinlay

The MIT Press
Cambridge, Massachusetts
London, England

© 1981 by
The Massachusetts Institute of Technology

All rights reserved. No part of this book may be reproduced in any form
or by any means, electronic or mechanical, including photocopying, recording, or by any information storage and retrieval system, without permission in writing from the publisher.

Printed and bound in the United State of America

Library of Congress Cataloging in Publication Data

Main entry under title:
Health care consumers, professionals, and organizations.

(The Milbank reader series ; 2)
Bibliography: p.
Includes index.
1. Medical care—United States—Addresses, essays, lectures. 2. Physi-
cian and patient—United States—Addresses, essays, lectures. 3. Physi-
cians—United States—Addresses, essays, lectures. I. McKinlay, John B.
II. Series. [DNLM: 1. Consumer participation—Collected works. 2.
Health facilities—Organization—Collected works. 3. Health occupations—
Collected works. W 84.1 H435]
RA395.A3H394   362.1′0973   81–12389
ISBN 0–262–63078–8 (pbk.)   AACR2
      0–262–13176–5 (hard)

Contents

v

Foreword

During 1973–74, the Milbank Memorial Fund, in conjunction with Prodist (New York), produced four edited volumes that drew together and organized published papers from the well-known and respected *Milbank Memorial Fund Quarterly*. In producing these four initial resource books (*Research Methods in Health Care, Politics and Law in Health Care Policy, Economic Aspects of Health Care,* and *Organizational Issues in the Delivery of Health Services*), the Fund had attempted to respond to heavy and continuing requests for accessibility and economy of the Milbank papers. The success of the four books exceeded even the most optimistic expectations, and all are now, unfortunately, out of print. They were adopted as course texts by many different health-related disciplines, were used widely throughout North America and abroad, were acquired by many university and professional libraries and were favorably reviewed in internationally respected professional journals.

The foreword to the earlier series noted that we always "planned to keep this series active and responsive to changing needs. Suggestions for future volumes will be welcome." Since their release, there have been numerous inquiries, requests, and suggestions for further volumes dealing with new and emerging issues concerning health care and social policy. The titles included in this second wave of edited volumes attempt to respond again to this widespread enthusiasm and need.

A venture of this nature has several obvious limitations. First of all, the universe from which the contributions were selected was limited to the *Milbank Memorial Fund Quarterly/Health and Society*, and to several books produced by the Fund as a result of roundtable meetings on particular health-care issues. However, more than enough rich material by eminent scholars was available for at least the present volumes. For the editor, a major problem was to decide which of several excellent papers had to be omitted (for reasons of economy, coverage, datedness, etc.) rather than what was available for inclusion in each volume. It should be emphasized that all of the authors represented here have progressed in their thinking and have advanced their work in other journals and books since original publication of the papers. Some have altered their theoretical orientation and some even their substantive interests. Wherever possible the editor has selected contributions published since the early 1970s. Indeed, most of the articles were first published within the last three or four years. Articles that were widely recognized as classic statements were selected from earlier years. Finally, several contributions dealt with a breadth of issues and were of sufficient quality to warrant their inclusion in more than one volume. Since each volume is likely to appeal to somewhat different readerships, this duplication was not considered problematic but rather enhanced the treatment of some health-care issues and the value of each volume.

It is hoped that this new series will help teachers, researchers, policymakers, public administrators, and especially students to overcome an ever-increasing problem: namely, how to gain easy and economical access to the rich resources contained in the recent Milbank Memorial Fund publications.

Introduction

The essays in this volume consider selected aspects of the interface between health care consumers, health professionals, and health care organizations. It is divided into three major sections. The first section is concerned with the consumers of health care—their role in policy formation, sponsorship of health programs, economic, social and psychological aspects of utilization, their relationship to health professionals and their role in the evaluation of health care activities. Rudolph Klein, in a reflection on Hirschman's influential *Exit, Voice and Loyalty* (Harvard University Press, Cambridge, Massachusetts, 1970), suggests that the challenge of health care policy is how to combine sensitivity to both consumer preferences (the economic model) and citizen wishes (the political model): What either wants the other may wish to deny him. Each model of man yields a different policy prescription. Adopting *homo economicus* tends to lead to the advocacy of competition in the health care market, unfettered by restrictive professional practices or distorting tax concessions. Adopting *homo politicus* tends to lead to the advocacy of institutional solutions to the problems of health care delivery—the use of planning and regulatory mechanisms. In the former case, it is competition that ensures responsiveness to consumer preferences. In the latter case, it is institutionalized political activity that guarantees responsiveness to citizen wishes. Klein's discussion provides an excellent background to the many issues raised in this volume.

Theodore Marmor and James Morone discuss how the health planning legislations of 1974, which established Health Systems Agencies (HSAs), had attempted to break patterns of decision making in public choices. It appears that one widely heralded strategy for controlling contemporary medical care—consumer involvement through accountability, representation and participation—is flawed by the failure to recognize that political markets are always imbalanced because of unequal interests and disproportionate resources. The authors ask how broad diffuse interests can be represented when all the incentives point to domination by a minority of intensely interested producers. They recognize that solutions favored at the local level may not best serve the entire nation. They suggest adjustment of mechanisms both internal and external to HSAs but fully recognize that their mandate reaches far beyond the possibility of accomplishment. Mark Pauly reviews and discusses a range of literature concerning economic influences on the demand for medical care and is particularly concerned with the influence that price exerts on individuals' behavior. He argues that in the field of medical care especially, price is not likely to be a pure incentive, that its interaction with other determinants of use subject to economic interpretation requires much more research and elaboration.

Ronald Anderson and John Newman present a theoretical framework for understanding medical care utilization that emphasizes, firstly, some characteristics of the delivery system; secondly, changes in medical technology and social norms relating to the definition and treatment of illness; and thirdly, some individual determinants of utilization. The authors attempt to demonstrate, through the use of empirical findings, how the framework proposed might be employed to explain some aspects of health care utilization behavior. John McKinlay and Diana Dutton attempt to move from a consideration of organizational, economic and demographic factors affecting consumer use of health services and extensively review a range of social psychological factors such as perception of need, recognition of symptoms, stress, ethnicity, stigma, alienation and aspects of the professional-consumer encounter. All of these factors appear to variously influence utilization behavior. Finally, on the basis of 1739 consumer-provider encounters in eleven ambulatory settings, Lawrence Linn investigates the relationships among characteristics of consumers, aspects of the health care encounter, and the consumers' evaluation of that encounter.

The second section of this volume includes seven papers concerning aspects of professional behavior. The first two deal with the apparent erosion of professional status. David Ermann subscribes to the view that the influence and autonomy of health care professionals have been declining in recent times—that the locus of much health care decision making has been slowly shifting from independent professionals to employed personnel of large scale governmental hospital insurance and research organizations. His concern is with what shall replace the previous reliance upon individual professional ethics to assure society that its newly powerful health care organizations are functioning in a desirable manner. The extent to which the erosion of professional authority observed in the United States is also occurring in Great Britain and the USSR is examined in the case of primary care physicians by Marie Haug. On the basis of informal interviews with health practitioners in three diverse societies, she argues that the model of the professions that bases physicians' autonomy and authority on the occupational characteristic of the monopoly of specialized knowledge is in need of some revision. Education of the patient emerged in Great Britain and the USSR as a critical factor in eroding physician authority in both countries, while patient age affected authority relations differentially in the two societies.

The next two papers deal with aspects of professional licensure. Harris Cohen analyzes the involvement of professional associations in the process of state licensure. He views licensure as an extension of the concern for self-regulation that characterizes professionalism and argues that, notwithstanding the mission of protecting public health and safety, licensure in many cases has provided a means of according status and recognition to a body of specialized knowledge resulting in a "state protected environment" wherein the profession is virtually autonomous. Odin Anderson's paper concerns Professional Standards Review Organizations as a deplorable form of "broad-side legislating," which has been introduced in advance of the development of a systematic methodology to monitor performance according to validated criteria. It is argued that this will lead to subtle sabotage of PSROs by the medical profession, justified by quality standards that are the profession's prerogative. Anderson views this as part of a move towards purely technical medical decision criteria, which ignores extenuating factors concerning the social, psychological and family environment of patients. Anderson suggests that PSROs will make medical practice even more technocratic and their alliance with administrative staffs of hospitals will allow patients even less to say about decision making. He is not sanguine about patient points of view being brought into the PSRO-type of decision monitoring.

The next three papers in this section discuss aspects of decision making. Paul Gertman considers some ways in which physician decision making may affect consumers' use of medical services. He argues that if there is some desire for control over utilization of health care then it is important to develop a better understanding of the mysterious behavior of the key decision maker—the physician—and the rationale he or she employs in guiding consumer use of health services. Jon Gabel and Michael Redisch suggest that physicians' decisions often influence the ways by which society's resources are used to achieve and maintain health. They recognize that physicians are social and economic beings, and that their behavior is in large part determined by the ways they are reimbursed. Reimbursement methods and physician preferences interact on important medical care variables: utilization of services, treatment setting, practice location, specialty choice and the efficiency of an individual physician practice. Finally, Diana Crane provides evidence that physicians respond to the chronically ill or terminally ill patient not simply in terms of physiological definitions of illness, but also in terms of the extent to which they are actually capable. Her unique study is concerned not with what physicians *should* do for the critically ill patient, but with their *actual* attitudes and behavior. The implications of the study's findings for those concerned with formulating policy and with developing ethical imperatives for research are discussed.

The third section of this volume concerns health care organizations and the way in which organizational characteristics influence professional behavior on the one hand and consumer behavior on the other. Many of the issues discussed in this third section therefore complement those already raised in the first two sections. Michael Redisch examines the physician's role in the hospital cost inflation process and the impact of hypothesized physician behavior on the expected relative success of alternative policies for containing hospital costs. He argues that the search for a single panacea to contain hospital and other health care costs is likely to be a futile one. Instead, the problem is one that will have to be solved or at least partially alleviated through a number of small discrete steps. Utilizing the physician as a lever to help contain hospital costs is one of those possible steps. Rockwell Schulz and his colleagues discuss the considerable participation of physicians in health service management that resulted from the reorganization of the British National Health Service in 1974. These authors believe that the experiences in Britain and other nationalized systems became more pertinent as the United States moves towards a governmentally financed and regulated health care system. In a careful study of seventeen hospitals, W. Richard Scott and his colleagues relate hospital characteristics to measures of services, outcome, and costs. The authors believe that their general research approach, which combines measures of organizational structure, processes and outcomes into a single design and which attempts to adjust process and outcome measures for differences in the types of clients served, is a promising new direction for future research. They caution, however, against generalizations based on their own small sample of hospitals. The concluding paper by Eliot Freidson brings us back to some consumer considerations. His paper discusses the ways in which a prepaid service, contract and closed panel practice brings a new dimension into the consumer-practitioner relationship and how physicians respond to it. Unable to manage unreasonable demands for service by use of a fee barrier, or encouragement to "go elsewhere," as in traditional solo people service practice, physicians were disturbed by a new type of demanding patient who claimed services on the basis of contractual rites and threatened appeal to higher bureaucratic authority. Here we see organizational considerations influencing the behavior of both consumers and health care professionals.

John B. McKinlay

Economic versus Political Models in Health Care Policy

RUDOLF KLEIN

School of Humanities and Social Sciences,
University of Bath, England

S TALKING THE DEBATE ABOUT HEALTH POLICY IN the United States are two models of man. The first is that of *homo economicus*: a lonely, self-regarding and rational shopper in the marketplace. The second is that of *homo politicus*: a social animal whose habitat is the world of political activity. In turn, each model of man yields a different policy prescription. Adopting the economic model of man tends to lead to the advocacy of competition in the health care market, unfettered by restrictive professional practices or distorting tax concessions. Adopting the political model of man tends to lead to the advocacy of institutional solutions to the problems of health care delivery: the use of planning and regulatory mechanisms. In the former case, it is competition that ensures responsiveness to consumer preferences. In the latter case, it is institutionalized political activity that guarantees responsiveness to citizen wishes.

Instinctively most of us probably feel somewhat uneasy about this dichotomization of man. Applying either model to the problems of health care policy seems, in many ways, unsatisfactory. The rational shopper model may capture some aspects of the health care consumer, but does not begin to incorporate the very complex patterns of behavior or the relations between providers and consumers in this field. Nor is the political model entirely satisfactory. It assumes that political

Milbank Memorial Fund Quarterly/*Health and Society*, Vol. 58, No. 3, 1980
© 1980 Milbank Memorial Fund and Massachusetts Institute of Technology
0160/1997/5803/0416-14 $01.00/0

Originally titled: Models of Man and Models of Policy: Reflections on *Exit, Voice, and Loyalty* Ten Year Later activity is a natural way of life, when we know that in fact political apathy tends to be the norm. Consequently the assumption of producer responsiveness—implicit in both models—is highly questionable. The economic model, it may be argued, neglects issues of professional dominance. The political model, it may be said, neglects issues of bureaucratic dominance. Moreover, health care has some of the characteristics of both a private and a public good: that is, it affects both those individuals actually receiving it and society at large. Thus a hospital not only benefits the patients (and staff) but also brings contingent reassurance to the surrounding population. The challenge of health care policy is therefore how to combine sensitivity to both consumer preferences (the economic model) and citizen wishes (the political model): what the consumer wants, the citizen may wish to deny him, or vice versa.

It is problems such as these that may help to explain the impact of Hirschman's (1970) *Exit, Voice, and Loyalty* since it was published ten years ago. On the face of it, the subsequent infiltration of this book into the intellectual repertory and footnotes of the health care literature may seem odd: there is no explicit discussion of health care in the book, and Hirschman has made no extended attempt to apply his insights to this particular field in his later reflections on his original work. In practice, however, the importance of his book lies in its pioneering endeavor to bring together the two models of man within the same framework of analysis: to rub together the intellectual sticks provided by two disciplines—economics and politics. If the resulting fire still burns, it is because the debate about health care policies continues to revolve—as I have sought to argue—around competing models of man. This, indeed, is why a discussion of Hirschman's work remains as relevant today as when his book was first published.

Hirschman's book starts with a puzzle. In the economist's paradigm, the response to deteriorating performance by a firm (or public service organization) is exit by the consumers. That is, consumers take their custom elsewhere, so giving the required alarm signals to the firm (or organization) to improve its product or service. If the alarm signals are heeded, then the performance will pick up again. If they are ignored, the firm or organization will go out of business, and its products or services will be provided by others. All will be for the best in the most efficient of all worlds. In reality, as Hirschman (himself an economist) points out, things do not work out so neatly or conveniently. Firms (or organizations) may actually welcome the exit of particularly demanding customers, and may tacitly conspire with each other to shuttle such troublesome customers back and forth between them. Exit may, in other words, inhibit complaints. The signals provided by exit may be ambiguous, in the sense that they may not give a precise message as to what it is that actually disgruntles customers. Such signals may therefore not provide the information required to adjust performance to consumer preferences.

So we come to voice, or what might be called political activity. In Hirschman's analysis, this is an essential complement to exit: the two models of man join hands, and the trick is to find (for any relevant area of policy) the best combination of voice and exit. Voice, in contrast to exit, is rich in information. It denies firms (or organizations) the easy and inviting option of getting rid of the most demanding customers. In turn, decisions by individuals as to whether to employ the exit or the voice option will depend on the degree of loyalty that they feel to the firm or organization in question: a high degree of loyalty is likely to inhibit exit and may encourage voice.

The optimal mix of exit and voice will, naturally, depend on the precise nature of the situation at issue. At one extreme, imagine a highly competitive market in which firms manufacture virtually identical products. In such a situation, exit may well be the response best calculated to convey the appropriate warning signals to the firm whose product is deteriorating in quality. At the other extreme, imagine (to take an example discussed by Hirschman) the public school system. Here, exit, such as switching children from the public to the private school system or moving to the suburbs, may simply reinforce the trend towards deterioration. If the most articulate parents, most sensitive to issues of quality, vote with their feet instead of engaging in voice—that is, traditional pressure group activities—then, Hirschman argues, there will be no incentive to those responsible for the public school system to try to arrest or reverse the process of deterioration. The policy implication is clear. Relying on policy models based on *homo economicus* may bring about perverse results in certain conditions, and it may be necessary to invoke *homo politicus* to redress the balance.

There are a number of problems about Hirschman's conceptual framework (Barry, 1974), and in applying it to specific policy areas. Some of these he has himself identified in subsequent reflections on his book (Hirschman, 1974, 1975). For example, the original argument tended to assume that exit would be costless and that voice would be expensive, and that there would be a consequent asymmetry in the likely reactions to deteriorating performance. But, as he himself has pointed out since, this is an over-simple view. Exit carries costs, such as the search for information or breaking the mold of existing habits (as in the case of divorce, or exit from marriage). Conversely, voice may be valued as an activity in its own right—setting aside any costs—in the sense that Aristotelian man engages in political activity because this represents his fulfillment as a human being.

More seriously, perhaps, Hirschman's neat antithesis between exit and voice does not—as Barry has pointed out—capture all the available options. It is possible to exit and, having done so, either to complain (i.e., use voice) or to remain silent. Similarly, it is possible to reject the exit option out of loyalty, but to reject voice also and remain silent. Further, Hirschman's analysis is applied to a very specific kind of situation: the *deterioration* in the quality of a product or service. But, as I shall try to argue in discussing the application of his ideas to health, it is important to bear in mind that—especially when it comes to heterogeneous services—discontent may stem from dissatisfaction not with falling quality but with the mix of types of product offered. Again, Hirschman's treatment of loyalty is somewhat sketchy: it is treated as a residual, to explain what otherwise cannot be accounted for in his analysis. Yet, and again this is highly relevant when it comes to health, the deliberate manufacture of feelings of loyalty might well be considered as a defensive strategy by threatened producers: certainly the doctor-patient relationship is highly charged with emotion and is manipulable (indeed, it could be argued that we need a model of *homo sociologicus* to complete the picture convincingly). Many services have symbolic outputs whose function is precisely to reinforce loyalty (Edelman, 1971).

These are important criticisms but, in a sense, they are beside the point when it comes to assessing Hirschman's influence. If, a decade after the publication of his book, his ideas are still bubbling away through the literature, the explanation does not lie in the formal rigor of his analytic method. His influence stems, I would argue, from the style of thought he introduced into the discussion of a wide range of issues, including health policy; he prompts interesting questions rather than providing ready-made solutions. Overall, the significance of his work has been admirably summed up by Young:

4

Hirschman's contribution to a dynamic theory of public service organization is several fold. First, he teaches us to combine our consideration of political and economic forces. Second, he isolates the key mechanisms—exit and voice—and, in so doing, puts the focus on the *clients* or *consumers* as the key element for controlling organizational performance. Third, he identifies the essential channels through which organizations receive information about, and incentives to improve, their performance. Fourth, he instructs us that when these channels are not properly structured, organizational behavior can be expected to deteriorate. (Young, 1974:52)

So it seems eminently worthwhile to make use of the insights provided by Hirschman by applying them to the field of health care policy. Specifically, to return to the point made at the beginning of this essay, what does his analysis imply for the continuing debate over whether a competitive or an institutional model is most appropriate for the organization of health care? Which market—the economic or the political—offers the best deal?

In the first place, asking such questions in the context of Hirschman's conceptual framework compels further analysis of just what we mean when we talk about "consumers" and the "product" in the field of health care. The health care market (Stevens, 1974) is characterized by a high degree of uncertainty about the product, "about which diagnostic and treatment procedures are most apt to prove efficacious." Moreover, the standard consumer strategy of seeking information through a process of trial and error may not always be appropriate in the health care market. Trading in a Ford for a Chevrolet may be a reasonably satisfactory way of obtaining information about the comparative performances of two cars; shopping around from doctor to doctor is somewhat less satisfactory, since the performance of the first physician may actually affect what the second one can do. (To take an extreme case, the freedom to shop around in order to find the most competent physician is hardly relevant to the patient who has not survived the operation by the first surgeon consulted). Lastly, the search for medical care tends to be contingent on something happening to us: so, at least in the case of sudden, acute illness, the incentives to seek information may be greatest at precisely the time in our lives when we are physically least able to shop around.

From this, it follows that—to the extent that we are concerned with exit as a corrective mechanism in the health care market—we should also be concerned to minimize the information costs or, to put it positively, to equip the shopper with the evaluative know-how required to make a sensible choice. This would suggest either more emphasis on "full disclosure" (Stevens, 1974:38) or using proxy consumer groups to generate relevant information (Young, 1974:54).

But there are a number of problems about this approach. For example, the question of how to assess the quality of medical care is notoriously contentious. There is little agreement even among the experts (e.g., McAuliffe, 1979), so that equipping the consumer with adequate information is no easy task. More centrally still, it is not self-evident that exit is necessarily an effective corrective mechanism, because of the heterogeneous, complex character of health care, which consists of delivering not only a number of very different technical procedures, but also of an environmental package (waiting rooms, hospital rooms, etc.). A consumer might well be satisfied with the technical treatment provided, but highly incensed about the quality of the environment in which it has been provided. If, then, he or she chooses to protest by using the exit option, the consequent signal to the producer is ambiguous. Exit, as Hirschman rightly stresses, is poor in information: in complex services, it provides little or no guidance as to the precise nature of the dissatisfaction. Moreover, any system of health care tends to shape the expectations of its own consumers: cross-nationally, there is some evidence (Kohn and White, 1976) that health care consumers tend to be satisfied with what they get, however different the nature of the delivery system. This reinforces the point made earlier about the capacity of health care systems to generate loyalty, and helps to explain why silence is so often the norm.

But it could still be argued that exit plus voice might provide both the incentives and the information required to persuade producers to respond to consumer wishes. Are there any mechanisms, in short, that could allow consumers both to vote with their feet and, having done so, to continue to exert pressure? The classic example of exit followed by voice in the health care market is, perhaps, the malpractice suit. However, this is generally not felt to be a very satisfactory mechanism because of its arbitrary character and its perverse effects on medical practice. For example, one study has shown that there is little correlation between the number of malpractice suits a hospital attracts and such measures of quality as are available (Department of Health, Education, and Welfare, 1973). An alternative approach might therefore be to argue for forms of consumer participation (Stevens, 1974): the deliberate creation of channels of influence through which consumers, having chosen to exit, can transmit information about the precise nature of their dissatisfaction.

The creation of such mechanisms of consumer representation may help to meet some of the difficulties inherent in relying on a strategy of exit followed by voice. But such strategy, it might be said, requires a considerable degree of altruism on the part of the disgruntled consumer: having made his exit, why should he bother to press for improvements that will benefit others? To the extent that representative bodies lower the cost of voice, by acting as proxy political activists, this objection may be weakened. Conversely, however, it could equally well be argued that the mere existence of such bodies will paradoxically weaken the incentive to exert voice because of the well-known free-rider problem inherent in all collective action (Olson, 1965). If we know that others are taking action anyway—and suspect, furthermore, that adding our voice will make little or no difference to the likely outcome—why bother to do anything, particularly when we have already made our exit? Economic man, balancing the costs and benefits, almost certainly would remain silent, though political man, with a regard to the public interest arguments involved, might decide otherwise. Consequently, it does not seem that creating new mechanisms for articulating consumer voice will necessarily solve the problems created by exit followed by silence.

So far, the discussion has been in terms of an atomistic market for health care: the implicit assumption has been that individual consumers deal with individual producers. Now let us complicate this picture (and make it more realistic) by introducing institutional providers. Imagine a city where three health maintenance organizations (HMOs) control the market and are competing for customers. Imagine also a family of three: the husband worried about a possible coronary, the wife expecting a baby, and a three-year-old child suffering from chronic asthma. The first HMO has a high reputation for the quality of its coronary and maternity care, but the pediatrician is notoriously unwilling to turn out at nights in emergencies. The second HMO has excellent maternity services and a responsive pediatrician, but its coronary care facilities are suspect. The third HMO scores high on acute and pediatric services, but low on maternity.

What, then, are the choices for the family faced with such a di-

7

lemma? If they exit from one HMO, they will only solve one problem at the price of creating another. In this situation, the consumer has a direct incentive to use voice in order to try to correct a deficiency (not, it must be stressed, necessarily to be equated with a deterioration in service provision). Unfortunately, as Hirschman points out in a different context, it does not follow that producers have an incentive to respond: a circular, and self-balancing, procession of consumers in search of the ideal package may suit all three HMOs very well. In this instance, introducing an element of consumer representation or participation into the governance of each HMO may indeed be the most effective solution: i.e., the implication would seem to be that creating mechanisms for articulating voice may be most important in those situations where exit does not provide a satisfactory option for the consumer. As this example would suggest, the problems of finding an appropriate balance between exit and voice in health care spring from the fact that consumers are not purchasing a product but a complex and heterogeneous package of very different services.

A further peculiarity of the health care market must be noted here, if only as an aside. Most consumers in the United States do not pay directly for the product or package, an obvious fact that raises an intriguing question, in the context of the kind of analysis prompted by Hirschman's approach. The literature generated by *Exit, Voice, and Loyalty* has produced, as noted above, a number of suggestions for strengthening the opportunities for voice by individual consumers. Yet this is to ignore the fact that most consumers are already collectively organized as members of insurance schemes such as Blue Cross. One of the missing elements in the American debate about health insurance, insofar as a transatlantic spectator can judge, is any discussion of the consumer *qua* consumer of insurance policies: why, in fact, insurance schemes are not considered as a mechanism for transmitting voice. If one of the problems of health care is the need for some kind of proxy organization to evaluate services and to articulate consumer voices, why not use existing organizations? The obvious answer may be that membership in insurance schemes tends to follow employment rather than individual choice. Even this answer, however, leaves the puzzle as to why there have been no suggestions, in the American context, for using insurance schemes as mechanisms of voice. Certainly the European experience would suggest that there is some scope for introducing an element of consumer representation in such schemes: for example, in both Germany and France there is a system of elections to the boards of the *kassen* or *caisses* that operate the insurance system.

To return to the main theme, however, there is a third model of health care organization that requires analysis. So far, we have considered an atomistic market of individual consumers and producers and a market with competing institutional providers. But the Hirschman framework of analysis would seem to provide a strong case for creating a monopoly provider of health care, something along the lines of Britain's National Health Service (NHS). This assertion follows from his discussion of the public school system, already cited. If a health care system combining public and private provision permits easy exit, then the result will be (as in the case of schools) to encourage precisely those with the most demanding standards to leave the public domain. Consequently, there may follow a process of self-reinforcing deterioration in the public sector—a prediction, drawn from Hirschman's analysis, that is certainly not falsified by American experience. In short, a pluralistic system will encourage self-regarding economic man to consult only his own interests, with perverse effects for the collectivity at large. In contrast, a monopolistic organization locks consumers into the system, and forces them to engage in voice—to act as political animals—whether they want to or not, pursuing the collective welfare. Moreover, voice provides the information that is essential in such a heterogeneous service as health, where the producers require signals not only about deterioration in quality but also about the appropriateness or adequacy of what is being provided.

Is the inference from this type of analysis that the United States should be moving toward the adoption of something like Britain's NHS? Not quite. For at this stage in the argument we meet again the peculiar paradox of health care: that, by and large, people like what they get, and what they are accustomed to. Despite its obvious shortcomings—poor physical conditions in hospitals, long waiting lists for some conditions—the NHS is extremely popular (Klein, 1979a). As this would indicate, it is possible not only in theory but also in practice to generate loyalty. In the case of the NHS, it could be argued that its most important symbolic output is equity—i.e., perceived fairness in dealing with people, regardless of their financial circumstances—which inhibits both voice and exit.

In turn, this would suggest that when quality deteriorates, one possible reaction is for consumers to rally to their organization. Certainly there was no evidence of an increase in exit from the NHS—i.e., an increased number of subscribers to private insurance—in Britain during the mid-1970s (Klein, 1979b) when there was much talk of a crisis of morale and declining standards (Royal Commission, 1979). Indeed, the prevailing rhetoric of crisis during this period suggests another intriguing application of the Hirschman thesis: it indicates that exit and voice may be options for service providers as well as for service consumers. In particular, a near-monopoly service like the NHS may give a greater incentive to service providers than to service consumers to use voice to articulate their grievances, a strategy frequently pursued by Britain's doctors (Powell, 1966). Such an outcome is even more likely in the circumstances of the 1980s when the choice of exit through emigration seems likely to be increasingly limited, and therefore service providers will increasingly be locked into the system. The point explains why one of the characteristics of all national health services, in all nontotalitarian countries, is a periodic confrontation between public authorities and the medical profession. Voice, in the sense of political or industrial action, becomes the main weapon of service providers.

Of course the NHS is not a total monopoly. There is, in Britain, a small private sector: about one in twenty of the population is covered by private insurance. It could therefore be argued that it is precisely the existence of this safety valve that accounts for the lack of voice from consumers, the conclusion that would be drawn from Hirschman's illustrative example of the public school system. If the most demanding health care consumers can exit, why be surprised that there is so little voice? This indeed is the view taken by the Labour Party, and explains its hostility to private practice. As against this, it has also been argued (Birch, 1975) that the possibility of exit is a necessary condition for the exercise of voice. The more tightly the consumers of any service are locked into the system, the more inhibited they will be in voicing their grievances, for fear of retaliation from the service providers; even if they are dissatisfied with the quality of the service provided, they are likely to take refuge in silence in such circumstances. One conclusion that might be drawn is that the more the health service organizations acquire a monopoly, albeit perhaps only a local monopoly, the more important it becomes to have proxy bodies capable of exercising voice on behalf of consumers who may be afraid of articulating their own grievances.

But the Hirschman thesis helps to explain at least one feature of the British NHS to which American critics (for example, Lindsay, 1980) frequently draw attention: the persistence of queues. Waiting lists are predominantly, though not exclusively, for nonurgent, elective procedures. In contrast, there is no queueing for acute conditions. And this is precisely what would be expected, on the basis of the Hirschman analysis, from the special characteristics of the private sector. The private sector in Britain does not offer a comprehensive alternative to the NHS: it concentrates overwhelmingly on precisely the kind of conditions for which there are waiting lists in the NHS, so giving paying customers a chance to circumvent the queue. It is therefore not surprising that the incentives to the NHS to get rid of waiting lists are blunted: the most exigent consumers have no reason to use voice, since they can buy exit. In contrast, there are fewer opportunities for exit in the case of life-endangering illness, and (predictably therefore) the NHS offers a better service in such cases. Also in conformance with Hirschman's thesis, the NHS is extremely poor in the provision of privacy and comfort within the acute sector; this, again, is what might be expected from the fact that those who put a high value on privacy and comfort can exit to seek them in the private market.

Using this kind of analysis also raises some troublesome questions of equity. The apparent inequity of the exit option is self-evident: it seems to provide a built-in bias toward the better off, who can buy improved services for themselves at the cost of those who cannot afford to leave the system. But the voice option does not guarantee equity, either. As Hirschman has pointed out, the ability (and willingness) to use voice may not be distributed equally among all consumers. Indeed, there is ample evidence to be drawn from the political science literature to show that willingness to engage in political activity, or to participate in civic affairs, tends to be associated with such factors as education, income, and age. So a system designed to encourage voice may have its own built-in biases as well, a conclusion that is of special relevance to health care policy, given the fact that the interests of consumers may often be in competition with each other.

The problem is, essentially, that a given population of consumers is not homogeneous but comprises four groups, with differing potentials for exit and voice:

Group 1: Voice potential high, exit potential high.
Group 2: Voice potential low, exit potential high.
Group 3: Voice potential high, exit potential low.
Group 4: Voice potential low, exit potential low.

This situation suggests that different kinds of institutional arrangements may be appropriate for different sectors of the health care system, depending on the characteristics of the consumers who use them.

Specifically, this very simple scheme shows why there are certain health service clients in group 4—such as the mentally handicapped or the elderly infirm—who appear to get a rough deal in *all* health care systems, whether the American or the British. Given the low voice and low exit potential of this group, it is inevitable that resources will be directed disproportionately to those consumers who rank high on both counts: hence, no doubt, the international phenomenon of high expenditure on the acute hospital sector and high technology to the neglect of other areas. There is no need to invoke, as so often happens, a medical conspiracy to explain this; the phenomenon is adequately explained by Hirschman's framework of analysis.

The puzzle, rather, is to explain why those in group 4—the most disadvantaged, those lacking in both market and political power—get any resources at all. To ask this question is to underline a curious gap in Hirschman's approach. The value of *Exit, Voice, and Loyalty*, as I have tried to show in these variations on Hirschman's theme, is that it is enormously stimulating, that it sparks off illuminating questions. But its limitation is that its focus is the behavior of *consumers* within specific organizational settings: economic man dominates even in political behavior (Barry, 1974)—the reconciliation of the two models of man remains somehow incomplete, even though Hirschman has used his approach to analyze the behavior of voters and governments. Yet, as argued earlier, we are interested in health care not only as consumers, actual or potential. We may also be interested as citizens who happen to believe that adequate and comprehensive health services for all sections of the population are a public good. In a sense, therefore, although Hirschman allows us to understand better the politics of the health care arena, he does not help us as much to understand the political market in which decisions about health care are taken. Yet, in many ways, this is the crucial issue. Hirschman's work has sensitized us to the problems involved in designing the mechanisms required within the health care arena, or any other organizational arena. But the introduction of those mechanisms will depend on political decisions taken outside the health care arena. So perhaps we still need another volume from Hirschman: the politics of exit, voice, and loyalty.

References

Barry, B. 1974. Review article: *Exit, Voice, and Loyalty*. *British Journal of Political Science* 4:79–107.

Birch, A.H. 1975. Economic Models in Political Science: The Case of *Exit, Voice, and Loyalty*. *British Journal of Political Science* 5:69–92.

Department of Health, Education, and Welfare. 1973. *Medical Malpractice: Report of the Secretary's Commission on Medical Malpractice*. Washington, D.C.: U.S. Government Printing Office.

Edelman, M. 1971. *Politics as Symbolic Action*. New York: Academic Press.

Hirschman, A.O. 1970. *Exit, Voice, and Loyalty*. Cambridge, Mass.: Harvard University Press.

———. 1974. *Exit, Voice, and Loyalty:* Further Reflections and a Survey of Recent Contributions. *Social Science Information* 13(1):7–26.

———. 1975. Exit and Voice: Some Further Distinctions (unpublished). A shortened version appeared as "Discussion," *American Economic Review* 66(2) (May 1976):386–389.

Klein, R. 1979a. Public Opinion and the National Health Service. *British Medical Journal* (12 May):1296–1297.

———. 1979b. Ideology, Class and the National Health Service. *Journal of Health Politics, Policy and Law* 4(3):464–490.

Kohn, R., and White, K.L., eds. 1976. *Health Care: An International Study*. Oxford: Oxford University Press.

Lindsay, C.M. 1980. *National Health Issues: The British Experience*. New York: Hoffmann-La Roche, Inc.

McAuliffe, W.E. 1979. Measuring the Quality of Medical Care.

Milbank Memorial Fund Quarterly/Health and Society 57 (Winter): 95–117.

Olson, M. 1965. *The Logic of Collective Action.* Cambridge, Mass.: Harvard University Press.

Powell, E. 1966. *Medicine and Politics.* London: Pitman Medical.

Royal Commission on the National Health Service. 1979. *Report.* London: Her Majesty's Stationery Office.

Stevens, C.M. 1974. Voice in Medical-Care Markets: "Consumer Participation." *Social Science Information* 13(3):33–48.

Young, D.R. 1974. Exit and Voice in the Organisation of Public Services. *Social Science Information* 13(3):49–65.

Address correspondence to: Professor Rudolf Klein, School of Humanities and Social Sciences, University of Bath, Claverton Down, Bath, BA2 7AY, England.

Representing Consumer Interests: Imbalanced Markets, Health Planning, and the HSAs

THEODORE R. MARMOR and
JAMES A. MORONE

Center for Health Studies,
Yale University;
Center for Health Administration Studies,
University of Chicago

THE PASSAGE OF THE NATIONAL HEALTH PLANNING and Resources Development Act of 1974, PL93-641, set in motion the establishment of 205 health systems agencies (HSAs) across the country. The aims of the legislation were ambitious—to produce planning "with teeth," to cut the costs of medical care, to rationalize access, and to do so with more attention to consumer interests than was the case under earlier health planning. Many commentators expected these efforts to produce little change. Yet in some state and local areas the tasks of health planning have been taken up with fervor. Our interest is the connection between consumer representation and these health planning institutions. Our focus is on the conceptual, legal, and administrative questions raised by efforts to create HSA boards dominated by actors "broadly representative" of the constituents of each local HSA. Our aim is to untangle some of the theoretical and political difficulties that have bedeviled PL93-641's efforts to improve consumer representation.

We first set a broad theoretical background, and show why concentrated interests (such as medical-care providers) dominate the politics of most industries. Representing consumers is cast as an important attempt to break this recurring pattern in decision-making about public choices.

In the core of the paper we analyze the concept of representation

Milbank Memorial Fund Quarterly/*Health and Society*, Vol. 58, No. 1, 1980
© 1980 Milbank Memorial Fund and Massachusetts Institute of Technology
0160/1997/80/5801/0125-41 $01.00/0

and such associated notions as accountability and participation. Understanding these concepts is important in explaining why the law's clumsy efforts at representing consumers have fostered legal challenges and will almost certainly continue to fail. We describe a number of these failures and prescribe in brief outline a remedy that seems conceptually more defensible and legally more practical.

It would be naive, nonetheless, to expect the Health Planning Act to achieve a major reorientation in American medicine, even if consumer representation were successfully instituted. We suggest reasons why this should be so, emphasizing the wildly inflated expectations characterizing PL93-641 and its rhetorical promises about planning's high technology and regulatory "teeth."

Our effort throughout is to describe, illuminate, and appraise one widely discussed policy strategy for controlling contemporary medical care: local planning agencies dominated by consumer representatives. While we discuss consumer representation, its potential and limits, current pitfalls and proposed adjustments, we are keenly aware that the health planning law is in flux, that we are appraising, so to speak, a moving target. But, if our analysis is correct, the movements toward controlling medicine through planning and consumer control are crippled by flaws in both the statute and the regulations. Explaining why that is so constitutes this paper's aim.

Representation and
Imbalanced Political Markets

The puzzles of representation are exacerbated in circumstances that stimulate representation without explicitly structuring it—when there are no elections, no clearly defined channels of influence, or only murky conceptions of constituency. The politics of regulatory agencies or regional authorities provide examples. Though representatives of groups commonly press their interests within such contexts, there are no systematic canvasses of the relevant interests, such as geographically based elections provide. It is unclear who legitimately merits representation, how representation should be organized, or how it ought to operate.

Interest-group theorists address the problems of representation in precisely such political settings. In their view, interests that are harmed coalesce into groups and seek redress through the political system. Despite the absence of electoral mechanisms of representation, their conception of representation is systematic; every interest that is strongly felt can be represented by a group. At their most sanguine, group theorists suggest that "all legitimate groups can make themselves heard at some crucial stage in the decision-making process" (Dahl, 1964:137). Politics itself is characterized by legions of groups, bargaining on every level of government about policies that affect them. Government is viewed as the bargaining broker, policy choices as the consequences of mutual adjustments among the bargaining groups (Bentley, 1967; Truman, 1951; Dahl, 1961; and Greenstone, 1975:256).

The group model is now partially in eclipse among academic political scientists (McFarland, 1979; Salisbury, 1978). One criticism is significant here: groups that organize themselves for political action form a highly biased sample of affected interests. This argument recalls Schattschneider's (1960:34) classic epigram: "The flaw in the pluralist heaven is that the heavenly chorus sings with a strong upper-class accent. Probably about 90 percent of the people cannot get into the pressure system." Furthermore, that bias is predictable and recurs on almost every level of the political process. We refer to it as a tendency toward imbalanced political markets.

Political markets are imbalanced in part because organizing for political action is difficult and costly. Even if considerable benefits are at stake, potential beneficiaries may choose not to pursue them. If collective goods are involved (that is, if they are shared among members of a group, regardless of the costs any one member paid to attain them, like clean air or a tariff), potential beneficiaries often let other members of the collectivity pay the costs, and simply enjoy the benefits—the classic "free-rider" problem.

Free riders aside, the probability of political action can be expected to vary with the incentives. If either the benefits or the costs of political action are concentrated, political action is more likely. A tax or a tariff on tea, for example, clearly and significantly affects the tea industry. To tea consumers, the tax is of marginal importance, a few dollars a year perhaps. Clearly those in the industry, with their livelihood at issue, are more likely to organize for political action. And even such concentrated interests are not likely to act if the expected benefits do not significantly outweigh the costs. As Wilson (1973:318) has phrased it, "The clearer the material incentives of the organization's member, the more prompt, focused and vigorous the action." (See also Marmor and Wittman, 1976.) From de Toqueville to David Truman, observers of American politics have argued that threats to occupational status are the most common stimulants to political action. If the group model overstated the facility and extent of group organization, some of its proponents isolated the most significant element: narrow, concentrated, producer interests are more likely to pay the costs of political action than broad, diffuse, consumer interests.

Not only do concentrated interests have a larger incentive to engage in political action, but they also act with two significant advantages. First, they typically have ongoing organizations, with staff and other resources already in place. This dramatically lowers the marginal cost of political action. Second, most economic organizations have an expertise that rivals that of other political interests, even government agencies and regulators. Their superior grasp (and sometimes even monopoly) of relevant information easily translates into political influence. The more technical an area, the more powerful the advantage, but it is almost always present to some extent.

In sum, two phenomena work to imbalance political markets: unequal interests and disproportionate resources. The two are interrelated: groups with more at stake will invest more to secure an outcome. However, the distinction warrants emphasis for it has important policy implications. Attempts to stimulate countervailing powers, by making resources available to subordinate groups, are doomed to fail if they do not account for differing incentives to employ them. For example, even a resource such as equal access to policy makers—now the object of considerable political effort—is meaningless if the incen-

tives to utilize it over time are grossly unequal. The reverse case—
equal interests, unequal resources—is too obvious to require comment. But that clarity should not obscure the fact that imbalanced
markets pose an even greater dilemma than the obvious inequality of
group resources.

Naturally, diffuse interests are not always somnolent. There are
purposive as well as material incentives to political action. A revolt
against a sales tax might necessitate cuts in programs that benefit
specific groups—scattered taxpayers defeating concentrated beneficiaries; tea drinkers may be swept into political action (even to the
point of dumping the tea into Boston harbor). Both are examples of
diffuse interests uniting for political action. Such coalitions tend to
be loosely organized and are characterized by a grass-roots style of
politics. Since sustained, long-term political action requires careful
organization, they tend to be temporary. With the end of a legislative
deliberation, the group disbands or sets out in search of new issues.
Concentrated interests, however, carry on, motivated by the same
incentives that first prompted political action.

The conception of imbalanced political markets is relevant to any
level of government, but it is particularly appropriate in considering
administrative agencies and bureaus. The problem is less nettlesome
for legislatures. On a practical level, lobbying legislators appears only
marginally effective; analysts have generally found that politicians are
more likely to follow their own opinions or the apparent desires of
their constituency (Schattschneider, 1935; Bauer et al., 1963; Marmor,
1973; Eulau and Prewitt, 1973). More important, there is at least a
formal representation of every citizen. Of course, this does not minimize the complexities of electoral representation. But elective systems do afford a systematic canvass of community sentiment, however
vague a guide it may be to concrete policy.

The advantages of organized groups—whatever their extent in legislative politics—increase after a policy's inception. Such groups can be
expected to pursue the policy through its implementation and administration. Administrative politics are far less visible; they are not
bounded by clear, discrete decisions, and are cluttered with technical
details rather than with the symbols that are more likely to arouse

diffuse constituencies. The policy focus of program administration is dispersed—temporally, conceptually, even geographically. Only concentrated groups are likely to sustain the attention necessary to participate.

Furthermore, when a bureau deals with a group or an industry over time, symbiotic relationships tend to form. A considerable literature documents the range of these clientele relationships and offers the following account of their life cycle: The industry groups typically have information vital to governing; their cooperation is often necessary to program success; and, as a bureau loses public visibility, the groups with concentrated stakes form a major part of its environment, applying pressure, representing their interests, interacting regularly with the agency (Bernstein, 1955; Noll, 1971).

In extreme cases, groups with intense, concentrated stakes can use a friendly agency to recoup legislative defeats. Important decisions are made in agencies and bureaus that define, qualify, even subvert original legislative intent. Administrative processes may even grow biased to the point that other affected parties are shut out from deliberations that concern them. For example, Congress included a consumer-participation provision in the Hill-Burton Act, but the implementing agency never wrote regulations for it. When consumers overcame the imbalance of interests and sued for participation, they were denied standing. Since the regulations had never been written, consumer representatives had no entry into the policy-making process (Rosenblatt, 1978).

As governmental administration becomes more important, the imperative of balancing political markets becomes more pronounced. The difficulties of doing so are intensified by the disaggregated character of the American political process. In contrast to the British case (McConnell, 1966; Lowi, 1969), congressional oversight of the regulatory and administrative agencies has in the past been uneven and often quite loose. This pattern illustrates imbalanced political markets and its extreme manifestation, agency "capture." The notoriously weak and undisciplined political parties in America contribute to this centrifugal tendency of authority within national government (Burnham, 1978).

The issue we address is how to balance political markets in administrative politics. How do we represent broad, diffuse interests, when all the incentives point to domination by a minority of intensely interested producers? The following discussion analyzes the details of the effort to achieve this balance in local health planning according to the strictures of the 1974 law and subsequent regulation: agencies governed by representative boards ostensibly dominated by consumers. We suggest how clearly understanding and properly institutionalizing the concept of representation can help formulate measures to overcome the tendencies toward imbalance that would normally subvert such efforts.

Consumer Representation and HSAs

The Health Planning Act addressed the issue of interest imbalance by mandating consumer majorities on HSA governing boards: between 51 and 60 percent of each board must be composed of "consumers of health care. . . broadly representative of the social, economic, linguistic, and racial populations" and of "the geographic areas" of the health service area.[1] The rest of the governing board is to be composed of health care providers. There was no means specified for conforming to this mandate in either the law or the regulations.

Administrators quickly discovered that achieving meaningful consumer representation requires considerably more than simply calling for it. Within two years of the law's enactment, a spate of lawsuits had been filed as various groups contended that they were not being represented; the law's ambiguity lent some plausibility to the claim of almost every group. Equally problematic was the question of who should count as representative of whom. And there were reports of public meetings attended only by providers, of consumers shut out of all meaningful deliberations, and of representatives overwhelmed by technical details (Clark, 1977). Such difficulties in the efforts to represent consumers were a major factor in the unexpected delays in certification ("full designation") of most agencies; confusion about or

---

[1] PL93-641 §1512(b)(3)(C)(i).

repudiation of consumer dominance has actually led to decertification in several instances. Not all the agencies have experienced such troubles, but where HSA success has been achieved, it occurs despite the federal law and its regulations.

Establishing representation requires making fundamental choices. Decisions must be made about the selection of representatives, what those representatives should be like, and the expectations that govern their behavior. Furthermore, the governmental structures within which representatives operate must be considered. Do they encourage or impede effective representation? Is the tendency toward political imbalance redressed? Finally, there is the issue of who is to be represented, a question particularly significant when geographic representation is supplemented or abandoned.

The character and success of consumer representation is contingent on how these questions get answered. Indeed, many of the difficulties that plague the Health Planning Act follow from a failure even to consider most of them.

Conceptual Puzzles and Consumer Representation

Three factors, central to consumer involvement in PL93-641, have been conceptually muddled, both in the law itself and in the analysis and litigation surrounding it. They are accountability, participation, and representation.

Accountability. Put simply, accountability means "answering to" or, more precisely, "having to answer to." One must answer to agents who control the scarce resources one desires. In the classic electoral example, officials are accountable to voters because they control the scarce resources officials desire. Public officials are accountable to legislatures, which control funds; to pressure groups, who can extend or withdraw support; or even to medical providers, who can choose whether to cooperate with an official's program.

The crucial element in each case is that accountability stems from some resource valued by the accountable actor. Accountability is thus not merely an ideal—such as honesty—that public actors "ought" to strive toward. Rather, the resources one cares about hang in the balance, controllable by the relevant constituency.

We call the means by which actors are held to account "mechanisms of accountability." These mechanisms can vary enormously in character and in the extent of control they impose on an actor. For example, voters can occasionally exert control with a "yes" or "no" decision, whereas work supervisors can regularly monitor a subordinate's work, enforcing compliance with specific demands.

There is often, to be sure, a give-and-take process in which actors try to maximize their freedom of action within the constraints of the formal mechanisms and thus minimize accountability. And those indifferent to the scarce resources in question (e.g., an official who has no desire to be reelected) are not, strictly speaking, accountable. But this illustrates the crucial point: in speaking of accountability one must be able to point to specific scarce resources, particular mechanisms that hold representatives to account.

Many of the HSA requirements that are touted as increasing accountability to the public are, in fact, irrelevant to it: a public record of board proceedings;[2] open meetings, with the notice of meetings published in two newspapers and an address given where a proposed agenda may be obtained;[3] an opportunity to comment, either in writing or in a public meeting, about designation,[4] or health system plans (HSPs)[5] or annual implementation plans (AIPs).[6]

These requirements might be said to facilitate public accounting, not accountability. Public participation and information can inform the exercise of accountability but, without formal mechanisms that force boards to answer to consumers, there is not what we call direct public accountability.

Well-defined mechanisms of accountability are central to the idea of

[2] 41 Federal Register 12812 (March 26, 1976) §122.114.
[3] 41 Federal Register 12812 (March 26, 1976), §§122.104(b)(1)(viii) and 122.109(e)(3).
[4] 41 Federal Register 12812 (March 26, 1976), §§ 122.104(a)(8) and 122.104(b)(7).
[5] 41 Federal Register 12812 (March 26, 1976), §122.107(c)(2).
[6] 41 Federal Register 12812 (March 26, 1976), §122.107(c)(3).

holding leaders to account. Propositions that substitute such notions as "winning over" or "working with" the community for an identifiable mechanism are much weaker, conflating the common-language usage of accounting for action with accountability to a constituency, a distinction pointed out by our colleague, Douglas Yates.

Suggesting that health systems agencies would be ineffective without public support is an equally weak conception of accountability to consumers. Every agency of every government expresses these expectations and fears. What is unique about representative government is that the citizenry—not the government agencies—is given the final say. And that say is not expressed by "inhospitality" or "lack of trust" or "written protests" but by an authoritative decision. What we term mechanisms of accountability are the institutionalization of that authoritative decision.

Accountability can be to more than one constituency. As health planning is now structured, the Department of Health, Education, and Welfare (HEW), state governments, local governments, consumers, providers, and numerous other groups can all attempt to hold an HSA accountable. These competing agents introduce significant tensions. One especially difficult problem is the conflict between accountability to local and to national government. There are indications that precisely this conflict is asserting itself as HEW, for example, drafts guidelines, and local communities protest that they do not apply in their specific situations. (Rudolf Klein [1979] has elaborated this argument in the British context, with elegant insight on the question of consumer participation.)

The emphasis on community control rests on Jeffersonian traditions, and has been seized upon by opponents of big government and centralized bureaucracies. Local communities, according to this view, understand their own needs best and ought, therefore, to be responsible for the policies by which they are governed.

The opposing position draws from sources as disparate as Marx and Weber, Madison and Hamilton. National needs require national solutions. What is good for individual communities (e.g., the best hospitals) may not sum to what is best for the entire nation (lower medical costs). This conception typically expresses egalitarian values—only a national policy can redistribute costs and benefits among states and regions.

Accountability in the Health Planning Act is only partially delineated, and is therefore geographically ambiguous. Since local communities establish their agency's modus operandi, the potential for local accountability is present. However, insofar as the law takes up the issue explicitly, it presses accountability to HEW.

HEW is responsible for reviewing the plans, the structure, and the operation of every designated agency at least once every twelve months (sec. 201515 [c] [1]). Presumably, renewal of designation (an important resource that HSA boards desire) is at stake. This is accountability in every important sense. But it can be traced to the public only through the long theoretical strand leading through the presidency. From this perspective, HSA boards are no more accountable to the public than is any other executive agency—certainly a far cry from the rhetoric that accompanied the enactment of PL63-641. As the law now stands, accountability to the public (either directly or through states and localities) is not prohibited or rendered impossible. But neither is accountability to the public instituted or even significantly facilitated.

Participation.   In classical political thought, self-government meant direct participation by the citizenry in public decisions. In this context, Plato envisioned a republic small enough for an orator to address; Aristotle, one in which each citizen could know every other. Rousseau argued that democracy ended when participation did. For obvious reasons, such formulations are generally considered anachronisms in modern industrial societies. Representation has replaced direct participation as the institutionalization of the idea that "every man has the right to have a say in what happens to him" (Pitkin, 1967:3). From a theoretical perspective, it is surprising that a law as concerned with consumer representation as PL93-641 articulates so few guidelines regarding representation, and so many regarding direct public participation.

The earlier discussion of imbalanced political markets suggests why direct participation provisions tend to favor providers over consumers. First, their interest in health planning is far more concentrated and obvious. Planning decisions can directly affect their livelihood. Hospital administrators, officials of state medical associations, and other employed medical-care personnel are far more likely to pay the costs of participating in open HSA meetings. The general public—"the consumers"—are not likely to do so. After all, their stake in the proceedings is much smaller; planning does not usually affect their livelihood in as obvious a way.

Furthermore, the difficulties of fostering direct consumer participation are aggravated by the nature of health issues. Health concerns, though important, are intermittent for most people. They are not as clearly or regularly salient as the condition of housing or children's schools—situations that citizens confront daily. Consequently, it is far more difficult to establish public participation in HSAs than in renter's associations or school districts (Marmor, 1977).

We are not suggesting that provisions for participation are objectionable or should be stricken from PL93-641. Rather, without being carefully tied to some mechanism of accountability or broader view of representation, the provisions are, at best, marginally useful to consumers. They are most likely to be utilized by aroused provider institutions.

Representation.   Representation is necessitated by the impossibility of direct, participatory democracy in modern society. The entire population cannot be present to make decisions. Hence, institutions must be designed to "represent"—literally, "to make present again" or to "make present in some sense something which is nevertheless not present literally or in fact" (Pitkin, 1967:8).

Three aspects of representation are usually considered in the appraisal of representative institutions: formal, descriptive, and substantive features, a formulation originated by Griffiths (1960), and refined and popularized by Pitkin (1967).

By *formal representation* we mean the institutionalization of representation—the specific mechanisms by which representatives are selected and controlled. The mechanisms need have nothing to do with what representatives should be like (descriptive), or the way in which they should act (substantive). Yet they are crucial in defining the process of representation. They are the structure through which representation is established and carried on; they define constituencies and link representatives to them. Institutionalizing accountability rests in large measure on formal requirements.

One commonsense definition of representation is purely formal. Birch (1971:20), for example, suggests that "the essential character of political representatives is the manner of their selection, not their behavior or characteristics or symbolic value." To him, elections equal representation. Few theorists would agree to so starkly formal a view. More commonly, elections must not merely be held but must offer significant "choice"—they must be "free" (Swabey, 1969; Friedrich, 1950:266 ff.). Although empirical referants are often noted (elections in the UK, not in the USSR), theorists have had difficulty in specifying precisely what constitutes "free" elections.

The most important issue of formal representation relevant to PL93-641 is whether representatives should be selected in general elections, by organized groups, by officials, or by self-selection. Though in many cases accountability to the community is increased by general elections, we do not believe that is the case for HSAs.

The Health Planning Act leaves most formal representational questions to be answered on the local level. This is not necessarily unfortunate, as long as the applications for designation are carefully reviewed regarding the issues of formal representation. These issues can be stated in broad terms by asking what constituency a representative is tied to, and by what institutional arrangements.

Descriptive representation refers to the characteristics of representatives. Early formulations of representation held that, since constituencies could not be present themselves to make public choices, they should be "represented" by a "body which [is] an exact portrait, in miniature, of the people at large." The reasoning is straightforward. Since not all the people can be present to make decisions, representative bodies ought to be miniature versions or microcosms of the public, mirroring the populations they represent. The similarity of composition is expected to result in similarity of outcomes; the assembly will "think, feel, reason (and, therefore) act" as the public would have (John Quincy Adams, cited in Pitkin, 1967:60).

A number of difficulties confront this formulation. First, "the public" is a broad entity. What aspect of it ought to be reflected in an assembly? The map metaphor is telling in this regard: Do we want the kind of map that shows rainfall, or altitudes? Topography? Trade regions? Dialects?

John Stuart Mill argued that opinions should be represented; Bentham and James Mill emphasized subjective interests; Sterne, more ambiguously, "opinions, aspirations and wishes"; Burke, broad fixed interests. Swabey suggested that citizens were equivalent units, that if all had roughly equal political opportunities, representatives would be a proper random selection and, consequently, would be descriptively representative. Whichever the case, a failure to specify precisely what characteristics are mirrored reduces microcosm or mirror theories to incoherence.

Even when the relevant criterion for selecting representatives is properly specified, mirroring an entire nation is chimerical. Mill's "every shade of opinion," for example, cannot possibly be reconstructed in the assembly hall on one issue, much less on all. One cannot mirror a million consumers, no matter which sixteen or eighteen consumers are representing them on the HSA governing board. Competing opinions or interests can of course be represented. But the chief aim of microcosmic representation is mirroring the full spectrum of constituencies. Pitkin notes that the language in which these theories is presented indicates the difficulty of actually implementing them. The theorists constantly resort to metaphor—the assembly as map, mirror, portrait. They are all unrealistic in more practical terms.

Mirroring the populace may be as undesirable as it is infeasible. Many opinions are idiotic. The merriment that followed Senator Hruska's proposal that the mediocre deserved representation on the U.S. Supreme Court suggests a common understanding of the foolishness of baldly descriptive views.[7]

Furthermore, if representatives are asked merely to reflect the populace, they have no standards regarding their behavior as repre-

[7] For notable formulations of this common idea, see Edmund Burke, "The English Constitutional System," in Pitkin (1969); or James Madison, "The Problem of Faction in a Republic," in *The Federalist,* Modern Library edition, 1937.

sentatives. Descriptive representation tells us only what representatives are, not what they do. Opinion polls would be more appropriate mechanisms for identifying public views.

Though microcosm theories are neither realistic nor achievable, descriptive (if not precisely mirror) views are relevant to the operation of modern legislatures. Legislators are commonly criticized for not mirroring their constituents' views or interests. In fact, Adams's formulation might be recast as one guideline to selecting representatives—members of the public vote, essentially, for candidates who appear to "think, feel, reason, and act" as they do. Thus, descriptive qualities inform the operation of formal mechanisms. But surely such very generally conceived descriptive representing is entirely different from the utopian endeavor of forming a microcosm of the populace in the assembly hall.

One contemporary manifestation of microcosm views is what Greenstone and Peterson (1973) refer to as "socially descriptive representation." Rather than mirroring opinions or interests, this conception proposes mirroring the social and demographic characteristics of a community's population. A precarious link is added to Adams's already rickety syllogism: If people a) share demographic characteristics, b) they will "think, feel, and reason" like one another and, consequently, c) act like one another. This is both bad logic and pernicious to the substantive representation of consumer interests.

The problems with mirror views, enumerated above, are all relevant to this version. Demographically mirroring a populace in an assembly is even more unlikely than mirroring their opinions. Obviously, not all social characteristics can (or ought to) be represented; the problem of discriminating among them is particularly vexing. Common sense rebels at representing left-handers or redheads. What of Lithuanians? Italians? Jews? The uneducated? Mirror views provide no guidelines for drawing such distinctions. Their central conception—the microcosm—is flawed, impossible. It is necessary to look beyond the logic of descriptive representation to choose the social groups that ought to be represented.

Even when the categories to be mirrored are specified, problems remain. Not all individual members of a social group will, in fact, "think, feel, and reason" alike; and they will not act with equal efficacy. Yet, in itself, mirror representation does not distinguish among members of a population group—one low-income representative, for example, is interchangeable with any other. As long as the requisite number of a population group is seated, the society is represented—mirrored—in the appropriate aspect. Such actors are not truly representatives but are mere instances of population groups.

Socially descriptive representation is pernicious because it removes the necessity of recourse to the constituency. The need for formal selection mechanisms and accountability is obviated. Skin color or income, for example, marks a representative as acceptable or not acceptable, regardless of what the constituency thinks. The result is that any member of the group is as qualified a representative as any other. This is a situation that almost begs for "tokenism." If the only requirement is that a fixed percentage of the board must be drawn from a certain group, there is nothing to recommend blacks, elected by fellow blacks or selected by NAACP, or women, elected by women or selected by NOW, over blacks and women "drafted" onto a board because they will "not rock the boat." Precisely this logic operated in New York litigation (*Aladmuy* v. *Pirro,* discussed below), where the judge found that, as long as the "quota" of minorities and poor was filled, there was nothing for him to do. He would not distinguish among them.

It has been suggested that socially descriptive representation might be effective if the representatives were tied to the groups they represented by some kind of pressure, some sort of oversight. Such representation then moves beyond mere socially descriptive representation. The selected agent is then a representative, not merely as an instance of a group's features, but because he or she is acceptable to that group. Thus, we return to a formal conception of representation—the constituency selecting a representative who "thinks, feels, reasons, and acts" as it does.

PL93-641, as it currently stands and has been interpreted in the New York and Texas district-court cases, does not provide for this. It requires only that the composition of the board be a statistical microcosm of the constituency's racial, sexual, and income distribution. The Health Planning Act does attempt to expand the health role of often overlooked groups. But, to be successful, it must mandate more than proportional representation on the HSA board; it must require that groups select and monitor their representatives.

Still, for all its difficulties, there is a kernel of truth (as Birch points out) within the theory of socially descriptive representation. Often social categories are related to interests; and, as we will argue in the following section, interests are what ought to be represented. Thus, religious affiliation bespeaks definite interests in Northern Ireland, race affects interests in America, poverty defines specific interests everywhere. And although the actual representation of interests may be subtle and complicated to evaluate, the social categories that are attached to them are almost correspondingly easy.

The choices regarding formal and descriptive representation must be made with the objective of furthering genuinely representative behavior, or *substantive representation*. This is an analytic category by which representatives can be guided and evaluated.

The central question about representative behavior is whether it is in the interest of the constituency. This raises the hoary problem of defining "interest" (Barry, 1965; Balbus, 1972; Flatham, 1966). Is it to be understood as objective fact or subjective choice? The answer determines whether representatives should be considered "messengers," simply conveying constituent desires and acting on constituent requests, or "guardians," doing what the representatives consider to be in the constituents' interest, without consulting them. Substantive representation fits neither of these extremes. Though certain choices are surely in a constituency's objective interest, regardless of their opinions, liberal institutions are ultimately structured on consent. Representatives may pursue their own understanding of constituent interest, but at some point the constituency must make a judgment. The directness of the judgment depends on the formal representation mechanisms, but that there is judgment is crucial.

There is always a danger of drift from substantive representation to simply a guardian or messenger role. In PL93-641, the former can occur, for example, when an organized group selects a representative and exerts too much control over his or her behavior. But drifting toward the guardian role is the greatest danger for consumer representatives.

Health issues are often viewed as technically complex; PL93-641 encourages that view in its emphasis on expert scientific planning. If consumer representatives are to be successful, they will need to develop expertise regarding health and planning issues, either through interaction with the HSA staff or by other means. However, as consumer representatives become sophisticated, their tendency may be to drift toward a guardian role, defending a consumer interest that is thought to be incomprehensible to the consumer constituency. This development may be aggravated when the perception of crisis gives representatives more latitude, at the expense of representational ideals such as accountability.

A related issue is the identity of the constituency. Should governing board representatives be working for the good of the community as a whole? Of the consumers as taxpayers? Of all black (female, poor) consumers? Some answers may be implicit in the formal mechanisms. The general model underlying HSA boards implicitly follows the liberal ideal of getting all the narrow, self-interested parties together and making them thrash out policy choices among themselves. Each representative works for his narrow interest group; yet, through the compromise and bargaining necessary to get his group anything, answers acceptable to all will emerge. If this is the model, then it is important that all groups be in on the bargaining process.

When, for example, lawyers for one HSA emphasize the importance of getting a board that is not segmented, they are incorrect. Ironically, the model calls for a highly segmented, even contentious, board, for a board on which every health interest is vigorously represented will be more contentious than one that is captured or dominated by a single interest.

It is also important that representatives affect policy outcomes. All representatives have some symbolic function; but insofar as they have no other, they are not substantively representative, for they give the public they represent no say over policy (Edelman, 1967; Pitkin, 1969: n.10, chapter 10).

By this logic it is clear how some representatives can represent their constituency better than others: they not only perceive what is good for—in the interest of—their constituency, but also have the ability to act successfully on that perception. An eloquent speaker, a successful operator, a person who is not easily duped, an individual with important contacts or serving on important committees, therefore provides more substantive representation than one with the same opinions but without the same capacities. There are many relevant examples from the community action programs (CAPs) of precisely this phenom-enon—boards that were relatively more successful because of the political skills, experience, and intelligence of some of their members (Greenstone and Peterson, 1973).

A representative's effectiveness, then, generally flows from a mixture of position and ability. An able person may affect policy, even from a relatively weak position. An incompetent one may fail to do so, even in a position of authority. The point is that substantive representation necessitates both knowing and successfully pursuing the constituents' interests.

Conceptual Puzzles Reconsidered. Substantive representation is the effective pursuit of the interests of the constituency. Ultimately it is the goal of all democratic representation. However, the final judge of representation must be the represented; either directly or indirectly the represented must control some scarce resource their representative wants (e.g., votes). Only then can we properly speak of a governing board as accountable to its constituency.

The Health Planning Act gives these issues little consideration. There is no systematically mandated accountability and little evidence of it as a concern. A representative's orientation is considered only in terms of socially descriptive representation. This approach patronizes the relevant groups. It will ineffectively advance consumer representation unless it is linked to effective mechanisms of accountability by which the members of those groups can evaluate the substantive quality of the representation received.

Effective Consumer Representation

This section suggests ways in which adequate consumer representation can be facilitated and effective mechanisms of accountability created. The task, as pointed out earlier, is balancing the health-planning political market, rather than just getting consumers on boards.

The HSA staffs are one resource that could help consumers

achieve political parity. Staffs generally have considerable expertise in issues of medical care and health. Occupying full-time positions in health planning, they have a concentrated interest in the industry. Is there any reason to believe that they will typically support consumers when there are conflicts of interest?

The evidence thus far shows wide variation in staffs' views. In New England, some play an outspoken proconsumer role (Codman, 1977). In many other areas they have allied with providers, often seriously undermining consumer representatives who cannot match the combined expertise of providers and staff (Clark, 1977:55). Generally the support of the staff appears to be essential to an active consumer role on HSA boards. The problem is systematically harnessing the staffs' market-balancing potential to consumer interests.

The most direct approach is to restructure the health systems agencies so that part of the professional staff is placed under consumer control—to be selected by and accountable to them. The staff's tasks could be specified in any number of ways, but its critical function would be providing professional (i.e., expert, full-time) support to the consumer effort.

Another potential for balancing the health planning market lies in organizations that already exist within the consumer population. Political scientists generally agree that the "basic units . . . of polity or political process are groups formed around interests" (Schmitter, 1975). The very existence of these groups attests to a commitment to improve the life circumstances of some part of the population. Furthermore, they have already paid the costs of organizing. We can expect their attention to issues to be high and relatively sustained. They can often overcome lack of expertise by redeploying their staff (Berry, 1977; Nadel, 1971; McFarland, 1976).

Organizations can meet a problem with more resources and in a more sustained way than isolated individuals. It is telling that much of the litigation challenging HSA boards comes from organizations formed to further the rights or general circumstances of certain disadvantaged groups within the consumer population. Existing "reform" organizations have potential, then, for balancing the health-care political market; we believe that they can play an effective role in selecting and monitoring consumer representatives.

The experience of the community action program (CAP) provides some support for this claim. Selection by groups tended to produce the most independent and competent boards. Moreover, where more than one organization wanted to select representatives for the same population or interest, elections were held among the groups. Organizations representing the poor in parts of New York City, for example, competed fiercely to gain support of the community—a far cry from the apathy that greeted general elections, and the alienation and cynicism that accompanied selection of representatives by officials (Greenstone and Peterson, 1973).

We recommend, therefore, that those charged with selecting members of consumer boards select not the members themselves, but groups organized around health-care interests. If more than one group seeks to select a representative for the same interest, a special election would be called. It is crucial that the interests themselves (e.g., poverty, race) be specified by HEW. Competition among groups representing an interest is acceptable, even desirable; competition among interests to be represented is not. (The logic of choosing what interests merit representation on HSA boards will be discussed below.)

A potential gap always exists between an interest felt and a group's articulation of that interest; however, groups that have overcome the obstacles to organization are the most likely promoters of a particular interest. Representatives from these groups will have clearly defined constituencies, experience in organizational politics, and resources at their disposal. These attributes will help them both in identifying group interests and in pursuing them, regardless of their other characteristics. (Even minorities suing for represention in Texas were willing to accept whites to represent blacks, for example, if the NAACP selected them.)

The experience of the CAPs indicates that representatives selected in this way tend to be the most able, show a universalistic orientation, and are least likely to be co-opted.

A group can be expected to monitor its representatives more carefully than will the general public. Thus, as long as the representatives are chosen for a fixed term, accountability is increased. Representatives should be allowed to serve out their term (without recall) so as not to bind them too tightly to the selecting organization (Lipsky and

Lounds, 1976:107); they should be permitted reelection so that they are not bound too loosely.

Ideally, then, the imbalanced political market in health planning will be tempered by two mechanisms, one internal to the health systems agency (staff assigned to the consumer representatives), the other external (selection of representatives by groups). We expect the former to facilitate organization and expertise among the consumer representatives, the latter to improve representation and heighten their accountability.

Of course, in some locations and for some interests it will be impossible to find appropriate groups. In these cases, another, less desirable, mode of selection (or formal representation) will be necessary. We evaluate two others: general election, and selection by officials.

General Elections.   Various reform groups have called for election of consumer representatives in a model roughly based on that for the selection of school boards. The surface plausibility of the proposal should not be permitted to obscure its difficulties. One problem with direct election of representatives to HSA boards stems from the failure of most Americans to consider themselves part of an ongoing health-care community. They typically seek care sporadically, and do not conceive of health care in terms of local systems. Both factors distinguish health planning from education or housing issues, where specific elections may be more effective.

Evidence from the CAP poverty programs supports the view that elections are problematic; fewer than 3 percent of the eligible population voted for local CAP boards in Philadelphia, fewer than 1 percent voted in Los Angeles. Those who did vote were moved to do so by personal, not policy, considerations. Overwhelmingly, they voted for their neighbors and, presumably, personal acquaintances. The consequent policy formulated by these representatives was, predictably, overwhelmingly particularistic. It helped their friends, not the community or the interests they ostensibly represented. Representatives generated little community interest or support. They tended to be ineffective advocates and operators.

Since the public chooses its health planning representatives directly, the representatives can theoretically be held accountable with relative ease. However, in practice, low incentives and marginal visibility will undermine elections.

It is important to note that "antiparticipation" city officials, who could not control the selection of CAP boards, preferred elections as the alternative. They apparently felt that this formal mechanism would not threaten their interests by generating energetic, aggressive representation of the interests of poor people—an outcome they feared from selection by groups.

Selection by Local Officials. This mechanism leaves accountability to the public very tenuous. The constituency is left with no direct control over its representatives, but must hold the selector of the representatives to account. In the worst cases, the selector is not directly accountable to the public either. Boards selected by local officials are accountable to, and presumably controlled by, local government; they will be as accountable as any other local agency. Yet they operate within a program that promises direct consumer participation. When a health planning issue becomes highly visible, we expect this mismatch of rhetoric and reality to cause public frustration and alienation.

Since officials can choose whichever member of a group they desire, many will choose ones that "make no trouble." Thus descriptive representation (what representatives "think, feel, and reason") will probably be low even when socially descriptive representation is high.

Substantive representation will generally be low. The HSA, over time, will become indistinguishable from other agencies in the local health-care bureaucracy.

Who Should Be Represented?

We now turn from the means of securing effective consumer representation to the issue of who should be represented. Which elements of the consumer population merit health representation?

The notion of dividing up the consumer population for the purpose of representation implies that there are subgroups of the consumer population with distinctive health care interests that ought to be represented.

Only one subcategory has been precisely delineated in PL93-641—those individuals who live in nonmetropolitan areas. Their representation on the board must reflect the proportion of nonmetropolitan residents in the health service area.[8] As for the rest, PL93-641 says only that consumers should be "broadly representative of the social, economic, linguistic, and racial population" of the area.[9]

Unscrambling the present confusion about representation requires an assessment of what consumer involvement is intended to accomplish. Presumably, the goal is to facilitate the articulation and satisfaction of the health care needs in American communities. If so, what is required is substantive representation, not hollow tokenism. Different health care interests in the area must be identified and selected for special attention through representation. The reason for including such groups as minorities, low-income persons, and women on the board should not be to mirror the community's population on the boards; that, we have argued, is foolish and impossible. Rather, certain groups—minorities, low-income people, and women—should be included insofar as they have different and important health interests that the political system ought to consider. The argument is most compelling when it refers to interests that are often overlooked in local political processes. Moving from mirror representation to the effort to improve representation of specified interests requires changing the language of the law requiring that consumer representatives be "broadly representative of the . . . populations" of the health service area, to language requiring them to be "representative of consumer health interests" of the health service area.

The obvious question, then, is what specific consumer health interests should be represented? The answer is not easy because interests vary by issue. Regarding questions of access to health care, the current debate has identified various groups with legitimate claims. For example, access problems are different for rural and for urban populations, or for the chronically as opposed to the intermittently ill. At the same time, there are groups that, while part of the population (and therefore potentially included on a board constituted on the microcosm principle), do not genuinely have health care interests peculiar to their own group. For example, it is not clear that those with little formal

[8] PL93-641, §1512(b)(3)(C)(iii)(II).
[9] PL93-641, §1512(b)(3)(C)(i).

education have specific health care needs or interests in the same way as the low-income or the aged populations.

As issues change, so do the interests that claim the right to a spokesman. The infirm could claim a representative for every type of disease, when the issue of new facilities arises; so could every ethnic group with specific genetic diseases that disproportionately or exclusively afflict them (blacks, Jews, Italians, for instance). The possible list is very long. However, to avoid an infinite round of litigation, HEW must make the difficult choices and specify the various consumer subgroups with recognizable health care interests that ought to be represented on the HSA boards. In this way, the present, almost infinitely broad, mandate would be replaced by one that is highly specific.

To illustrate, HEW could specify that groups reflecting the following interests be provided representation on the HSA board in approximate proportion to their number in the health service area: a) the poor; b) women; c) the aged; d) racial or linguistic groups comprising significant portions of the population; e) area of residence (the Codman Report [1977] breaks health service areas into hospital service areas—essentially, these are large catchment areas corresponding to the distribution of hospitals within a health service area. We suggest such a division of all health service areas, getting representatives from each subdivision in approximate proportion to its percentage of the total population of the health service area; f) groups that pay for medical care, such as insurance companies or unions; g) other identifiable groups that the secretary of HEW recognizes as having a health care interest and forming a significant segment of the population. Examples are migrant workers, black-lung victims, persons exposed to occupational hazards. These groups should be specified by the secretary either on the recommendation of the state or by appeal of that group.[10]

The specification of interest we propose will not only curtail the

[10] For a similar list, see Georgia Legal Services Program, "Proposed Amendments to PL93-641," Dec. 9, 1977, #3. To avoid litigation, regulations should make clear that this is a residual category to be filled at the discretion of the secretary, not a sweeping general provision mandating representation slots for all identifiable groups having significant health care interests.

stream of litigation that has sprung from the microcosm view, but will also help insure the representation of important interests. As the law stands, a great deal of discretion regarding who is represented is left to state and local political games. And while it is appropriate to maximize the competition among groups on the board regarding health care issues, it is important to minimize the competition over which interests get on the board in the first place to compete over these issues. The danger is that groups will try to take over the boards, shutting out other legitimate interests. The vagueness of the current law and regulations as to who is to be represented increases the possibility of conflict—and some of the litigation indicates that fear of further conflict is not groundless.

While the preceding discussion resolves a practical problem, it introduces a theoretical one: there is no systematic rationale by which HEW can make those "difficult choices" among affected interests. No matter which interests are selected, not all individuals are equally represented, or even equally enfranchised. How, under such conditions, can HSAs claim legitimacy as authoritative community decision-makers?

The answer is clear when there is a macrotheory of objective interests spanning the entire citizenry, such as class analyses include. However, liberal theory offers no comparable vision of fixed systematic interests. Pluralism brilliantly avoided the issue by assuming the link between subjective interest felt and group formed. Bentley is clear and adamant on this issue: "To state the raw materials of political life [—] the groups directly insisting on [a policy] . . . those directly opposing it, and those more directly concerned in it—is much more complete than any statement in terms of self-interest, theories or ideals" (Greenstone, 1975:244). Market conceptions provide little help. Although the populace is, theoretically, divisible into consumers and providers, regarding any functional area, those labels press a horde of often competing interests under a single label. As shown earlier, seating "consumer" representatives is a difficult mandate, regardless of the infelicitous mandate that boards be "broadly representative." Finally, the choices we have urged HEW to make are plausible, not Platonic ones.

This does not mean that we are without a rationale for selecting interests. Emerging groups can be legitimated or strengthened as political actors by this type of quasi-corporatist program. The most important of these may be advocacy groups speaking for broad consumer constituencies and organizations such as unions and industrial associations. They are organized and have a clear, relatively concentrated interest in the politics of medical care. Such groups are promising market balancers. Other interests (minority groups, poverty groups) can be included for similar reasons, or because it is reasonable, necessary, or prudent to include them, given the objectives of the program. Anderson's (1977) elaboration of this argument helps clarify the problem of the legitimacy of the HSA boards.

For various reasons, HSAs are structured to improve public accountability and representation. However, that structure is not relevant to the legitimacy of these agencies qua governmental units. HSAs must be viewed as a supplement to, rather than a substitute for, geographic representation. As administrative agencies, their legitimacy flows not from representational schemes, but from a legislative mandate—from Congress.

Litigation and Representation

PL93-641 was enacted in January 1975. By December 1977, it was the subject of eighteen lawsuits, five of which included the issue of consumer representation. These five cases are analyzed below in light of the preceding discussion of representation and accountability.

> *Aladmuy, et al. v Pirro, et al.,* C.A. No. 76-CV-204 (N.D., N.Y., April 7, 1977). The plaintiffs were dissatisfied with the minority representation on the Syracuse-Onandaga County (N.Y.) Planning Agency. The court ruled against plaintiffs because the representation of minorities was numerically adequate. With respect to the selection of certain minority members over others, the court stated that it would not find an abuse of discretion by the secretary of HEW except where the secretary's action was "so arbitrary as to be clearly wrong."

The case is an illustration of the application of the view of mirror representation. The court found no criterion in either the law or the regulations by which to judge representatives except for descriptive characteristics (in this case, "minority" status). Since both the representatives selected for the HSA board and their challengers satisfied that criterion, there was no way to choose between them. It was not possible to select one minority group member as any better, or more "representative," than any other. Since PL93-641 and its regulations say nothing about formal representation, challengers have no recourse and courts have no reason to insist on accountability if the criterion of socially descriptive representation is minimally satisfied.

Three companion cases can be considered together:

The Louisiana Association of Community Organizations for Reform Now (ACORN), et al. v New Orleans Area/Bayou Rivers Health Systems Agency, et al., C.A. No. 17-361 (E.D. La., filed March 15, 1977). ACORN is an association of low- to moderate-income citizens claiming that the New Orleans HSA is not "socially or economically" representative of the area. ACORN states that of thirty-nine consumer members of the board, only four have incomes under $10,000.

Rakestraw, et al. v Califano, et al., C.A. No. C77-635A (N.D. Ga., Atlanta Div., filed April 22, 1977). Plaintiffs assert that there is inadequate representation of low-income individuals and families as well as of the handicapped and women.

Califano is cited, not only for conditionally designating a board with inadequate representation of the above-mentioned groups, but for failing to "propose and promulgate regulations dealing with the composition . . . and selection process" of HSA boards. The court is asked to require Califano to devise a method of selecting consumer representatives that renders them accountable to the public.

Texas ACORN, et al. v Texas Area V Health Systems Agency, et. al., C.A. No. S-76-102-CA (E.D. Texas, Sherman Div., March 1, 1977). The plaintiffs argued that only three of the forty-one consumer representatives have incomes below the median for the area ($10,000). They argued that if people with income above the median are to represent lower-income consumers ("under specific circumstances"), then the burden of proof is on the defendant HSA to indicate how some or all of the board members with over $10,000 incomes would represent the poor.

They contend that representatives of the "public at large" do not count as representatives of the poor; this is a consequence of the model underlying their notion of HSAs, one of pluralistic bargaining among interests.

The federal defendants replied that it is not necessary to be poor to represent the poor; but they conceded that the federal regulations were inadequate, with regard both to the selection of the consumer representatives and to the representation of consumers on the board. (Note that these are precisely the charges in *Rakestraw*.)

The district court a) enjoined the defendant HSA from acting as an HSA or expending HSA funds, and b) ruled that between sixteen and twenty-five of the forty-one representatives must have incomes below the mean. Thus a strictly mathematical delineation was made, with a little "give" in it to make it "broadly" rather than "precisely" representative.

Defendant HEW has asked for a stay in the case until regulations can be developed; it will then be determined whether the Texas HSA conforms to the regulations.

Once again we find HEW mired in attempts to enforce socially descriptive representation. In bringing suit, the ACORN organizations use the mirror conception of representation to their advantage. But they recognize that it alone will not suffice to produce adequate representation of consumer interests over the long run. This realization—although present in all three cases—is most explicit in *Rakestraw*. There, HEW is sued not only regarding the "composition" but also regarding the "selection" of boards. The suit asks HEW to consider what we describe as the formal aspect of representation. Furthermore, plaintiffs demand not mere specification of a formal mechanism, but a mechanism that guarantees accountability to the public. They are, to some extent, willing to waive socially descriptive requirements in favor of accountability engendered by the selection process. The trade-off is illustrated in the Texas ACORN brief, with the suggestion that a white selected by the NAACP would be acceptable from the perspective of black interests.

Texas ACORN et al. v Texas Area Health Service Area, et al., 559 F2nd 1019 (U.S. Court of Appeals, 5th Cir., Sept. 23, 1977). On appeal, a broader view of the case was taken. The district court's undifferentiated mirror view was rejected and a full evidentiary hearing, in which HEW demonstrated precisely how board members were representative of the low-income or demographic population, was mandated. The view that one must be a member of those groups was explicitly rejected.

This ruling shows a far greater sensitivity to the issues of representation. There is cognizance of questions regarding the representatives' relations to their constituencies and the necessity of various skills relevant to achieving substantive representation. In sum, there is awareness that a mindless adherence to the mirroring ideal can undermine the effective (or—in our terms—substantive) representation of a constituency's interests.

Amos, et al. v Central California Health Systems Agency, et al. C.A. No. 76-174 ci (E.D. Calif., filed Sept. 10, 1976). Plaintiffs charged that Whites were underrepresented on the board because Fresno and Kern counties were underrepresented. HEW has sent the defendant agency a letter, noting that its governing board is not composed in conformity with the requirements of PL93-641, so this case will probably not be settled in court. The race issue was not directly dealt with by HEW but subsumed under the criticism that the representation of metropolitan and nonmetropolitan areas was not fixed in exact proportion to the population. About race, HEW said only: "The ethnic representation on your board can be reasonably readjusted when you correct its composition in terms of nonmetropolitan/metropolitan distribution."

The *Amos* case illustrates two other difficulties. First, the charge that minorities "captured" this HSA board, as the plaintiffs claimed, points out the distinction between a) giving contending groups a place on the board to dispute policy questions, and b) letting groups contend for the places on—or control over—the board. The latter defeats the purpose of representative boards: to allow local consumer interests to thrash out local health issues with each other as well as with providers.

A second difficulty follows directly from the first. Precisely who is being represented is not made clear by a law and regulations that merely mandate broad representation of the "social, economic, linguistic, and racial populations" of the health service area. Who is to determine what is "broadly representative"? We have argued that the concept of "broadly representing" (i.e., mirroring) a community is a meaningless guide to consumer representation. Instead, the interests or groups that merit representation must be specified precisely. That specification must be made with a fuller understanding of representation than is at present evident in PL93-641.

Health Policy, Health Plans, and the HSAs

HSAs face insurmountable problems completely apart from that of representing consumers. The Health Planning Act has generated expectations for reshaping American medicine that no HSA can meet. The health systems agencies are simply not equipped to control inflation, solve problems of inadequate access, or rationalize the health services of a community. In discussing why, we shall point particularly to the factors that were expected to distinguish this planning effort from previous ones—"teeth" and sophisticated technology.

Authority and Health Planning

Serious planning involves choosing goals for the future and the ways of arriving at them. One must distinguish between this sense of planning—manipulating a system toward particular goals in a specified fashion—and the writing of (often unreadable) documents termed "plans." The former requires the capacity for authoritative decisions about the allocation of resources.

How nations in fact plan for health—that is, make allocative decisions regarding future goals—is not exhaustively illuminated (indeed, sometimes not seriously touched on) by studies of how official planning bodies operate. Put another way, we have two subjects: the process of operational health planning, and the process of health planning organizations (Marmor and Bridges, 1980). The key element is the connection between choosing goals and the capacity to pursue or "implement" them. When the connection is loose—when plans are isolated from the process of resource allocation and, more generally, from authority—planning can become a smokescreen, a symbol, or simply frustrated wheelspinning.

At the same time, de facto plans will be either the choices of those who in fact allocate resources (the connection between authoritative choices based on financing arrangements and system control holds true under most conditions—including laissez-faire), or a result of the incentives operating within ongoing arrangements. The latter may be termed "change without choice" (Marmor, 1976), but it ought not be confused with the "change without influence" that is implicit in homeostatic—antiplanning—market conceptions. Such arrangements tend to be characterized, not by the theory's self-regulating market, but by the domination of identifiable actors—hospitals, nursing homes, physicians—with an unrelentingly clear incentive: "more." Thus, the well-known incentives of an American hospital are more high technology, more modernization, a fuller range of services and, therefore, more prestige, more first-class physicians, and so on. The consequences of this system are impressive technologies, rising costs, and a frustrating lack of corresponding change in health status indicators (Sidel and Sidel, 1977; Marmor and Morone, 1979). An HSA that overcomes some of the problems described above and plans for "less," will need more than its "plan" to deflect that hospital from the incentives that ideology, financing, and provider expectations have generated.

The American suspicion of centralized authority is well documented (Hartz, 1955; Shonfield, 1965). Even the sweeping expansion of government legitimacy in the 1930s included only fleeting relaxation of this resistance. Intellectually, the hostility has been expressed in two major ways: in arguments that authoritative planning or control is tyrannous (Friedman, 1962; Hayek, 1944; von Mises, 1962), and that it is not realistic (Lindblom, 1959). The Health Planning Act and its HSAs fit obviously into this tradition. Their mission is overstated, their role ambiguous, their authority and political capacity highly circumscribed. They are certainly no match for the grandiosity of their plans. Most of what occurs in local health markets is beyond their jurisdiction: the terms of reimbursement, the closing of facilities, the positive choices of places to expand. The powers they are given are widely qualified: they review certificates of need, but can only make recommendations; they are supposed to conduct "appropriateness review," but the sanctions of inappropriateness are unclear (indeed, the regulations guiding this task remain unpublished).

In sum, HSAs do not have the authority—"teeth" is the current metaphor—necessary for the tasks, such as taming medical inflation, that have been assigned to them.

The difficulties of limited authority are compounded by the uncertain relation between HSAs and the rest of government. Indeed, the brief history of the law reads like a catalogue of contemporary confusions in American federalism: local governments are spurned for the—partially new, partially redundant—HSA structures; states and counties fight for influence within the framework of the law (Iglehart, 1973). Federal guidelines are promulgated with little clarity about how seriously they will (or indeed ought to) be taken in the communities. To the confusion of the now traditional "marble cake" metaphor (M. Grodzins, cited by Sundquist and Davis, 1969:7) we can add the impermeability of "picket-fence federalism" (Hudson, 1979). Unclearly stated regulations, interagency jealousies, lack of hierarchical support, and a growing, bureaucratic, self-generating political sector (Beer, 1978) lead to confusion, and ineffective governance and planning. Within the confusion, both governmental accountability and authority are dissipated.

We are not sanguine about the HSA successes that have been reported. Logic rebels at the peculiar idea that a planning agency without sufficient authority can scheme, scold, and cajole a dynamic system into compliance with plans that run contrary to all that system's incentives. On their own terms, HSAs will achieve varying levels of success. But they will not achieve the foolish expectations that have been thrust upon them. They simply do not have the authority or the resources.

The Technological Fix

The present health planning effort promised more "teeth" than its failed predecessor (comprehensive health planning), but added few. Another well-publicized innovation was scientific planning. The Health Planning Act was presented as the marriage of community participation and scientific planning. The success of the law was seen to hinge to a large extent on the latter.[11]

The reliance on the technology of planning is the most recent manifestation of a recurring alchemy in American politics: the effort to derive objective solutions from political choices. This impulse was very much a part of the Progressives' search for the "public interest"; relatedly, the "best way" was a kind of grail for scientific managers preoccupied with achieving measurable efficiency (McConnell, 1966; Taylor, 1971).

There are of course legitimate—perhaps pressing—data needs in health delivery. Indeed, data are notoriously poor, and tend to be monopolized by provider institutions, which are predictably reluctant to share them with regulators. And, clear data sometimes have clear policy implications. For example, one Philadelphia study showed that people admitted on Fridays have longer hospital stays than those admitted on Mondays and Tuesdays with the same ailment. Furthermore, a quarter of the hospital days in the same sample were taken up by patients suffering from alcoholic and nervous disorders, both more effectively (and economically) treated on an outpatient basis (*Business Week*, 1979).

The policy implications of such findings are relatively clear, but difficult to implement. Furthermore, there generally remains the policy leap between facts and political choices—where to build a hospital, how to allocate limited resources, or, more dramatically, "who shall live." Even problems that seem objectively solvable (where to close down hospital beds) are intensely political. Ignoring the realities of political interests and value choices without some fundamental—and unlikely, undesirable—system changes is a naiveté that will result in irrelevant plans and frustrated planners.

The difference between data analysis and political choices is reflected in the odd disjunction of commentary on health planning: from Washington and academia flows an apparently steady stream of

---

[11] See, for example, the report by the Committee on Interstate Commerce and Foreign Commerce on the National Health Policy, Planning and Resources Development Act of 1974. Report No. 93-1382, Washingtin, D.C.: Government Printing Office, Nov. 26, 1974.

methodologies, simulations, and data processing advice. At the same time, reports from the HSAs deal with the different world of power struggles, influence peddling, and political choices. The language of science seems strikingly distant from the realities of local health planners.

There are some fundamental political and philosophical conflicts that the language of technology obscures. Two such conflicts are apparent in the Health Planning Act.

Federalism. The conflict between national demands and local desires was referred to earlier. When a national program invites local participation, the community will generally want to make alterations. Local residents see a different set of needs, for their perspective is different, and community politics—to recall a classic variant—involves a different cast of political actors. The conflict is resolved neatly when de facto responsibility for each part of the program is fixed at one level of government, however much the symbols or rhetoric of the program may distract attention from the outcome.

The structure of the Health Planning Act exacerbates this tension rather than resolving it. The law stimulated wide-ranging community participation, local discretion in agency design, and goals and purposes so vague that they appeared to promise significant local autonomy. However, set expectations, fixed goals, and stringent guidelines followed. With it came a furor that reflected the conflict between local participation and national goals.

Scientific planning cannot relieve this tension. Selecting problems requires choosing between values, as does the series of increasingly narrow decisions that follow. And participants on various levels of government must hammer out agreement about what those choices are. The vision of objective solutions, replicable from place to place (in the manner of scientific experimentation) is, in this context, a vacuous one.

Efficiency. A second formidable conflict lies between representing community interests and program efficiency. The constant juxtaposition of representation and scientific planning reiterates the hope that representative boards can somehow be made efficient with an infusion of "science." In reality, the phrase is an oxymoron—the juxtaposition of opposites.

The point is illustrated nicely by the Common Cause official (cited by McFarland, 1978) who was told that his organization was not sufficiently democratic and participatory. He responded that if it were any more so its efficiency at achieving policy objectives would be hampered. He was correct for a number of reasons.

First, inducing wider representation introduces conflict. This may be desirable, indicating the articulation of various interests and perspectives, but it is not administratively efficient. And much of the conflict is irrelevant to the agency's tasks, often reflecting long-standing community animosities, personal agendas, and the like.

Second, the essence of administrative superiority is the skillful gathering, use, and even monopolization of information. The resulting expertise and technical skills are complicated—often undermined—by the introduction of nonprofessional participants, particularly when they are accountable to outside constituencies rather than to agency superiors. The logic of representation emphasizes a principle directly contrary to the logic of efficient organizational management on this point.

Third, administration will be more time-consuming. Representatives reexamine first questions and basic values; they may need to consult with constituencies, delaying the decision-making process. Such problems particularly complicate long-term planning where objectives must remain fixed over time. The starts and stops of a volunteer-governed agency can make the planning process considerably rougher than one run by professional staff.

The result is that representative institutions are inherently less efficient than bureaucratic ones, even when they are properly institutionalized. In the case of HSAs, the inefficiency is more apparent because amateurs are asked to plan and regulate a technical system that has been highly resistant to almost every sort of government intervention. The litany about marrying representation and science is useless in this regard. And it even undermines the HSA effort. For each argument against the efficiency of representation is a hurdle that must be overcome if representation is to survive. And insofar as the myth of science distracts from serious consideration of a proper volunteer role, it contributes to the antirepresentational impulse grounded in the exigencies of efficient administration and planning.

Though expanded interest-representation makes administration less efficient, it is worth pursuing. There are numerous reasons for this choice, though all finally point to the permeability of policy-making institutions by the public.

First, Weber's efficient bureaucracy may not be desirable for policy bodies. The reevaluation of fundamental values, the limitations on technical vocabularies, the brakes on routinization and standard operating procedures, all make such agencies more accessible to public groups.

Furthermore, when limits to bureaucratization are removed, imbalance is facilitated. Bureaucratic agencies tend to tug issues out of politics and resolve them administratively. The bargaining process remains, but entry qualifications grow so high that only concentrated interests are likely to meet them. Administrators, with their expertise and their specialized vocabulary, grow inscrutable to any but provider (expert) groups. Public accountability is difficult, legislative scrutiny unlikely.

Finally, an open process makes it less likely that groups will be completely shut out—like the consumers suing by participation in Hill-Burton. A market open to all health system actors is more difficult to manage because conflict is introduced; the planning process grows more complicated and time-consuming. However, in a time of dwindling resources, forging a consensus among all health system actors is important to planning success.

In an increasingly bureaucratic age, representation is a more fragile value than efficiency. If the Health Planning Act accomplishes nothing more than introducing and legitimating potential market balancers on an ongoing basis, it will have achieved considerable success.

Conclusion

The vision of representation in the National Health Planning and Resources Development Act is impossibly flawed, but not irretrievably so. We have suggested one plan for achieving reasonably effective consumer representation and balancing provider dominance. But representing consumers, overcoming imbalance, even discerning the public interest on HSAs will not alter the American health system in any profound fashion. The HSA mandate—limiting costs, expanding access, and improving the quality of health—reaches far beyond the agency's capabilities. Measured by these standards, the act's program is trivial, more symbols and rhetoric than significant improvement.

Rather, the law's significance lies in its stimulation of a broad range of consumer interests. Viewed as an effort to organize communities into caring for their own health systems, it is the largest program of its kind. And one that could influence health politics long after its particular institutional manifestations—HSA planning boards—have been forgotten.

References

Anderson, C. 1977. Political Design and the Representation of Interests. *Comparative Political Studies* 10 (April):127–152.

Balbus, I. 1972. The Concept of Interest in Pluralist and Marxian Analysis. In Katznelson, I., et al., eds., *The Politics and Society Reader.* New York: David McKay.

Barry, B. 1965. *Political Argument,* chapter 10. London: Routledge and Kegan Paul.

Baur, R.A., Pool, I., and Dexter, L.A. 1963. *American Business and Public Policy.* New York: Atherton Press.

Beer, S. 1978. Federalism, Nationalism and Democracy in America. *American Political Science Review* 72 (March):9–21.

Bentley, A. 1967. *The Process of Government.* Cambridge, Mass.: Harvard University Press.

Bernstein, M. 1955. *Regulating Business by Independent Commission.* Princeton, N.J.: Princeton University Press.

Berry, J.M. 1977. *Lobbying for the People.* Princeton, N.J.: Princeton University Press.

Birch, A. 1971. *Representation.* New York: Praeger.

Business Week. 1979. August 6:54.

Burnham, W.D. 1978. American Politics in the 1970s: Beyond Party? In Fishel, J., ed., *Parties and Elections in an Anti-Party Age.* Bloomington, Ind.: Indiana University Press.

Clark, W. 1977. Placebo or Cure? State and Local Health Planning

Agencies in the South. Southern Governmental Monitoring Project, Southern Regional Council, Atlanta.

Codman Research Group. 1977. The Impact of Health Planning and Regulation on the Patterns of Hospital Utilization in New England. Executive Summary, DHEW Contract 291-76-0003. Final Report, Year 1, September.

Dahl, R. 1961. *Who Governs?* New Haven: Yale University Press.

———. 1964. *A Preface to Democratic Theory.* Chicago: University of Chicago Press.

Edelman, M. 1967. *The Symbolic Use of Politics.* Urbana: University of Illinois Press.

Eulau, H., and Prewitt, K. 1973. *Labyrinths of Democracy.* Indianapolis: Bobbs-Merrill.

Flatham, R. 1966. *The Public Interest.* New York: Wiley.

Friedman, M. 1962. *Capitalism and Freedom.* Chicago: University of Chicago Press.

Friedrich, C.J. 1950. *Constitutional Government and Democracy,* 266 ff. New York: Blaisdell.

Greenstone, J.D. 1975. Group Theories. In Greenstein, F., and Polsby, N., eds., *The Handbook of Political Science,* vol. II. Reading, Mass.: Addison-Wesley.

———, and Peterson, P.E. 1973. *Race and Authority in Urban Politics: Consumer Participation and the War on Poverty,* chapter 6. Chicago: University of Chicago Press.

Griffiths, A.P. 1960. How Can One Person Represent Another? *Aristotelian Society,* supplementary vol. 34 (6):187–208.

Hartz, L. 1955. *The Liberal Tradition in America.* New York: Harcourt, Brace, and World.

Hayek, F. 1944. *The Road to Serfdom.* Chicago: University of Chicago Press.

Hudson, R. 1979. A Bloc Grant to the States for Long Term Care. Waltham, Mass.: University Health Policy Consortium, February 2.

Iglehart, J. 1973. Health Report: State, County Governments Win Key Roles in New Program. *National Journal,* November 8.

Klein, R. 1979. Control, Participation, and the British National Health Service. *Milbank Memorial Fund Quarterly/Health and Society* 57 (Winter):70–94.

Lindblom, C.E. 1959. The Science of Muddling Through. *Public Administration Review* 19 (Spring):79–88.

Lipsky, M., and Lounds, M. 1976. Citizen Participation and Health Care: Problems of Government Induced Participation. *Journal of Health Politics, Policy, and Law* 1 (Spring):106–109.

Lowi, T. 1969. *The End of Liberalism.* New York: Norton.

Marmor, T.R. 1973. *The Politics of Medicare.* Chicago: Aldine Press.

———. 1976. Welfare Medicine: How Success Can Be a Failure. *Yale Law Journal* 85 (July):1149–1159.

———. 1977. Consumer Representation: Beneath the Consensus, Many Difficulties. *Trustee* 30 (4):37–40.

———, and Bridges, A. 1980. Comparative Policy Analysis and Health Planning Processes Internationally. Prepared for the director of the Bureau of Health Planning and Resources Development, DHEW, May 1977. Revised for *Journal of Health Politics, Policy, and Law.* In press.

———, and Morone, J.A. 1979. Innovation and the Health Service Sector: Notes on the U.S. In Altenstetter, C., ed., *Innovation in Public Services.* Berlin: Internationales Institut für Management und Verwaltung.

———, and Wittman, D. 1976. Politics of Medical Inflation. *Journal of Health Politics, Policy, and Law* 1 (Spring):69–83.

McConnell, G. 1966. *Private Power and American Democracy.* New York: Knopf.

McFarland, A. 1976. *Public Interest Lobbies.* Washington, D.C.: American Enterprise Institute.

———. 1978. "Third Forces" in American Politics: The Case of Common Cause. In Fishel, J., ed., *Parties and Elections in an Anti-Party Age.* Bloomington, Ind.: University of Indiana Press.

———. 1979. Recent Social Movements and Theories of Power in America. Paper delivered at the American Political Science Convention, August. Washington, D.C.

Nadel, M.U. 1971. *The Politics of Consumer Protection.* Indianapolis: Bobbs-Merrill.

Noll, R. 1971. *Reforming Regulation.* Washington, D.C.: Brookings Institution.

Pitkin, H.F. 1967. *The Concept of Representation.* Berkeley: University of California Press.

———, ed. 1969. *Representation.* New York: Atherton Press.

Rosenblatt, R. 1978. Health Care Reform and Administrative Law: A Structural Approach. *Yale Law Journal* part 2:264–286.

Salisbury, R. 1978. On Centrifugal Tendencies in Interest Systems:

The Case of the U.S. Paper delivered at the International Sociological Association, Uppsala. August 17.

Schattschneider, E.E. 1935. *Politics, Pressures and Tariff.* Englewood Cliffs, N.J.: Prentice-Hall.

———. 1960. *The Semisovereign People,* 34. Hinsdale, Ill.: Dryden Press.

Schmitter, P.C. 1975. *An Inventory of Analytical Pluralist Propositions.* Unpublished monograph. University of Chicago.

Shonfield, A. 1965. *Modern Capitalism.* New York: Oxford University Press.

Sidel, V., and Sidel, R. 1977. *A Healthy State.* New York: Pantheon Press.

Sundquist, J., and Davis, D. 1969. *Making Federalism Work.* Washington, D.C.: Brookings Institution.

Swabey, M.C. 1969. The Representative Sample. In Pitkin, H.F., ed., *Representation.* New York: Atherton Press.

Taylor, F. 1971. Scientific Management. In Pugh, D.J., ed., *Organizational Theory.* New York: Penguin Books.

Truman, D. 1951. *The Governmental Process.* New York: Knopf.

Von Mises, L. 1962. *Liberalism and Socio-Economic Exposition.* Kansas City: Sheed, Andrews, and McMeel.

Wilson, J.Q. 1973. *Political Organizations.* New York: Basic Books.

Acknowledgments: We want to thank Brian Barry particularly for his careful reading and constructive criticisms. Various other colleagues at the Institution for Social and Policy Studies, Yale University, and the Center for Health Administration Studies, University of Chicago, have been challenging, and helpful. And our thinking was advanced, particularly at the outset, by the writings and comments of Rudolf Klein and Charles Anderson. Julie Greenberg deserves great credit for improving the successive drafts of this article.

Earlier versions of the paper were presented at seminars at Yale, Harvard, and the University of Chicago; the penultimate draft was read at the American Political Science Association's Convention, 1979. The topics here discussed are more fully dealt with in part of Morone's forthcoming dissertation on "Consumer Representation, Public Planning and Democratic Theory."

Address correspondence to: Theodore R. Marmor, Ph.D., Chairman, Center for Health Studies, and Professor of Public Health and Political Science, Yale University, 15A Yale Station, 77 Prospect Street, New Haven, Conn. 06520; or James A. Morone, Bustin Research Fellow, Center for Health Administration Studies, 5720 South Woodlawn Avenue, Chicago, Illinois 60637.

Economic

Aspects of

Consumer Use*

MARK V. PAULY

The task of explaining the economic factors affecting the use of medical care would, in principle, be equivalent to the task of explaining all the economic influences in the medical-care market. To explain or predict use, one must know everything that determines what people will demand and everything that determines what providers will supply. Only satisfied demand and utilized supply result in actual use.

This paper does not take on the prodigious task of explaining everything but attempts instead the possibly more manageable task of summarizing and commenting on what we know and do not know about economic influences on the demand for medical care. In theory, whatever the difficulty in practice, the separation of knowns and unknowns is feasible for most consumer purchases. When we ask about demand we want to know what other factors affect the quantity the consumer would demand at a particular price. We also want to know how he changes the quantity he demands when prices change but the other factors do not. Then his use is that quantity at which, given a particular price, he demands exactly the same quantity that suppliers are willing to supply.

But with medical care the separate specification of demand influences is much more difficult, for two reasons. First, the price that

* The author benefited in writing this paper from the helpful comments of David Salkever, Jon Joyce, and Joseph Newhouse.

In *Consumer Incentives for Health Care*, edited by Selma J. Mushkin. New York: PRODIST, 1974.

is relevant to determining an individual's use, the marginal user price, is not taken by him as given, as it would be in a competitive market, nor is it even a datum to be manipulated unconstrainedly, as in a monopsony. Instead, the consumer can vary the user price he pays by purchasing customary forms of insurance. But, one way or another, he pays for price cuts in his insurance premium. Thus the user price is not parametric, nor is it necessarily equal to the price producers receive. To explain demand for care, then, one must also explain demand for insurance, for it is the latter that determines the user price.

The second difficulty arises because there is reason to suspect that the supplier can manipulate demand relationship. In the more typical economic model of an undifferentiated good, the only way a provider of a good can increase the amount that people are willing to buy from him is by lowering the price. When goods are differentiated, it may be worthwhile for a provider to advertise, though advertising is costly and not always effective. It is also an influence not well incorporated into economic theory.

But it is alleged that availability of medical care—unfilled hospital beds, physicians seeing fewer patients than they would like—affects the quantity of care a person is willing to pay for. It has that effect not because price falls, but because the physician, in his role as advisor to the patient on the usefulness of care, can almost costlessly shift the patient's willingness to pay for care, perhaps within rather wide limits. For purposes of explaining demand, we must therefore know something about the extent of persuasion or advocacy by physicians. That means that, in a very critical sense, consumers' demand for care may not be independent of physicians' willingness to provide care. So in what follows insurance and supply must be discussed to explain demand.

Taxonomy of Economic Influences

To classify economic influences on the use of medical care, it will be helpful to begin with the paradigm of consumer choice that the economist employs in analyzing the demand for other goods and services. The paradigm does more than indicate which are important independent variables; it also indicates, for some of them, the direction of their effect. One purpose of this paper will be to examine the extent to which studies of empirical reality seem to fit the "economic man" paradigm.

In a sentence, the economist's model is one of an individual who maximizes his utility subject to a budget constraint. That constraint equates his money income to his expenditures on all goods, and those expenditures in turn are the products of multiplying quantity by price. The model implies that there are four main influences on demand for any good:

(1) things that determine the "shape of the utility function," called "tastes," and are assumed to be given,

(2) money income,

(3) the price of the good, and

(4) the prices of closely related goods, either substitutes or complements.

More sophisticated versions of the model differ in several ways. First, they recognize that income is more than just money income; in addition to a money-budget constraint, a person may face a time-budget constraint. Second, and similarly, not all prices are money prices—some services have time prices and inconvenience prices, which affect demand. Third, it is sometimes useful to view the household itself not as a final consumer but as a producer whose inputs are purchased goods, services, and time of household members and whose outputs are useful characteristics. In the case of medical care, for example, one useful characteristic may be "health," and medical care may be but one input into its production. Fourth, if a good adds to an individual's ability over time to earn income, in a human capital sense, the utility of the good is the present value of the extra income it permits a person to earn.

But these extensions are fully consistent with, though they are improvements upon, the simpler model described earlier. Consequently, in what follows, influences will be characterized as having predicted effects on use that are "price-like," "income-like," "taste-like," and so on.

Are there any peculiar characteristics of medical care that do not fit in this framework? One characteristic is uncertainty—uncertainty about the incidence of illness. In the case of medical care as in other contexts, the response of the risk-averse consumer is to purchase insurance. In its purest form, insurance affects only the money-income constraint, in effect transferring income from one possible state of the world to another. The insurance premium reduces income in no-loss states, but insurance benefit payments raise income in states that are insured against. Unfortunately for simplicity of analysis, typical medical insurance does more than transfer income. It also reduces the user price of some kinds of care. The implication of these remarks is that neither money income nor the price of the good is parametric when the consumer can choose his insurance coverage.

A second problem is that "tastes" for medical care may not be fixed. The most striking illustration is in the incidence of illness. One's "taste" for an appendectomy will vary, depending on whether or not he has abdominal pain. The problem could be handled with an ad hoc rule relating "tastes" to illness, or by defining health as the output and illness as a random reduction in the stock or flow of health. A second serious analytical problem is that consumers may be persuaded by physicians or by others to like or dislike various kinds of medical care. Unless such changes can be predicted, the explanatory power of the economic theory of demand is much reduced. To the extent that physicians are economically motivated, it may be possible to predict the effect of their advice on tastes.

Finally, the market for medical care may be such that demands are not fully satisfied. Then the pattern of use may be affected little, if at all, by demand elements and may simply reflect the curious behavior of suppliers.

In the following pages each of the influences on demand—income, prices, and tastes—will be examined, with comment on the normative implications of the findings for "appropriate" incentives to seek. An area of considerable importance, and one that is as yet relatively sparsely investigated, is that of interaction effects (the point has recently been made most strongly by David Salkever, of Johns Hopkins University). At question here is not the influence of prices when income, tastes, and illness incidence are held constant, but rather how responses to price changes vary with different incomes or tastes or illness states.

We might also wish to ask whether income affects use differently at high user prices than it does at low ones. So after indicating what we know and need to know about the direct effects on use, we shall consider interaction effects as well. Perhaps the omission of interaction effects, in most empiricial work, is the result of the multivariate regression analysis customarily used by economists; that analysis typically picks up the independent effect of one variable with the others held constant, but in doing so gives no information on interaction effects.

Effect of Income on Demand

A proper definition of income would distinguish between transitory and permanent income, with the latter being a measure of the true wealth constraint implied by theory.

Even if it were possible to measure permanent income, there are additional reasons why the "pure" effect of income on demand for medical care is difficult to estimate. The incidence of illness itself may be related to income (positively or negatively), and the existence of illness surely affects income. To get a pure income effect, we would have to determine the effect of income on use for given states of health, and that effect should be separated from any effect of income on health status. In principle, some of those separations can be made by using the concept of time. Income presumably affects health not instantaneously, but with a lag (as yet not too well known). Thus, two individuals with the same present income but with unequal income in the past should differ in their use of care. Illness may, of course, have the effect of reducing permanent income more or less immediately.

Pure Effect of Income

Why should we expect income to have an effect on use for a given condition? There are two reasons, but they point in opposite directions. First, there may be a time cost whose value varies directly with income, since the opportunity cost of time would be roughly proportional to income. Opportunity cost would, however, be even more appropriately measured by the wage rate, but no study has looked at the effect severity of illness has on the response of use for persons with different wage rates. Second, as income increases, persons have more to spend. One of the goods on which they spend more could be medical care. The only goods for which use actually declines with income are those goods for which higher priced substitutes exist, e.g., steak and hamburger. There does not seem to be a higher priced substitute for medical care in general, although the use of some kinds of care—clinics, physician—substitutes—may decline with income.

Relatively few studies have used data on state of health or illness as well as income. In one study, Richardson (1970) showed that income did indeed affect use, and in the expected way; the poor tended to use less care for a given state of health. A second study by him gave less conclusive results but looked at the effect of income with only seriousness of illness held constant, and did not control for other variables (Richardson, 1971). A study by Andersen, Anderson, and Smedby (1968) also indicated that income did affect use, and more strongly in the United States, where user prices are mostly positive, than in Sweden. Unfortunately, the only indicator of health used in the study was whether a person had a symptom; the seriousness of the symptom was not considered.

Surprisingly, there seems to be no large-scale, definitive data on the use of hospitals by individuals with given symptoms that would shed light on the effects of income. While there have been some studies of the variation of use with income by diagnosis, the severity of illness for a given diagnosis has not been considered, perhaps because of the difficulty of getting an independent measure of severity. An unpublished study in Rhode Island indicates that, for some kinds of illness, low income is likely to lead to more frequent hospi-

Mark V. Pauly

talization (e.g., for pneumonia and bronchitis) because desirable home-care alternatives are less readily available (see Scott, 1973). Moreover, the effect of income on care is obscured in simple cross-tabular analysis by the positive relationship between income and insurance coverage.

When medical condition is not included as a control variable, the effect of income on use becomes twofold. It affects both health and use.

Effect of Income on Health

There are at least four separate ways in which income might affect health, where health is defined as a stock that accumulates or depreciates over time. First, and most obviously, if income positively affects the use of medical care in each time period, and if additional medical care adds to the stock of health, rich people will be healthier. Second, other goods whose consumption increases with income—good housing, good food—may improve health. Third, still other goods may not affect health directly but may improve the efficiency by which health is produced; education is the prime example, although in theory it could also be considered as an input, like entrepreneurial capacity in the theory of the firm. Finally, other goods whose consumption increases with income may reduce the health stock at any point in time—goods such as rich food or liquor or even habits, such as reduced physical exercise.

Michael Grossman's recent work (1972) and that of his colleagues at the National Bureau of Economic Research, has shed light on the relationship between income and health (see, also, Auster et al., 1972; Silver, 1972). Surprisingly, Grossman's work indicates that income in itself does not affect the stock of health and that it affects the flow of health services negatively. What does affect both measures in the appropriate way is not total income but the wage rate, which is positively and significantly related to health.

Grossman interprets that finding in the context of an investment model. Since the wage is the "cost" of workdays lost, the higher the wage the fewer workdays a person will want to lose. Consequently, he will choose a larger stock of health and the flow of healthy days from that stock. Of course, wage income and total income are likely to be correlated, since the bulk of most peoples' income is from wages. But Grossman says that in his data "these variables are not so highly correlated that the results are dominated by multicollinearity." When wages are left out of the equation, income is positively related to health.

What do these results suggest about behavior patterns? Grossman's answer is that the negative relationship between income and health may be due to the fact that higher income induces people to buy more "bads" as well as "goods" and that the former dominate. He interprets the results as indicating that health is not mainly wanted as a consumption good but as an investment good.

Taken literally, Grossman's results indicate that transfers of income (e.g., family assistance to the poor) that do not depend on work effort or that reduce the net wage rate will worsen health. Extra income allows people to buy things that are bad for them, at least those who are in the labor force, are white, and who have a record of not using sick time.

Grossman's results have two alternative explanations. The first is that those persons who have large nonwage components of income —the self-employed, moonlighters, etc.—may be in situations tending to affect their health adversely. The second is that a work-loss day provides leisure time. If leisure is a normal good, an individual will buy more of it as his income rises. Hence work-loss days will rise as income rises for a given "price" of a lost day of work. The rise occurs even if a work-loss day does not represent perfect leisure, in the sense that some illness is needed as a psychological excuse for staying home from work.

Grossman did not estimate the effect of income on the demand for medical care with health status held constant. Instead, he estimated an equation in which use of medical care was regressed on income, wage rates, age, sex, and family size. Note that no price variable was included. Here the wage rate is not significant, nor is education. Income has a significant positive effect, as it does in the "health demand" equations if the wage rate is left out. Insignificance of the wage rate probably stems from its two conflicting ef-

Mark V. Pauly

fects: A higher wage rate makes health more valuable and so induces a person to buy more care, but it raises the time cost of care, which tends to reduce use.

When Grossman estimates a "production function" for health, medical care has the right sign, it does contribute to health. But its significance is sensitive to the measure of health and to the particular set of variables excluded or included.

Measuring "Total Effect" of Income on Use

The permanent income elasticity of demand was the subject of an estimation attempt by Andersen and Benham (1970). Theory suggests that permanent income elasticity should be greater than transitory income elasticity, and their results confirm the theory. When a measure of quality is included, income elasticity of demand for physicians' services is 0.17 (i.e., a 10-percent increase in income increases use by 1.7 percent, but it is not significantly different from zero). When quality is excluded, the measure for income elasticity is 0.24.

In a study by Morris Silver (1972), the medical expenses of only currently employed persons are studied. The limitation should reduce some of the income-health relationship, since persons in very ill health (because of previously low income, for example) would not be included. Paradoxically, Silver found a high income easticity of demand in the range 1.2 to 2.0 for care as a whole, with lowest values for hospital and physician expenditures and highest values for dental expenditures. When Silver includes the earnings rate as well as income (though in his data the two valuables are highly correlated), income elasticity drops to the lower portion of the range. But because of data limitations, Silver was unable to separate out the effect of insurance, and insurance tends to be positively related to income.

Richard Rosett and L. F. Huang (1973) also estimated income elasticities that differ by income classes. They obtained measures for insured households ranging from 0.25 for those with incomes of four thousand dollars a year to 0.45 for those with ten thousand dollars a year. Feldstein (1971a) has estimated an income elasticity of demand for hospital bed-days of 0.54, using cross-section, state-aggregated data.

The results of the studies suggest that a good guess, if we had to pick a single number, would be an income elasticity of 0.5 or a little less. Note, however, that this is a "combined" or "total" income elasticity. If income does affect health status adversely (either in itself or as a proxy for wages), these measures overstate the pure or instantaneous effect of income on demand for care.

What we do not know is how the interactions occur. Theory would predict, for example, that the effect of income on use would decline as the user price declined. At the zero price extreme, people with the same utility functions would be likely to use about the same amount of care. Only Rosett estimated a "cross effect" term, which was positive and significant, suggesting the opposite. On the other hand, a study by K. Roghman and his associates (1971) indicated that differences in use remained even after people received Medicaid, indicating that full-coverage insurance did not remove all differences in use. Likewise, Andersen, Anderson, and Smedby (1968) found that income was more important in the United States, where the population is not fully insured, than in Sweden, where it is close to being fully insured. Another interaction effect is that of income and seriousness of illness. Richardson (1971) found, as we might expect, that the less serious the illness, the stronger the effects of income (and other economic influences).

Future Research

We are still ignorant about the relationship between income and the use of medical care. It appears that, as Paul Feldstein (1966) conjectured in 1965, the use of medical care does increase with income. Yet we are woefully ignorant of the pure effect of income on health, and Grossman's work is one of the few studies indicating that it may be wages, not income, that governs the relationship. There must be a more serious look at the effect of income on health, of medical care on health, and of income on use, given health status. What is clear, however, is that income transfers would affect the incentives people have to use health services.

The most important policy implications of findings about the disincentive effect of low income on use of care relates to some national health insurance proposals. One possible rationale for government interference in the financing of care is that some subsidization of care for the poor is necessary to make sure that the poor get what people in general regard as appropriate or needed care. To deal with presumably less use by the poor, several plans (Pauly, 1971b; Feldstein, 1971b) suggest arrangements in which reductions in user price via increased insurance coverage are used to offset the inability of the poor to afford care. The plans are appropriate only if lower income in fact leads to less use, and the subsidy depends in part on the extent to which use varies with income. The subsidy also depends on the responsiveness of use to price cuts. If there is no relationship between income and use, or if it is only a weak relationship, there would by that argument be no or almost no rationale for subsidization.

Tastes as a Determinant of Use of Care

The interest here is in those determinants of taste that are capable of direct economic interpretation. In this sense, they are taste-like variables, rather than the pure residual influences that the economist usually calls "tastes."

Education

Why should education affect the use of medical care? First, it may make consumers more aware of the utility and limitations of health care. The direction its effect will have on use is therefore unpredictable, since ignorance can lead to either too little or too much care. Second, education may enhance the value to the consumer of health. If he believes that care affects health, it may increase his use of care. If adjustment is made for wages, the only effect would be on consumption. Finally, as Grossman has suggested, education may enhance the "efficiency" with which the family produces health. Here its effect could be negative; education could make the family so efficient in producing health that it would use less medical care.

In most empirical studies, education and income are highly correlated, and education is perhaps better correlated with permanent income than with present income. When the wage rate was included, Grossman found that education had little effect on use. It is safe to say that we still do not know much about the pure effect of education on use.

Family Size and Composition

An individual's use of care will be affected by the kind of family of which he is a member. Although that influence is included here as a demographic determinant of "tastes," recent research suggests that in its economic influence it resembles both income and prices. If the family is viewed as a production unit that produces useful attributes employing goods as inputs, it does so constrained by the total amount of resources it has available. Those resources are obviously total family money income (and indeed family income rather than individual income or even family income per capita has customarily been employed in use or demand studies), but they also include the total amount of time available to the family and the total amount of human capital (e.g., education) available to the family as a whole. Similarly, the "price" of a unit of a family member's time in producing care for himself or others will vary with the alternative uses of his time.

The critical empirical question is whether alternative family configurations involve budget and price effects, and demand effects too, that will influence an individual's use, as suggested by a considerable amount of casual and less casual empirical evidence. Individuals who live alone, for example, use more care than others. That is doubtless because, in two-person families, one individual can produce care for the other that would otherwise have to be sought from the formal medical-care system. Other family characteristics, involving which person in the family is ill, whether the wife works and at what wages, and so on, are also relevant.

Recent economic research has begun to emphasize the "economics of the family," but relatively little has been done in health care. (The only research of which the author is aware is some yet unpublished work by Jon Joyce of Wesleyan University.) Even descriptive empirical work in the area might be very useful and have important policy implications. To give one example: There is a fair amount of evidence that hospital stays can often be shortened without adverse medical consequences and that many procedures can be done on an outpatient basis. Since such steps reduce costs incurred within the system, it is natural that many people consider desirable those arrangements that appear to produce these results, such as health maintenance organizations (HMO's). Yet in reckoning the true social cost of care, it is clear that the extra implicit costs imposed on the household must be considered. What does the household lose by virtue of the fact that it must produce care? Home care is desirable only if it "costs" less than institutional care. In the empirical studies of the advantages and disadvantages of reimbursement arrangements that reduce use, the offsetting cost imposed on the household is rarely considered.

Price and Price-Like Incentives

The economist naturally thinks of price as an incentive to encourage or discourage use. In a normative sense, the "wrong" price may provide an incentive to use too much or too little of a good. Conversely, given a definition of what constitutes appropriate use and given enough information, it is possible, at least theoretically, to design a price system that will induce individuals to choose that level of use.

While the role of price as an incentive has sometimes been recognized by noneconomist specialists in health care, there appears to be a curious sort of schizophrenic conventional wisdom in much of the policy-oriented work. Thus it is sometimes maintained that positive prices are likely to be bad because they discourage needed care, and at the same time there is an unwillingness to believe price has much effect on decisions to seek care. Recent research by economists and others has, however, increased our knowledge of the potential magnitude of price effects and has also provided some analysis of the appropriate use of prices. In both cases, research has served mainly to suggest that there are many more unanswered questions.

Why Price Might Affect Use

Price can affect use in two ways: First and most obvious is in the individual consumer's decision whether to seek care. If additional care has a positive cost to him, he will seek care only as long as he values the care he receives more than the other goods and services he might have purchased. The second way is in the effect the price paid by the consumer may have on the physician's decision about how much and what kind of care to render. The physician, acting properly in his role as proxy decisionmaker for the consumer, may decide that some kinds of beneficial care are not worth their cost to the consumer. Or a physician's orders for care may meet resistance from consumers who must pay the user price and acquiescence from those whose insurance pays the price. Even if the physician does not know the net or user price paid by a particular patient, he may adjust his behavior to an average level of the price that prevails among all his patients.

All this discussion is frankly speculative, since we know little about the precise way in which price affects the physician-patient decision nexus. In large part, our lack of knowledge is the result of a more basic ignorance about the way in which physician prices are set and the extent to which nonphysician charges affect the price the physician can get. We do not know, for example, whether a scheme in which physicians, rather than patients, were billed for hospital services would affect use and total cost to the consumer.

Mark V. Pauly

Concepts of Price

The true concept of the price that affects demand is broader than that of simple transfers of money. Obviously, what is relevant to a consumer's use of care is not the price charged for the services but the price he has to pay for them, the "user price." The higher the price charged or the greater his insurance coverage, the higher will be his premiums, but the effect of higher premiums in reducing spendable income will be spread over all his purchases and affect his purchases of medical care only slightly.

Prices can be paid in ways other than money. For many types of medical care price is the sacrifice of time, either in getting care or in traveling to a source of care, and psychological and physical pain and discomfort may be more important than money price. (Since medical insurance does not usually provide pain and suffering benefits, use is likely to be less than infinite even at a zero money price.) The cost of time is the value that time would have had in its next best use. Here again, we know relatively little about the effect of time on use, although Grossman's result of a zero wage elasticity of demand for care is suggestive, and there is currently some research being done on the effect of time costs on use.

Finally, a change in the price of a good affects more than just the demand for that good; it affects the demand for closely related goods. In the most extreme case, competition can be defined as an infinitely great cross-elasticity of demand between the price charged by one seller for a given good and the quantity demanded from another seller for the same good. Thus, the price charged by one physician or hospital might affect the demand for other physician or hospital services, and the user price in the outpatient department might affect the use of care in physicians' offices.

Effect of User Charges on Use

Common sense suggests that the more "discretionary" the type of care, the greater the effect of user charges. It is probably lack of data that accounts for the fact that most documentation of the effect of user charges is on inpatient hospital care, probably the most non-discretionary sort of care. In addition, many studies have looked at the effects that represent combinations of incentives to consumer (user charges), incentives to physicians and hospital administrators (reimbursement mechanisms), and organizational form (solo practice, multi-specialty group). As a result, it is hard to isolate the effect of charges on demand.

The difficulty is particularly marked in a series of studies begun in the mid-1950s and continued up to the present. The earlier studies have been summarized by Klarman (1965) and Donabedian (1969). Their main message was (with some exceptions) that prepaid group practices had lower levels of hospital utilization and lower inplan costs than did insurance plans that provided mainly fee-for-service coverage for inhospital procedures.

But only rarely was it possible to tell whether observed differences in utilization were the result of the way physicians were paid, the price incentives facing consumers, the mode of organization, or the characteristics of plan members. In some of the studies, plan members were matched to reduce the last problem, that of self-selection.

A more recent study of the same sort done at the University of California at Los Angeles has not been published, but some of the results were the subject of a statement by the study director before a congressional committee (Roemer, 1972). Extensive data on use and demographic characteristics were obtained on three types of plan (two examples of each): commercial indemnity, Blue Cross service benefit, and prepaid group practice. Group practices had the lowest hospital admissions, but the indemnity plan was a close second. The Blue Cross plans had the greatest use. The smallness of the gap between indemnity plans and prepaid group practice was attributed to the fact that indemnity plans covered better risks. Length of stay is, however, much lower in the group-practice plans, so that total hospital bed-days are much lower there. Ambulatory-care use is least for the commercial plans and greatest for the Blue Cross plans. Unfortunately, these gross findings have not yet been subject to multivariate analysis, so that their main cause is not known. And since only four noncomprehensive plans were studied, there will be at most only four possible values for user price.

Whatever the studies may tell us about the advantages of one particular plan over another, they do not provide answers to the general question of incentives. In addition to failing to separate effects, they are plagued by "small number" problems of two sorts. First, at best they compare half a dozen plans, surely a small sample. Second, they provide relatively few differential observations on alternative user prices. Consequently, some recent economic analyses have departed from the case-study approach in order to use larger or more diverse bodies of data.

Earlier work had indicated that higher levels of insurance coverage tended to be associated with greater expenditures in, and presumably greater use of, medical care. A recent, more sophisticated study by Martin Feldstein (1971a) used state-aggregated hospital admissions and mean stay as measures of use. Constructing a measure of user price by multiplying the gross price by an "average" measure of coverage for that state, he found that use was indeed responsive to coverage. An instrumental variable technique, not too clearly described, was used to avoid simultaneity problems.

Feldstein estimated that price elasticity of demand for hospital bed-days was about 0.67, with elasticity being somewhat greater for mean stay and less for admissions. All three are substantial elasticities and suggest that reduction from the present twenty percent to ten percent in the fraction of care costs would increase hospital expenditures by one-third. A somewhat similar estimate by Davis and Russell (1972), using similar data but a slightly different measure of insurance coverage and ordinary-least-squares regression analysis, estimated own-elasticity of demand to be 0.32 to 0.46.

A recent study by Richard Rosett and L. F. Huang (1973) used observations on coverage and total medical expenditures for individual spending units. Some ingenious methods of estimation were necessary to get around deficiencies in the data. Nevertheless, their estimates of elasticity range from 0.35 at a twenty percent copayment to 1.50 at an eighty percent copayment. Their figures suggest that, for example, going to zero copayment under a national health insurance plan from the present one-third level could as much as double expenditures.

Some other recent work, of a case-study nature, provides estimates of elasticity of demand for physicians' services (Scitovsky and Snyder, 1972; Phelps and Newhouse, 1972b). The work studied the effect of introducing a twenty-five percent copayment for physicians' services in one prepaid comprehensive group practice for employees of Stanford University. Imposition of the copayment reduced usage about twenty-five percent. The arc elasticity, using average price as a base, is calculated to be 0.14. A similar study of the introduction of a forty-one percent copayment in Saskatchewan indicated an arc elasticity of 0.13, although it is unclear whether this "use" elasticity is uncontaminated by supply as well as demand responses (Phelps and Newhouse, 1972a).

For the Stanford study, it is clear that results need not be comparable to what they would be in a more typical setting. Presumably there would already have been an incentive in that plan for physicians to keep physician use low (especially since hospital services were not obtained within the plan). Consequently, the possibilities for further reduction in use would have been limited. For the other studies, the low elasticities are a little more difficult to explain, although fixed prices might contribute to the Saskatchewan results. The results may also indicate rationing behavior by physicians, as Feldstein (1970) has suggested.

Finally, although one might have expected physician visits to be more price sensitive, the published results are certainly possible. Moreover, if the demand curve is linear rather than constant-elasticity, low levels of elasticity at low absolute prices are to be expected.

Can anything be said about the direction of bias in the Feldstein-Rosett-Huang-Davis-Russell estimates? The most serious aggregation problem arises because researchers have used an average rather than a marginal measure of insurance coverage. Since a typical policy will contain a deductible, the average fraction covered will ordinarily fall short of the marginal fraction covered. Thus, when a person with no insurance is compared with a person who has positive but relatively low average coverage but high marginal coverage, any increase in use will be attributed to the relatively slight increase in average coverage rather than to the large increase in marginal coverage. Consequently, estimates of the effect of coverage on use will be biased upwards.

The argument is correct as far as it goes, but it does not go far enough. An offsetting bias arises if it is true that marginal coverage is likely to remain high over a wide range of expenses. The change in marginal user price over such a range will be low or zero, while the change in average user price will be relatively greater. The change in expense associated with that change in average coinsurance will in fact reflect the zero or slight change in marginal coinsurance, and so a measure of the effect of coinsurance on use will be biased downward. The direction of bias in the estimate of the overall effect of coverage on use will depend on the strengths of the two effects, and there is no reason to suppose that the resulting bias will be necessarily upward.

A similar criticism is made in a paper by Newhouse and Phelps (1973); the results of Rosett-Huang's study are also properly criticized in it for omitting (because of data deficiencies) employer-financed coverage, leading to a large group of low-estimated coverage, low-estimated expenditure observations.

Insurance Effects

Another kind of omitted criticism is related to a problem endemic in all the studies of use so far completed. Results may be biased because the adjustment to user price caused by insurance is not exogenous. If individuals can choose their level of insurance coverage, potential expenditures and potential effects of coverage on use would affect the amount of coverage they buy. Even when obvious demographic characteristics are used to match populations, the fact that one individual chooses one form of coverage and another chooses a different form is evidence that they are not identical individuals. As long as insurance may affect use, the differences in individuals may likewise affect use.

There are no published studies that directly consider the simultaneity problem. Feldstein uses an instrumental variables approach rather than ordinary least squares, but it is not possible to tell whether the set of exogenous variables used to determine the instruments is the appropriate set. Attempts are presently being made, both at the RAND Corporation and elsewhere, to tackle the problem. It may be useful to consider the issues involved.

The endogenous nature of insurance can induce two sorts of bias into estimates of the effect of coverage on use. The biases arise from the problems of adverse selection and moral hazard.

Adverse selection occurs when premiums are not tailored to the expected losses of individuals. If, for example, all pay the same premium but have different expected losses (and hence different actuarially fair premiums), those for whom the premium charged is low in relation to what would be actuarially fair (the bad risks) will tend to choose high coverage, and those for whom the premium is high (good risks) will tend to choose low coverage. Coverage will then be related to losses, but the causal relationship runs from losses to coverage, not the other way around.

Adverse selection is less likely to raise estimation problems when geographically aggregated data are used. It arises when individuals have expected losses that differ from the average expected loss on which premiums are based. If a Blue Cross plan in a state is to break even, it must charge premiums that, on the average, cover its costs. If higher incomes increase medical-care expenses but premiums do not vary with income, and if other things (including risk aversion) are equal, higher income families would demand more insurance. But those are families with incomes higher than that of the average family on whose experience premiums are based, not necessarily families with higher absolute income. Families with high relative incomes may buy more insurance, but families with low relative incomes will buy less. The effect of income on insurance depends on the strength of the effects of each group's changes. This statement implies that one of Feldstein's reasons for attributing a possible positive effect to income in an insurance-demand equation was misleading (see Feldstein, 1973). So long as premiums are "experience rated" for a group, that group's average expenditure need not be affected by adverse selection. But unaggregated data, such as those used by Rosett and Huang, may give estimates that are biased upward.

Moral hazard will also affect the quantity of insurance bought. Families may differ in their responsiveness to user price changes. If so, families most responsive to price incentives will tend to purchase little insurance, because the "welfare cost" to them of such insurance will be relatively great. And families who do restrain use will purchase more extensive coverage (see Cummins, 1973). The differences would be accentuated if the marginal price of insurance reflected differential moral hazard, something that is plausible for experience-rated groups. If differential moral hazard does affect insurance choice, empirical estimates of the effect of additional coverage on overall use that ignore differential moral hazard will be biased downward. Families with little insurance are only those who, if given more coverage, would have much greater use than those who now have relatively extensive coverage.

In summary, it is fairly easy to come up with a number of reasons why existing estimates of the effect of insurance on use may be biased. Unfortunately, since even a guess at the direction of bias appears to be impossible, it seems appropriate to conclude only that prices do affect use.

Prices and Substitutes

Though a number of attempts have been made to relate the change in user price of a type of medical care to its use, there have been few empirical attempts to see whether changes in price can produce substitution between different types of care. It has always been an article of faith (or perhaps logic) that comprehensive coverage would reduce inpatient hospital use by reducing the user price of outpatient care to at least the level of inpatient care. (Indeed, the own-elasticity effects on outpatient care of such coverage changes have generally been ignored in policy-oriented discussion.)

That faith is confirmed in the study by Davis and Russell. Use of outpatient services is indeed affected by the price of inpatient care, with a cross-elasticity of 0.85 to 1.45. Outpatient care is also sensitive (elasticity = 1) to its own price. Since outpatient services are often very similar to the services a physician provides in his office, the numbers are also suggestive about own and cross-elasticities of demand for physician care.

There have been almost no estimates of the effect on use of prices charged for close substitutes, such as hospitals or physicians providing the same care. Although ostensibly similar hospitals may have very different charges, they do not necessarily have different user prices. A study by Newhouse (1970) in which he claimed that there was little competition between physicians was shown to be seriously flawed (Frech and Ginsburg, 1972). Lack of data on individual physician charges has prevented a direct approach to the problem. Yet if we are to determine if schemes that propose making the patient aware of differential hospital or physician charges are to be useful, we need to know more about the individual hospital or physician-level response of use to price.

Price as a Rationing Device

As noted above, there is now strong empirical evidence that user price is a feasible device for affecting use. The critical policy question is whether the device is desirable. It is commonplace to remark that, while price may discourage excess use, it may also inhibit needed care. But to make any sense out of the remark, we need a definition of "excess" and "needed."

There are at least three alternative notions of desirable levels of care: (1) medical necessity; (2) personal preferences; and (3) private and social benefits.

The notion of medical necessity as a method of specifying appropriate use is probably what most people have in mind. But it may not even be a feasible norm. It is clearly impossible to set up standards for appropriate treatment that apply to every individual case. Physical illnesses, patient personalities, and physician attitudes are too diverse. The most that could be expected is to set up standards for samples of identifiable diagnoses. While the appropriate length of stay for an appendectomy may vary, depending on the situation, the average length of stay (among a physician's patients, in a hospital) could be examined for conformance with a norm. Probably that is what the emerging professional standards review organizations will try to do, though it is not clear that sufficient agreement on proper care will be obtained.

Even if a consistent definition of medical necessity is possible, there still remains the question of whether it is a proper definition of appropriate levels of care. There are reasons to believe that it may not be. Within the scope of health per se, it is unlikely that what medical men are able to agree upon will correspond to that allocation which maximizes health. With limited resources, maximization of health implies care should be used only up to the point at which the health benefit (expected benefit, in an uncertain situation) from that care equals the benefit the same resources would produce if used for health elsewhere. In other words, care that may do an individual some good ought in some circumstances not to be given.

It is doubtful that the judgment of medical men will reflect that kind of thinking about trade-offs and cost, for their training is not usually in such terms. And if it is recognized that people have goals other than health, the appropriate question becomes the even more difficult one of whether extra medical care in a given situation provides as much benefit to the individual as would the same resources used for housing, for education, or even for entertainment. In summary, whether or not medical necessity in fact gets elevated to the status of a policy norm, there are important reasons to believe that it is not an appropriate norm.

A second kind of norm assumes that individual choices should determine the level of care. A rational individual will, of course, consult physicians and other experts to determine the possible benefits from care, but ultimately he will make a choice on whether to take care (or take a physician's advice about taking care) by considering both the costs and benefits to himself. Given such a norm, any reduction in user price caused by insurance is positively pernicious. It is likely to push price below cost and hence will induce the individual to use care which, as far as he is concerned, is worth less to him than its cost. Of course, he will have to pay the cost in the premium, so he is worse off with a reduction in user price than he would have been if his decision on use had reflected the full cost— that is, the full value of the alternative uses of his resources.

The dead-weight welfare cost of health insurance may, of course, be a necessary evil, in the sense that the individual may be willing to pay it in order to get coverage of risky expenditures, but the individual would still be better off if some way could be found to provide the same protection without reducing the user price. Indemnities of various sorts would be preferable to service benefits, and service benefits with some copayments would often be preferable to full coverage.

If an individual bought insurance at prices reflecting its cost, he would buy coverage up to the point at which additional risk-reduction benefits exactly offset additional welfare cost. In fact, various tax incentives are likely to induce the individual to buy too much insurance (Feldstein and Allison, 1972).

The thought here is that, by reducing insurance coverage, individuals are faced with a positive user charge, and the reduction in overuse may more than compensate for increased exposure to risk. The latter point should not be overemphasized, since much of present "first dollar" coverage does not cover very risky situations. But there is some additional risk of expense associated with reductions in coverage. Is there no way "to have the cake and eat it too," to retain both appropriate price incentives and coverage of risk?

There is another form of insurance, used extensively outside the medical-care area, that does preserve incentives. It is indemnity insurance, insurance that as far as possible makes the insurance benefit depend not on expense, which is manipulable by the insured, but on the occurrence of a loss-producing event. To take a concrete example, a pure indemnity insurance would pay a fixed amount if tonsillitis occurred, regardless of the amount of care sought. The user price would be unaffected by such an insurance payment. Indemnities have, of course, sometimes been used in medical expenses cases, mostly for physicians' fees, but their importance is diminishing. Pure indemnities may not be feasible because of the practical impossibility of determining "medical condition" with sufficient accuracy. But some forms of indemnity modified to preserve both price incentives and risk coverage may still represent improvement over customary forms of insurance. The author has discussed such forms of indemnity coverage elsewhere (Pauly, 1971a); on a priori grounds it appears that, for many medical-care situations, indemnity coverage would be both feasible and desirable.

One legitimate objection to the analysis of user charges, and to calculations that make them benefit measures, is that they assume that individuals' choices are in fact made with "appropriate" information (which is not necessarily complete information if information is costly). One rather cavalier though correct answer is that, if information is deficient because of monopoly restrictions on supply or competition, then the appropriate remedy is more information on the benefits of care. A more useful response for the purposes of this discussion is that, even if individuals had appropriate information, (a) there is no reason to suppose they would buy the quantities of care they are induced to buy by existing or proposed insurances and (b) in an ideal situation, user prices should still be as close to true factor opportunity cost as possible. In other words, prices might still be appropriate incentives. Indeed, if it were possible to determine what individuals would buy if fully informed of benefits and costs, it might be better to structure insurance so that user prices induce persons who are less than fully informed to buy the same quantities. Such user prices might be above as well as below market prices. In summary, given this view of appropriate norms, prices are not only desirable as incentives, they are probably essential.

The third norm recognizes that society, in the sense of other people, may be concerned about the level of care an individual receives. Medical care may well be one of those goods whose consumption generates a kind of "external benefit" and not only in cases of contagious disease. Altruistic or humanitarian motivation may make individuals willing to pay something for care for others when that care would relieve perceived suffering (Pauly, 1971b).

Not all care would generate such benefits, since there may certainly be cases in which an individual buys enough care on his own so that others would perceive no benefit from additional care. But for those individuals who, if faced with the full user price, would buy what others regard as too little care, some device to increase use would be desirable. One device would be to reduce user charges by providing or subsidizing an "insurance" that gives more coverage (lower user prices) than any amount of insurance the individual buys on his own. Since empirical studies of the effect of income on demand indicate that the poor will use less care, the rationale given above suggests that relatively extensive coverage should be provided to the very poor, and then the extent of coverage should decline with income.

Individuals' willingness to pay for the care of others is reflected via the political process. While the expert adviser cannot tell the politician-representative what portion of his constituents' incomes should be spent on subsidizing health care, possible "reasonable" norms and their costs could be suggested. It would be useful to know, for instance, the cost of a scheme of price cuts needed to bring the poor up to the median level of use for various illnesses. Information would also be useful on the consequences of price cuts on use for different kinds of individuals, different kinds of care, and different types of illnesses. Or it might be worthwhile to consider a kind of "original position" approach, in which individuals are thought of as asking themselves what kind of public medical care subsidy, if any, they would wish to see if they were completely ignorant of what was to be their status, income, or position in life.

For different kinds of care, we have already seen that in general the measured response to price changes differs. What is perhaps more important to know is how the use of various kinds of care responds to price incentives for different kinds of illnesses. Almost all the studies by economists, and many of those by others, have failed to look at the relationship of price response to price incentives for different kinds of illness.

The only exception in the former group is in the study of the Stanford group practice by Scitovsky and Snyder (1972). They find some suggestion that a greater share of use reduction occurred in "minor complaints." They also find a decline in physical examinations (by 18.7 percent), which fell short of the overall decline in use (25 percent), but for some groups was in excess of the average decline. For male nonprofessionals the increase in user price cut physical examinations in half (from an already low base). Though one need not agree with their judgment that this was probably a reduction in "needed" care (since they have no standard of need), such information is clearly useful for those who must make policy decisions. Of course, Scitovsky and Snyder were only looking at a price change over one range, for one type of care, and for the grossest illness categories. More detailed study, and a method of summarizing results, would clearly be desirable.

Whatever the level of information obtained, it will never be possible to design a system of prices that guarantees that every person will use the right amount of care. Ostensibly identical people may respond in different ways to the same price, and some of the factors that affect use (level of education, family size) might themselves be distorted if user price varied with them. At any price, therefore, there will be some underuse and some overuse. As user price is reduced from any level, overuse will decrease as underuse increases. A balance will have to be sought, and it is surely possible that underuse might be regarded as worse than overuse. But it is unlikely that balance will be achieved in a system in which everyone is faced with a zero user price for every type of care. And even if the money price of care were zero, the time, distance, and inconvenience costs would still be positive.

One final comment should be made on the relationship between changes in user prices and severity of illness. It has sometimes been suggested that severity of illness and response to changes in user price might be related in a nontautological way. Zola (1964) suggested, for example, that the extent to which illness interferes with activities might be a better measure of that severity which is related to use than type of symptom.

The relevant point here is that an economic approach may also be useful in generating hypotheses about interrelationships between illness characteristics, user, charges, and use or demand. To take the simplest case, consider the "investment" approach suggested by

Grossman, in which care is desirable only as it influences the stock of health and health is desirable only as it affects the ability to earn income. At any user price, care will be used for any illness up to the point at which the increment in earnings expected from the use of that care equals its user price. The expected increment in earnings can, crudely, be considered as the product of the effect that care has on illness and the effect that an illness change has on the ability to earn income. Only the latter second effect, the effect of illness on function, seems to correspond to Zola's measure of severity.

Now let the user price rise. By how much will care be reduced? It will be reduced relatively less for those kinds of illnesses for which an increase in illness severely limits activities and for which a small reduction in care use greatly increases the likelihood or severity of illness. Conversely, care will be reduced relatively more for those kinds of illness in which the marginal illness effect on income and the marginal care productivity of illness are low. Note that absolute severity of illness alone does not predict response; the marginal effect of illness on functioning and the marginal effect of care on illness must also be known. In principle, both concepts can be defined and measured empirically. A useful classification of illness might be based on this sort of analysis.

Supply Effects on Demand

Up to this point the author has tried to avoid discussing the effects on use of supply responses. But even though it was intended to discuss only demand effects on use, such a separation is not possible in any discussion of medical care. The reason is that there are strong theoretical and empirical grounds for believing that supply response affects demand directly, in addition to whatever other effects it may have on price or rationing or other determinants of use. The quantity of care people are willing to take at various prices may be affected by the incentives facing suppliers of care.

The theoretical reason is that people are sometimes unsure about the effects of medical care and tend to buy advice about how much care to use from the same persons or firms who supply that care. Especially if competition is not strong, it is possible that suppliers may be able to "shift" demand. One piece of empirical evidence to that effect is the substantial difference in use sometimes detected between prepaid group practice, where the incentive is to supply little care, and fee-for-service medicine, where the incentive is to supply as much care as yields the provider additional real income. Although some of the difference is undoubtedly due to self-selection in that the people who choose to belong to a prepaid group would have demanded a bundle similar to the bundle supplied, probably not all of it can be explained away. A second kind of empirical evidence, a little less substantial, is Feldstein's (1971a) finding that hospital beds, numbers of general patients, and numbers of specialists affect hospital use. The results are less substantial because the relationship could also reflect supply response to omitted demand parameters.

At the present time we know little about the extent to which suppliers can affect demand. It seems reasonable to conjecture that there are upper and lower bounds. Few people could be persuaded to have surgery for a cold or to take aspirin as a cure for a lacerated finger. It seems reasonable to suppose that the limits vary for the different kinds of illness or symptoms that individuals experience. It also seems reasonable to suppose that, within this range, incentives faced by providers will determine how much they shift or try to shift demand. Finally, one suspects that the effect of physician persuasion or other supply influences on an individual's demand should differ depending on the information he has; if more education really leads to more efficient production, for instance, it is likely that the demand of better educated people should be less influenced by supply influences. But other than these speculations and the gross empirical evidence mentioned above, there is little that we know.

Conclusion

In this essay I have discussed a number of economic or economically interpretable influences on use, but I have given the most stress to and spent the most space on the influence of user price. This emphasis is proper, since economics is, in a sense, about the influences price exerts on individuals' behavior. The general message is that, in medical care especially, price is not likely to be a "pure" incentive. Its interaction with other determinants of use, almost all of which are subject to economic interpretation, is an area in which both public policy and intellectual curiosity suggest that we should try to find out much more than we now know.

References

Andersen, R. J., O. W. Anderson, *and* B. Smedby
  1968   "Perception of and response to symptons of illness in Sweden and the United States." Medical Care 6: 18–30.
Andersen, R. J. *and* L. K. Benham
  1970   "Factors affecting the relationship between family income and medical care consumption." Pp. 73–95 in Klarman, H. M. (ed.), Empirical Studies in Health Economics. Baltimore: Johns Hopkins University Press.
Auster, Richard A., I. J. Leveson *and* D. K. Sarachek
  1972   "The production of health, and exploratory study." Pp. 135–160 in Fuchs, V. R. (ed.), Essays in the Economics of Health and Medical Care. New York: Columbia University Press.
Cummins, J. M.
  1973   Cost Overruns in Defense Contracting. Ph.D. dissertation, Northwestern University, Evanston, Illinois.
Davis, Karen A. *and* Lucille B. Russell
  1972   "Substitution of hospital outpatient for inpatient care." Review of Economics and Statistics 54 (May): 108–120.
Donabedian, Avedis B.
  1969   "An evaluation of prepaid group practice." Inquiry 6 (September): 3–27.
Feldstein, M. S.
  1970   "The rising price of physicians' services." Review of Economics and Statistics 52 (May): 121–133.
  1971a   "Hospital cost inflation: A study in nonprofit price dy-

namics." American Economic Review 61 (December): 853–872.

1971b   "A new approach to national health insurance." Public Interest 23 (Spring): 93–105.

1973   "The welfare loss of excess health insurance." Journal of Political Economy 81 (March/April): 251–280.

Feldstein, M. S. *and* E. E. Allison

1972   "Tax subsidies of private health insurance: Distribution, revenue loss, and effects." Boston: Harvard Institute of Economic Research, Discussion Paper No. 237.

Feldstein, P. J.

1966   "Research on the demand for health services." Milbank Memorial Fund Quarterly 44 (July): 128–165.

Frech, H. E. *and* P. B. Ginsburg

1972   "Comment." Southern Economic Journal 38 (April): 573–577.

Grossman, M. J.

1972   The Demand for Health: A Theoretical and Empirical Analysis. New York: Columbia University Press.

Klarman, Herbert E.

1965   "Effects of prepaid group practice on hospital use." Public Health Reports 78 (November): 955–965.

Newhouse, J. P.

1970   "A model of physician pricing." Southern Economic Journal 37 (October): 174–183.

Newhouse, J. P. *and* C. E. Phelps

1973   "On having your cake and eating it too: A review of estimated effects of insurance on the demand for medical care." Preliminary draft. Santa Monica: The RAND Corporation, October.

Pauly, Mark V.

1971a   "Indemnity insurance for health service efficiency." Journal of Economics and Business 32 (Fall): 53–59.

1971b   Medical Care of Public Expense. New York: Praeger Publisers, Inc.

1972   An Analysis of Alternative National Health Insurance Proposals. Washington, D.C.: American Enterprise Institute.

Phelps, C. E. *and* J. P. Newhouse

1972a   Coinsurance and the Demand for Medical Care. Santa Monica: The RAND Corporation, R-964-OEO/NCHSRD.

1972b   "Effects of coinsurance: Amultivariateanalysis."SocialSe-
        curity Bulletin 35 (June): 20–28.

Richardson, William C.
1970   "Measuring the urban poor's use of physicians' services in
        response to illness episodes." Medical Care 8: 132–142.
1971   Ambulatory Use of Physicians' Services in Response to Ill-
        ness Episodes in a Low-Income Neighborhood. Chicago:
        University of Chicago, Center for Health Administration
        Studies.

Roemer, Milton I.
1972   Testimony before the House Committee on Ways and
        Means, June.

Roghman, K. J. et al.
1971   "Anticipated and actual effects of Medicaid on the care pat-
        tern of children." Unpublished paper.

Rosett, R. M. *and* L. Huang
1973   "The effect of health insurance on the demand for medical
        care." Journal of Political Economy 81 (March/April):
        281–305.

Scitovsky, Anne A. *and* Nelda M. Snyder
1972   "Effect of coinsurance on the use of physician services."
        Social Security Bulletin 35 (June): 3–19.

Scott, H. D.
1973   "Uses of hospital discharge data for community planning
        and quality assessment." Providence Evening Bulletin
        (April 5).

Silver, Morris
1972   "An economic analysis of variations in medical expenses
        and work-loss rates." Pp. 97–118 in Fuchs, V. R. (ed.), Es-
        says in the Economics of Health and Medical Care. New
        York: Columbia University.

Zola, I.
1964   "Illness behavior and the working class: Implications and
        recommendations." Pp. 76–94 in Shostak, A. *and* W. Gom-
        berg (eds.), Blue Collar World. Englewood Cliffs: Pren-
        tice-Hall.

Societal and Individual Determinants of Medical Care Utilization in the United States

RONALD ANDERSEN

JOHN F. NEWMAN

A theoretical framework for viewing health services utilization is presented, emphasizing the importance of the (1) characteristics of the health services delivery system, (2) changes in medical technology and social norms relating to the definition and treatment of illness, and (3) individual determinants of utilization. These three factors are specified within the context of their impact on the health care system. Empirical findings are discussed which demonstrate how the framework might be employed to explain some key patterns and trends in utilization. In addition, a method is suggested for evaluating the utility of various individual determinants of health services utilization used in the framework for achieving a situation of equitable distribution of health services in the United States.

Analyses of the determinants of medical care utilization in this country are receiving increasing attention.[1] This attention seems to result from the emergence of a number of related societal values and perceptions including: (1) a growing consensus that all people have a right to medical care regardless of their ability to pay for this care[2]; (2) the general belief that certain population groups such as the "poor," blacks, Spanish-speaking Americans, American Indians, and inner city and rural residents, are not receiving medical care which is comparable in terms of quality and quantity that is available to the rest of the population[3]; (3) high expectations concerning the extent to which medical care can contribute

[1] For recent reviews of the growing health services utilization literature, see Aday and Eichhorn (1972); Anderson and Andersen (1972); Lohr (1972); and McKinlay (1972).

[2] In early 1971, 92 percent of a national sample of household heads agreed with the statement, "All people have a right to good medical care whether they can pay for it or not" (Andersen et al., 1971: 47).

[3] See, e.g., Richardson (1969). Recent studies have suggested, however, that actual differences in use of physician services according to socioeconomic status have diminished considerably. See Bice, Eichhorn, and Fox (1972).

Milbank Memorial Fund Quarterly, Winter, 1973.

to the general health level of the population[4]; and (4) public consternation over "the crisis in medical care" stimulated by rapidly rising prices and growing dissatisfaction about the availability of services.[5] Increased financial support of utilization studies in recent years by governmental and private sources is based on the expectation that research will contribute both to a better understanding of the processes through which medical care is currently distributed and to the development of new policies which will alleviate the perceived crisis in medical care.[6]

The utilization of health services can be viewed as a type of individual behavior. In general the behavioral sciences have attempted to explain individual behavior as a function of characteristics of the individual himself, characteristics of the environment in which he lives, and/or some interaction of these individual and societal forces (Moore, 1969). To date, most of the empirical studies and theories dealing with health services utilization have emphasized the individual characteristics while less attention has been paid to the societal impact.[7]

This paper outlines a framework for viewing health services utilization which takes into account both societal and individual determinants.[8] In addition we will present empirical findings which demonstrate how the framework might be employed to explain some key patterns and trends in health services utilization. Further with respect to patterns an assessment of the relative importance

[4] For example, over half of a recent national sample of household heads and their spouses agreed with the statement, "Modern medicine can cure most any illness." Unpublished data, Center for Health Administration Studies, University of Chicago.

[5] Three-quarters of the heads of families in the United States in 1971 agreed with the statement, "There is a crisis in health care in the United States" (Andersen et al., 1972: 45).

[6] For one view of the government role, see Fox (1972). Nongovernmental interest in utilization studies is exemplified by the recent statement of the Milbank Memorial Fund (1972), the highly respected, nonprofit corporation which for almost 70 years has supported a "diversity of programs and activities within the field of health and has chosen successive areas of concentration in response to the continually shifting patterns of the growth of knowledge, the emergence of new problems and public needs, the changing potentials for significant advances and the availability of resources . . . the fund will concentrate its efforts upon the exploration of more effective *utilization of health services by consumers,* with particular emphasis upon the

of the model components is presented for the different types of services. Finally, a method for evaluating the utility of various individual determinants of health services utilization used in the framework for achieving a situation of equitable distribution of health services in the United States is presented.

The Framework

Figure 1 shows the relationships of the main components of the framework. Societal determinants of utilization are shown to affect the individual determinants both directly and through the health services system. Various types of individual determinants then influence health services used by the individual. In subsequent sections, these determinants will be defined and data will be presented to illustrate some of the suggested relationships. Prior to such discussion the nature of the utilization variable itself needs to be considered.

Characteristics of Health Care Utilization

The last major component of the framework for viewing health services shown in Fig. 1 defines the unit of health service utilization to be analyzed. This is an important dimension because the configuration of the other components of the framework vary considerably, depending on special characteristics of the unit analyzed.

acquisition and application of knowledge about the accessibility and acceptability of such services to consumers."

[7] That is not to say that specific attributes of the community culture or delivery system have not been used to explain variations in individual behavior. See Aday and Eichhorn (1972), McKinlay (1972), and Lohr (1972). However, relatively few attempts have been made to systematically develop the relationship between general societal forces, the health service system, and the population's use of health services. Some recent attempts using a more inclusive systems approach include Sheldon et al. (1970: particularly chapters 3, 4, 5, and 7); Field (1971); Bice and White (1971); and Weinerman (1971). One of the few systems approaches which has attempted to incorporate empirical data into the scheme is provided by Anderson (1972).

[8] Our purpose is to integrate and further elaborate models developed in earlier works. The individual model was originally developed in Andersen (1968). Extensions of the model with specific application to dental services were presented in Newman (1971) and Newman and Anderson (1972). The systems model was first proposed in Andersen, Smedby, and Anderson (1970).

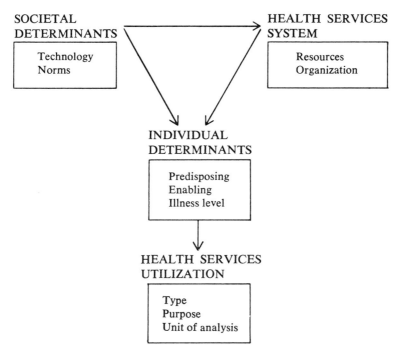

FIGURE 1.
Framework for viewing health services utilization.

The characteristics of prime importance as outlined in Fig. 2 include type, purpose, and unit of analysis.

With respect to type of health service we will subsequently argue that societal determinants have resulted in very different

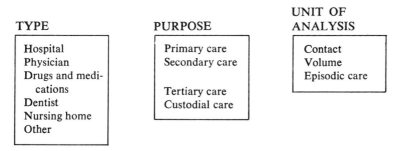

FIGURE 2.
Characteristics of health services utilization.

long-term trends for physician, hospital, and dental services. Further, the current individual determinants of hospital, physician, and dental services will be shown to vary considerably.

Utilization can also be characterized by purpose. Primary care has to do with stopping illness before it begins. Secondary care refers to the process of treatment which returns an individual to his previous state of functioning. Tertiary care provides stabilization for long-term irreversible illnesses such as heart disease or diabetes.[9] Custodial care essentially provides for the personal needs of the patient but makes no effort to treat his underlying illness conditions. The determinants of each type of care vary considerably. For example, factors related to use of preventive services such as general checkups, immunization and vaccinations differ from those related to diagnosis and treatment (National Center for Health Statistics, 1965: 8-10, 25-26).

A final characteristic describing the utilization to be studied is the unit of analysis. It makes considerable difference whether we are studying initial contact with a physician during a given period of time or whether we are studying the number of services received in a given period of time. For example, the characteristics of the individual might be of primary importance in explaining whether or not any services are received. However, characteristics of the physician and, indeed, of the total health service system in which the individual enters, might be expected to be decisive in determining the overall volume of services.

Another way of looking at the illness experience is through the episode concept.[10] It is an attempt to delineate a particular illness experience and all of the medical care associated with that experience. The episode approach is necessary if one is interested in studying important questions such as care associated with specific diagnoses, reasons for delay in seeking care, continuity of care received, level of patient compliance, and patterns of referral.

Societal Determinants

Definitions

Figure 1 suggests that the main societal determinants of health

[9] These distinctions were first made by the Commission on Chronic Illness in the United States (1957).

[10] The importance of the episode concept was developed by Solon et al. (1967). For a recent application of the episode concept to health survey research, see Richardson (1971).

service utilization are technology[11] and norms.[12] It should be noted that the postulated causal links between the societal factors and resulting utilization behavior discussed below, can only be inferred since the nature of our data and the state of our methods and theory generally preclude direct testing at this time.[13]

Figure 3 shows the skeletal structure of one conceptualization of a health services system.[14] The health care system structures the provision of formal health care goods and services in society. Formal health care goods and services include physician care, hospital care, dental care, drugs, and health appliances and services provided by other health care practitioners.[15]

A national health care system consists of two major dimensions, resources and organization. Together they shape the provision of health care services to the individual.

The resources of the system are the labor and capital devoted to health care. Included would be health personnel, structures in which health care and education are provided, and the equipment and materials used in providing health services. Organization describes simply what the system does with its resources. It refers

[11] The general definition of technology we shall use here is "a set of principles and techniques useful to bring about change toward desired ends" (Taylor, 1971: 3). One definition of medical technology might then be principles and techniques providing "tools for extending the physician's powers of observation and making more effective his role as a therapist" (Warner, 1972: 1).

[12] Norms, as used here, correspond to Wilbert Moore's description of social control as representing the spectrum of modes whereby social systems induce or insure normal compliance on the part of members (Moore, 1969: 300). As Moore points out, the concept is inclusive of Sumner's classic distinctions of degree of control and correlative degree of negative sanctions for violators: folkways (it is normally expected), mores (you ought to behave), and laws (you must comply).

[13] For a discussion of some methodological problems in applying a systems model, see Bice and White (1971: 263-268).

[14] The general concept of systems refers to "a set of units or elements that are actively interrelated and that operate in some sense as a bounded unit. . . . General systems theory is, then, primarily concerned with problems of relationships, of structure, and of interdependence than with the constant attributes of objects," Baker (1970: 4-5). This discussion of the health service system is based largely on Andersen et al. (1971: 5-9).

[15] The definition does not include provision of sanitary services or other general public health measures; nor does it include provision of necessities of life, which influence the state of health, such as food, clothing, or shelter. Also, informal health services such as care provided by the family of a

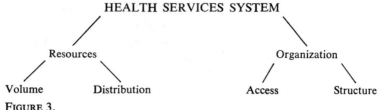

FIGURE 3.
The health services system.

to the manner in which medical personnel and facilities are coordinated and controlled in the process of providing medical services. Both resources and organization include two sub-components as illustrated in Fig. 3.

The resource component includes total volume of resources relative to the population served and the way in which the resources are geographically distributed within a country. Volume includes personnel/population ratios for various kinds of health related occupations (including physicians, nurses, dentists, etc.) actively providing medical care. Total amount of resources can also be measured by examining facilities which provide patient care. In this case, bed/population ratios for hospitals of various kinds, nursing homes, and other institutions providing inpatient care are common measures.

The importance of volume of resources is based on the rather obvious assumption that, as the resource/population ratio increases, the medical care consumed by the population will also increase. However, it is made on the premise that all other dimensions of the system are "equal," while these other dimensions are often not equal over time or from one system to another. Further, we know that there are other societal influences apart from the health service system which directly influence people's use of health services. Consequently, it is necessary to state the assumption explicitly and, when it is not borne out by the data, look for reasons why.

The second component of resources, geographical distribution, is important because the resources of the health system may not be homogeneously dispersed throughout the country. If such is the

patient are not included in this definition of formal health care services, although it should be remembered that such care has a direct influence on the amount of formal care provided by a doctor or hospital. For a more detailed discussion of services comprising the formal health services system, see Anderson (1972: chapter 2).

case, the resource/population ratio for the society as a whole will not reflect the availability of medical services accurately for persons living in areas with either more or fewer health resources than the national average. We might expect greater dispersion of resources to result in more equitable distribution.

The components of organization are called access and structure. Access refers to the means through which the patient gains entry to the medical care system and continues the treatment process. It specifies the requirements that must be met and the barriers which must be overcome before medical care is received. The degree of access of any system varies according to such things as direct out-of-pocket cost for medical care to the patient, length of the queue for various kinds of treatment, and general definitions concerning conditions which qualify the patient for treatment. Accessibility is assumed to increase as the proportion of medical care expenditures paid for by the government, voluntary health insurance, or other third-party payers increases; as waiting time for medical care decreases; and as the range of conditions accepted for treatment increases.

Structure, the second component of organization, deals with characteristics of the system that determine what happens to the patient following entry to the system. Of interest here are: the nature of medical practices of the primary practitioners who first see the patient in the system, the utilization of ancillary personnel, processes of referral to other sources of care, means of admission into the hospital, characteristics of hospital care, and the disposition and care of patients following hospitalization.

The structural component is the most difficult of the health services systems components to define as well as to relate to utilization patterns. The definitional problems result from the many facets of structure, only some of which are mentioned above. Also, the structure component is highly interrelated to the other components. Certainly, access as we have defined it depends in part on structure, and the structure of any system is dependent on the resources available to it.

Illustrative Trends and Relationships

Turning to examples of the impact of technology on the health service system and the utilization of health services, let us first consider one of the major trends in mortality since the beginning of this century: the rapid decline of deaths due to tuberculosis, influenza, pneumonia, and other infectious diseases. Since 1900 the mortality rate per 100,000 persons due to tuberculosis declined from 194 to a rate of 3 in 1969, while the rate from influenza and pneumonia for the same period declined from 202 to 35 (U.S. Bureau of the Census, 1965: Series B114-128; U.S. Bureau of Census, 1971: Table No. 77). This decline has generally been attributed to improvements as a result of public health efforts such as sanitation, comprehensive immunization programs, and development of new forms of antibiotics. Hence the utilization, for example, of tuberculosis hospitals has declined as a result of technology affecting illness levels which in turn influence utilization (U.S. Bureau of the Census, 1971:70, Table 100).

Other technological developments have increased the utilization of hospitals. It is argued that perfection of anesthesia and asepsis made the hospital a viable institution for providing medical care in the twentieth century and changed it from a custodial institution for the poor to a curative institution providing services for the total population (Anderson, 1968:26). More recently, developments in such fields as surgery, radiology, and nuclear medicine have significantly altered the patterns of care for hospitalized patients in terms of case mix and average length of stay.

While it is generally agreed that changes in technology have had considerable impact on the health services system and on utilization, less attention has been given to the effect of societal norms. The normative component of the societal determinant can be reflected through formal legislation as well as growing consensus of beliefs and homogeneity of values which pervade the society, thus shaping the health service system and utilization patterns. Changes in the treatment of mental illness provide an example of the joint impact of technology and norms. The development of new therapeutic drugs and changes in beliefs about site of treatment have resulted in a shift from largely custodial care to treatment on an outpatient basis. In fact, the proportion of mental patients who are treated in mental hospitals or in other inpatient settings has decreased from 77 percent to 47 percent in the time period from 1955 to 1968 with a concomitant increase in the proportion of persons seen on an outpatient basis (U.S. Bureau of the Census, 1971:73, Table 105).

Growing use of the hospital as a place to be born and to die is probably a more dramatic example of the major impact of changing social norms, with technological change of only secondary importance. Ninety-eight percent of all live births now occur in a hospital compared to 56 percent as recently as 1940 (U.S. Bureau of the Census, 1971: Table 59). In contrast even today in a technologically advanced country such as Holland, 70 percent of the births take place in the home (National Center for Health Statistics, 1968:2). It is also unlikely that technological change can account for the fact that in 1935, 34 percent of all deaths occurred in hospitals while by 1961 some 61 percent of all deaths took place in hospitals.[16]

Possibly, the societal norms which have the greatest effect on health service utilization have to do with how medical care is financed. Further, approaches to financing the various kinds of health services suggest that societal values attached to these services differ considerably. Presumably, the extent of voluntary health insurance coverage and government payment of medical care, as illustrated by the Medicare and Medicaid programs, are measures of the importance society attaches to a given service since third-party payments reduce the extent of financial hardship resulting from out-of-pocket expenditures for medical care and increase accessibility to that care in the population.

Table 1 shows a substantial growth in the proportion of the population covered by voluntary insurance over the past 30 years. The growth, however, has not been uniform among services so that while the major proportion of the population is currently covered for hospital and doctor costs, dental insurance is only now being made available to any significant proportion of the population.

Table 2 indicates that over the past 20 years there has been a continual decrease in the proportion of total personal health expenditures paid for directly by the consumer. Between 1950 and 1965 the reduced proportion of out-of-pocket expenditures was balanced by increased private insurance payments. Since 1965,

[16] 1935 estimate is based on 469,000 hospital deaths as reported in Lerner and Anderson (1963: 249) and 1,393,000 deaths (excluding fetal) as reported in U. S. Bureau of the Census (1965: Series B6-9). 1961 is abstracted from National Center for Health Statistics (1965b: Table 2).

TABLE 1
Private Insurance Coverage by Type: Selected Years

	Percentage of U.S. Population Insured		
Year	Hospital	Surgical-Medical	Dental
1940	9[a]	6[a]	[d]
1950	51[a]	51[a]	[d]
1953	57[b]	48[b]	[d]
1958	65[b]	61[b]	[d]
1962	[d]	[d]	2[e]
1963	68[b]	66[b]	[d]
1969	78[c]	76[c]	4[e]

[a] U.S. Bureau of the Census (1965); Series X 469-482; unduplicated total.
[b] Andersen and Anderson (1967), Table 41.
[c] Social Security Bulletin, 34 (February, No. 2), 1971: Table 1. The estimates for 1969 excluded.
[d] Not available.
[e] U.S. Bureau of the Census (1971: Table 706).

with the advent of the Medicare and Medicaid programs, the shift in payments has been from the consumer to public sources.

Table 2 also points out that the growth in third-party payments for medical care varies greatly accordingly to service. By 1970, most hospital care and well over one-half of physician services were paid for by government and private insurance while 90 percent of the costs of dental care were still borne directly by the consumer.

Changing technologies and norms over the past 40 years are assumed to be major causes of the large increases in the gross measures of health service use documented in Table 3, since it is unlikely that changes in the underlying illness levels independent of technology and norms could account for these trends. Table 3 shows rather consistent gains in the use of all services except mean number of physician visits per person which began to decline from the late 1950s to current times. Over the total period hospital admission rates and percentage of the population seeing a dentist more than doubled and the mean number of physician visits increased by 65 percent.

TABLE 2
Percentage of Personal Health Care Expenditures
Met by Various Sources: Selected Years

		Percentage of Total Expenditure			
Year	Service	Out Of Pocket	Private Insurance	Philanthropy and Other	Public
1950[a]	All types	65.5	9.1	2.9	22.4
1955[a]	All types	58.1	16.1	2.8	23.0
1960[a]	All types	54.9	21.1	2.3	21.8
1965[a]	All types	51.8	25.1	2.0	21.1
1970[a]	All types	37.7	25.5	1.5	35.4
1970[b]	Hospital	13.1	35.8	1.4	49.7
1970[b]	Physician	38.9	36.1	0.1	24.9
1970[c]	Dentist	90.7	4.1	—	5.2

[a] Cooper and Worthington (1972), derived from Tables 5 and 6.

[b] Cooper and Worthington (1972), derived from Tables 2 and 6.

[c] Cooper and Worthington (1972), derived from Tables 2, 3, and 6. The percentage estimate for private insurance is for all personal health care excluding hospital care and physician services. The out-of-pocket estimate is calculated by subtracting the public and private insurance estimates from 100 percent.

Individual Determinants

Definitions

In addition to societal effects we are interested in the individual characteristics of people which help to determine the health care they receive. It is necessary for such an analysis to develop a model which relates these individual characteristics to utilization patterns in some logical fashion. The model should also serve as a guide in the selection of relevant variables to include in the analysis. Finally, together with the systems components the model should suggest postulates concerning the differing impact of these variables (see Fig. 1). The purpose of this section is to describe one attempt at such a behavorial model of health services utilization which is depicted in Fig. 4.

The underlying model assumes that a sequence of conditions contributes to the type of volume of health service a person uses.

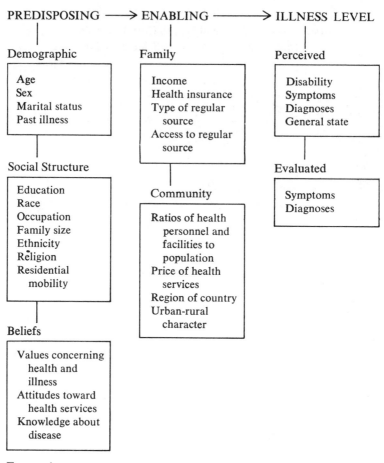

PREDISPOSING ⟶ ENABLING ⟶ ILLNESS LEVEL

Demographic

| Age |
| Sex |
| Marital status |
| Past illness |

Social Structure

| Education |
| Race |
| Occupation |
| Family size |
| Ethnicity |
| Religion |
| Residential |
| mobility |

Beliefs

| Values concerning |
| health and |
| illness |
| Attitudes toward |
| health services |
| Knowledge about |
| disease |

Family

| Income |
| Health insurance |
| Type of regular |
| source |
| Access to regular |
| source |

Community

| Ratios of health |
| personnel and |
| facilities to |
| population |
| Price of health |
| services |
| Region of country |
| Urban-rural |
| character |

Perceived

| Disability |
| Symptoms |
| Diagnoses |
| General state |

Evaluated

| Symptoms |
| Diagnoses |

FIGURE 4.
Individual determinants of health service utilization.

Use is dependent on: (1) the predisposition of the individual to use services; (2) his ability to secure services; (3) his illness level.[17]

[17] In addition to the framework proposed in this paper, other attempts at explaining utilization have focused on (1) the structure of social groups to which individuals belong as in Suchman (1965), (2) cultural norms as in Maclachlan (1958), (3) the perceived seriousness of illness balanced against the consequence of not seeking care as in Rosenstock (1966), (4) disease characteristics as in Greenlick et al. (1968), or (5) economic demand analysis such as Wirick (1966).

In the paragraphs following, we will briefly describe each of these components and suggest variables which operationalize them. The variables were chosen because of their correspondence to the model, because previous research has related them to health service use, and because experience has shown that they can be operationalized in social survey research.[18]

Predisposing Component. Some individuals have a propensity to use services more than other individuals, where propensity toward use can be predicted by individual characteristics which exist prior to the onset of specific episodes of illness. People with certain of these characteristics are more likely to use health services even though the characteristics are not directly responsible for health service use. Such characteristics include demographic, social structural, and attitudinal-belief variables. Age and sex, for example, among the demographic variables, are intimately related to health and illness. However, they are still considered to be predisposing conditions inasmuch as age per se is not considered a reason for seeking health care. Rather, people in different age groups have different types and amounts of illness and consequently different patterns of medical care. Past illness is included in this category because there is considerable evidence that people who have experienced health problems in the past are those most likely to make demands on the medical care system in the future.

The social structure variables reflect the location (status) of the individual in his society as measured by characteristics such as education and occupation of the family head. These characteristics suggest what the life style of the individual may be, and they point to the physical as well as social environment of the individual and associated behavior patterns which may be related to the use of health services.

Demographic and social structural characteristics are also linked to a third subcomponent of the predisposing conditions — attitudes or beliefs about medical care, physicians, and disease. What an individual thinks about health may ultimately influence

[18] For more complete descriptions of earlier versions of this model, hypotheses derived from it, and discussions of related literature, see Andersen (1968: 10-20, 78-86), and Andersen et al. (1972: 26-40). For a more recent review of the literature using components of this model to organize the findings, see Aday and Eichhorn (1972).

health and illness behavior. Like the other predisposing variables, health beliefs are not considered to be a direct reason for using services but do result in differences in inclination toward use of health services. For example, families who strongly believe in the efficacy of treatment of their doctors might seek a physician sooner and use more services than families with less faith in the results of treatment.

Enabling Component. Even though individuals may be predisposed to use health services, some means must be available for them to do so. A condition which permits a family to act on a value or satisfy a need regarding health service use is defined as enabling. Enabling conditions make health service resources available to the individual. Enabling conditions can be measured by family resources such as income, level of health insurance coverage, or other source of third-party payment, whether or not the individual has a regular source of care, the nature of that regular source of care, and the accessibility of the source.

Apart from family attributes, certain enabling characteristics of the community in which the family lives can also affect the use of services. One such characteristic is the amount of health facilities and personnel in a community. If resources are reasonably plentiful and can be used without queuing up, they might be used more frequently by the population. From the economic standpoint one might expect people experiencing low prices for medical care to use more services. Other measures of community resources include region of the country and the rural-urban nature of the community in which the family lives. These variables might be linked to utilization because of local norms concerning how medicine should be practiced or overriding community values which influence the behavior of the individual living in the community.

Illness Level. Assuming the presence of predisposing and enabling conditions, the individual or his family must perceive illness or the probability of its occurrence for the use of health services to take place. Illness level represents the most immediate cause of health service use. In addition to perception of illness by the individual or his family, a clinical evaluation is also included in the model since once the individual seeks care from the formal system the nature and extent of that care is in part determined by them.[19]

Measures of perceived illness include number of disability days that an individual experiences. Such days are those during which the individual is unable to do what he usually does be that go to work, go to school, take care of the house, or play with other children. Other measures of perceived illness include symptoms the individual experiences in a given time period and a self-report of general state of health, e.g., excellent, good, fair, or poor.

Evaluated illness measures are attempts to get at the actual illness problem that the individual is experiencing and the clinically judged severity of that illness. Under ideal circumstances included here would be a physical examination of the individual. Since this is often not practical given most research designs and, in addition, is exceedingly expensive, alternative measures are often used. In the most recent national survey by the Center for Health Administration Studies and National Opinion Research Center, the symptoms reported by the individuals have been weighed by a panel of physicians as to the probability of need for care for each symptom for each age group.[20] In addition, all reported care has been verified through the physician or clinic who provided services. From this verification more valid diagnoses are obtained which can be used in the analysis. Further, the diagnoses are rated according to clinical judgment as to probable need for service.

From a theoretical perspective the major determinants of health services utilization have already been defined, such that the need for new explanatory variables is minimal.[21] Methodologically a promising avenue appears to be a further specification of the

[19] It should be noted that those theories and/or models which emphasize health or illness levels as determinants of utilization such as Rosenstock (1966) or Greenlick et al. (1968) do not generally take into account what changes if any occur in the decision-making process from the individual's perspective once initial health service contact is made.

[20] This national survey of 3,880 families, conducted in early 1971, is the fourth in a series spanning almost 20 years, conducted to study the nation's use of health services and expenditures for these services. The current study is funded though a contract with the National Center for Health Services Research and Development (HSM-110-HSRD-58 (0)). Findings from the previous three studies are summarized in Andersen and Anderson (1967).

[21] An attempt has been made to operationalize most of the individual variables discussed in this paper in a recent national survey conducted by the

relative importance of the independent variables on utilization as improved measures of evaluated health are devised. The development of such measures together with multivariate techniques such as path regression analysis will eventually provide further specificity.

Illustrative Trends and Relationships

In this section which is concerned with empirical data on individual determinants, attention is given to a social structure variable, race, and to an enabling variable, family income, because these variables are important from a public policy perspective. Also, data are available over a considerable period of time, allowing us to make some inference about the effects of societal changes on the relative importance of race and income.

Table 3 shows major reversals in the relationship of income to the use of hospital physician services over time. In 1930 the high-income group had a third more hospital admisisons and almost twice as many physician visits as the low-income group. Following the trends over time, the poor consistently increased their utilization relative to the rest of the population, so that by the latter 1950s they were the heaviest utilizers of hospitals and by 1970 also had more physician visits, on average, than the other income groups. A corresponding increase in third-party payments over this period suggests that reduction of the out-of-pocket costs to the poor was an important reason for their increased utilization.

In contrast to the other services, the use of dental services was much higher for the upper income groups in the 1930s and continues to be so today. We suggest that dental care is viewed by society as much less necessary than the other services (Newman and Anderson, 1972). It is only recently that party payers are beginning to make inroads into the financing of these services. Consequently, the poor with limited resources and a relatively low priority assigned to dental care continue to lag far behind the rest of the population in their use of dental services.

Table 4 shows relationships between race and utilization over time although, unfortunately, the data only go back to the latter 1950s. The trends show that for each service utilization was
Center for Health Administration Studies and the National Opinion Research Center. Some preliminary findings from this survey are reported in Andersen et al. (1972).

TABLE 3

Trends in Hospital Admission Rates, Mean Number of Physician Visits and Proportion with a Dentist Visit by Family Income: Selected Time Periods

Period[g]	Family[a] Income	Hospital Admissions 100 Persons Per Year		Mean Physician Visits/Person Per Year		Proportion With A Dental Visit Within A Year	
1928-1931[b]	Low	(15%)	6	(15%)	2.2	(15%)	10%
	Medium	(73%)	6	(73%)	2.5	(73%)	20
	High	(12%)	8	(12%)	4.3	(12%)	46
	Total		6		2.6		21
1952-1953[c]	Low	(16%)	12	(16%)	NA	(16%)	17%
	Medium	(71%)	12	(71%)	NA	(71%)	33
	High	(13%)	11	(13%)	NA	(13%)	56
	Total		12		NA		34
1957-1959[d]	Low	(27%)	13	(16%)	4.6	(16%)	19%
	Medium	(51%)	13	(62%)	4.9	(62%)	36
	High	(22%)	10	(22%)	5.7	(22%)	54
	Total		12		5.0		37
1963-1964[e]	Low	(21%)	14	(28%)	4.3	(29%)	26%
	Medium	(57%)	14	(54%)	4.5	(55%)	44
	High	(22%)	10	(18%)	5.1	(16%)	64
	Total		13		4.6		42
1968-1970[f]	Low	(20%)	17	(18%)	4.7	(18%)	28%
	Medium	(58%)	13	(46%)	4.1	(46%)	40
	High	(22%)	11	(36%)	4.3	(36%)	59
	Total		14		4.3		45

[a] Numbers in parentheses indicate the percentage of the population represented for each income category.

[b] 1928-1931 from Falk, Klem, and Sinai (1933). Admission rates, p. 113; physician visits, p. 283. Dentist proportion as cited in Kriesberg (1963: 349).

[c] 1952-1953 from Anderson and Feldman (1956). Admission rates, Table A-84, p. 183; dentist proportion, Table A-99, p. 199.

[d] 1957-1959 hospital admissions per 100 person-years from Andersen and Anderson (1967), Table 17, p. 38. 1957-1959 physician visits from U.S. National Health Survey, Series B, Number 19, p. 29. 1957-1959 dentist proportion from U.S. National Health Survey, Series B, Number 14, p. 15.

[e] 1963-1964 hospital admissions per 100 person-years from Andersen and Anderson (1967), Table 17, p. 38. 1963-1964 physician visits from National Center for Health Statistics, Series 10, Number 18, p. 13. 1963-1964 dentist proportion from National Center for Health Statistics, Series 10, No. 18, p. 13.

[f] 1968-1970 hospital admissions per 100 person-years from Andersen et al. (1972). 1968-1970 physician visits, National Center for Health Statistics, Series 10, No. 70, Table H, p. 10. 1968-1970 dentist proportion, National Center for Health Statistics, Series 10,

No. 70, Table H, p. 10. 1968-1970 dentist proportion, National Center for Health Statistics, Series 10, No. 70, Table 16, p. 37.

ᵍ During a given time period the base year for the utilization rates varies depending on the source of the data.

TABLE 4
Trends in Hospital Admission Rates,
Mean Number of Physician Visits and Proportion with a Dentist Visit
by Race: Selected Time Periods

Period	Race	Hospital Admissions/ 100 Persons/ Year	Mean Physician Visits/Persons/ Year	Proportion With a Dentist Visit
1957-1960ᵃ	Nonwhite	9	3.5	17
	White	12	5.2	39
	Total	12	5.0	37
1963-1964ᵇ	Nonwhite	10	3.3	23
	White	13	4.7	45
	Total	13	4.5	42
1965-1967ᶜ	Nonwhite	10	3.1	d
	White	13	4.5	d
	Total	12	4.3	d
1968-1970	Nonwhiteᵉ	11	3.5	28
	White	14	4.4	47
	Total	14	4.3	45

ᵃ "Hospital admissions" for 1958-1960 are number of patients discharged/1000 population per year and do not take into account persons who died during the year. Source: National Center for Health Statistics, Series B, Number 32, Table 9, p. 22. Physician visits from National Center for Health Statistics, Series B, Number 19, p. 27. Dentist proportion from National Center for Health Statistics, Series B, Number 14, p. 4.

ᵇ 1963-1964 hospital admissions from National Center for Health Statistics, Series 10, Number 30, p. 17. This has been adjusted to exclude deceased patients' use multiplying rate given by .958; see p. 66. Physician visits from National Center for Health Statistics, Series 10, Number 18, p. 13. Dentist proportion from National Center for Health Statistics, Series 10, Number 29, p. 17.

ᶜ1965-1967 hospital admissions from National Center for Health Statistics. Rates were calculated by taking the percent white (10.2) and nonwhite (8.2) persons with short-stay hospital days (Series 10, Number 56, p. 20) and multiplying by the population ratio of discharges/100 population, 12.3, to the proportion of the population admitted, 9.8 (Series 10, Number 52, p. 22). Physician visits from National Center for Health Statistics, Series 10, Number 18, p. 13.

ᵈ Not available.

ᵉ 1968-1970 hospital admissions per 100 person-years from Andersen et al. (1972). Admission rates were adjusted to take into account the proportion 0.5% of the original sample which died during the year according to the following formula:

$$AR = \frac{(UR \times P) - (D \times ADR)}{P - D}$$

AR = adjusted rate for the population (13.6)
UR = unadjusted admission rate (138/1000)
  P = weighted sample size (56,815)
  D = deaths in weighted sample (297)
ADR = adjusted death rate from Series 22, Number 2,
       Table 1, p. 11. ADR = (5.5) (1024/1000)

Thus, the unadjusted admission rates for nonwhites (11.1) and whites (14.2) were multiplied by a constant (13.6/13.8) which is the ratio of the adjusted rate to the unadjusted rate.

Physician visits from National Center for Health Statistics, Series 10, Number 70, Table H, p. 10. Dentist proportion from National Center for Health Statistics, Series 10, Number 70, Table 16, p. 37.

considerably higher for whites in the earliest period and, while the relative differences decreased slightly over the last 10 years or so, the white rates continue to be significantly higher today. The differences in the findings for income and race suggest that the societal impact of increasing third-party payments may have been much greater for the low-income group as a whole than it has been for the nonwhite population — much of which is actually found in the low-income group. However, these diverse findings also indicate the need to take into account other societal forces and individual determinants of use if there is to be a significant improvement in the understanding of observed differences in utilization among various groups in the population.

While it is beyond the scope of this paper and, indeed, the state of the field to provide any sort of definitive analysis of the relative importance of the various determinants of use, we can begin to make some tentative generalizations. Table 5 shows our estimate of the relative importance of each major component of the individual utilization model. It is an overall assessment of the strength of the relationship between a given component and hospital, physician, and dental use, independent of the effects of other components of the model. The assessment is based on a general review of the literature in the field as well as those particular works cited in Table 5 and is an attempt to estimate the current situation for the United States as a whole.

Thus, it can be seen that illness level is "high" in relative importance for all three types of services and in fact is the major determinant of utilization. In contrast, community resources and attitudes are "low" in relative importance for the three services;

TABLE 5

Relative Importance of Subcomponents in Predicting Utilization for Hospital, Physician, and Dentist Utilization[a]

Component	Relative Importance		
	Hospital	Physician	Dentist
Predisposing			
Demographic	Medium	Medium	Medium
Social structure	Low	Medium	High
Beliefs	Low	Low	Low
Enabling			
Family resources	Medium	Medium	High
Community resources	Low	Low	Low
Illness level			
Perceived	High	High	High
Evaluated	High	High	High

[a] The terms "low," "medium," and "high" were selected because they indicate relative magnitudes which were consistent in an examination of three pieces of research using similar methods, analysis strategies, and variable definitions. The three studies and the data on which Table 5 are based are (1) Andersen (1968:49, Table 9); (2) Andersen et al. (1970:91, Table 46; 96, Table 47; 100, Table 48; 103, Table 49; 107, Table 50; 109, Table 51; 112, Table 52; 117, Table 54); and (3) Newman (1971:91, Table 6).

variables related to these components are the least important in terms of use.

Demographic variables appear to be of "medium" importance for all services, while social structure variables are more important in ascending order moving from hospital to physician to dentist use. Finally, while family resources are of "medium" importance with respect to hospital and physician use, the relative strong effect of resources remains for dental use.

Policy Implications

As the ability to measure the impact of various model components improves, we suggest the output might be used to operationalize the increasingly accepted but still vaguely defined public policy goal of "equitable distribution of services."[22] Table 6 provides a grid for such an undertaking.[23]

[22] An implicit assumption of a public policy of equitable distribution is that it will ultimately result in an improvement in the general health status of

TABLE 6
Evaluating the Intervention Potential of Model Components in Equalizing the Distribution of Health Services

Model Component	Goal	Current Weight	Intervention Properties			Intervention Potential[b]
			Mutability	Causation[a]	Interaction[a]	
Predisposing						
Demographic	Maximize		Low			
Social Structure	Minimize		Low			
Beliefs	Minimize		Medium			
Enabling						
Family	Minimize		High			
Community	Minimize		High			
Illness Level						
Perceived	Maximize		—			
Evaluated	Maximize		—			

[a] Illustrative examples are given in text.
[b] Summary evaluation to be based on previous characteristics.

The first column would ideally list all of the particular variables which might have a direct impact on the distribution of services. Since the approach is merely outlined here, only the main subcomponents of the individual determinants of use are listed.

Column 2 indicates what we would expect to happen to the relative importance of the model components in a situation of equitable distribution. Equitable distribution, rather than implying that all individuals receive the same amount of health services regardless of their characteristics, suggests that some characteristics should become important and others less so as equity is achieved.

Among the seven subcomponents, only the effects of the demographic variables and the two measures of illness level are clearly maximized in a system of equitable distribution. The remaining four subcomponents, social structure, beliefs, and family and community resources, should have minimum influence on the distribution of health services.

Demographic variables are important bases for distributing health services under a system of equitable distribution because of the well established relationships of age, sex, and marital status to physical need, disease patterns, health maintenance, and subsequent use of services. The influences of social structure and health beliefs are minimized because allocation on the basis of a man's education, color, or knowledge about disease, for example, is contrary to the underlying value that medical care should be distributed primarily according to his medical need.

The effects of family resources such as income and health insurance would also be minimized. Lack of these resources may represent financial barriers to medical care. Barriers to use cause differences which a policy designed to spread health services seeks to remove.

the population. There are many problems in measuring health status, but it is clear that reliable and valid measures must be developed both to aid in determining when services should be provided and to measure the impact of these services on the population receiving them. Measures of health status may be viewed as but one aspect of a more general trend towards the development of social indicators. For example, see Moriyama (1968) and Goldsmith (1972).

[23] An earlier version of this approach was first introduced in Andersen (1968: 58-64).

Community resources also differentiate individuals for reasons which are not compatible with the concept of equitable distribution. For example, the rural person may use fewer services than his urban counterpart because of the longer distance he must travel to a doctor.

Variation explained by illness is maximized. In fact, the concept of equitable distribution is based on the assumption that illness as defined by the patient and his family or the system should be the primary determinant of how services are distributed.

The intervention potential for a given component depends on the extent to which it is currently important in distributing services. Of course, the relative weight ultimately assigned in column 3 would depend upon the particular service being evaluated. The important point is that a component must actually account for some of the variation in use for it to be considered a likely candidate to reduce unwanted variation in the use of services in the system. For example, if we were to find that knowledge of disease has little impact on the services that people use, we might strongly question the value of a national health education campaign designed to increase the public's understanding of certain diseases to bring about more equity in the distribution of services.

The next three columns of Table 6 are subsumed under the heading of "intervention properties." These are important characteristics of the components which need to be taken into account in consideration of social change potential.

Mutability refers to the extent to which a given component can actually be altered to influence the distribution of health services.[24] For example, the demographic variables are rated low because it is obviously impractical to consider a major change in the age structure of the country as a potential method for reducing variance in the distribution of services. In general, it appears more feasible to bring about change through the enabling variables than through the predisposing variables. For example, in the short run it is much more feasible to consider an alteration in family income than it is to consider an alteration in the educational structure.

[24] Coleman (1971) distinguishes between policy variables and control variables. Policy variables are "those variables which can be or have been amenable to policy control." Control variables "play a part in the causal structure which lead to outcome variables, and thus must be controlled in the analysis or the design, but are not subject to policy control."

The column of Table 6 headed "causation" indicates the importance of causal relationships among the model components. The expectations about causal relationships among the predictors can have major implications for attempts at social change. For example, suppose we find both education and family income fairly highly correlated with utilization. Our goal under a system of equitable distribution is to reduce the magnitude of these relationships. Changing educational levels is a long-term process and consequently not a promising approach for attaining short-term goals. However, if we find education and family income are accounting for the same variance in utilization, then we might focus on changing the income distribution without too much concern about the variance accounted for by education.[25]

The third intervention property in Table 6 emphasizes the need to consider the possibility of interaction effects between two or more variables in planning for social change. For example, the influence of health insurance benefits varies considerably according to the illness level of the group. For people who are very ill, the nature of health insurance benefits seems to be relatively less important than for populations in relatively good health. This suggests that an increase in the comprehensiveness of health insurance benefits is likely to result in a greater relative use increase for the healthy than for the people in ill health.

In the last column in Table 6 we would, ideally, sum up the overall intervention potential of each component in order to determine which might be best suited to bring about change. In general, the best candidates are those which we wish to minimize, have a relatively high current weight, are mutable, and—in the causal sequence of events—are expected to be closest to the actual utilization of services. It is painfully obvious that at this point our theoretical and empirical sophistication are such that we lack the ability to fill in much of the information that the grid in Table 6 calls for. Much work remains to be done before approaches such as this one will be truly effective. In the meantime, however, policy decisions will continue to made, often with very limited information. In such cases even an admittedly preliminary framework

[25] The assumption is that education influences income, which in turn influences the distribution of services. By altering the income variable we could also expect to reduce the variance related to education.

which calls attention to the relative importance of various societal and individual determinants might prove helpful.

Ronald Andersen, PH.D.
Associate Professor
Center for Health Administration Studies
University of Chicago
5720 Woodlawn Avenue
Chicago, Illinois 60637

John F. Newman, PH.D.
Research Associate
Center for Health Administration Studies
University of Chicago
5720 Woodlawn Avenue
Chicago, Illinois 60637

This Study was funded in part through Contract HSM 110-70-392 with the National Center for Health Services Research and Development, Department of Health, Education, and Welfare.

References

Aday, Lu Ann *and* Robert L. Eichhorn
  1972   The Utilization of Health Services: Indices and Correlates. Lafayette, Indiana: Purdue University.

Andersen, Ronald *and* Odin W. Anderson
  1967   A Decade of Health Services: Social Survey Trends in Use and Expenditures. Chicago: University of Chicago Press.

Andersen, Ronald
  1968   A Behavioral Model of Families' Use of Health Services, Research Series No. 25. Chicago: Center for Health Administration Studies, University of Chicago.

Andersen, Ronald, Bjorn Smedby, *and* Odin W. Anderson
  1970   Medical Care Use in Sweden and the United States: A Comparative Analysis of Systems and Behavior, Research Series No. 27. Chicago: Center for Health Administration Studies, University of Chicago.

Andersen, Ronald, Joanna Kravits, *and* Odin W. Anderson
1971   "The public's view of the crisis in medical care: An impetus for
changing delivery systems?" Economic and Business Bulletin 24
(Fall): 47.

Andersen, Ronald, Rachel McL. Greeley, Joanna Kravits, *and* Odin W.
Anderson
1972   Health Service Use: National Trends and Variations—1953–1971.
Washington: U. S. Department of Health, Education, and Welfare,
DHEW Publications No. (HSM) 73–3004 (October).

Anderson, Odin W. *and* Jacob J. Feldman
1956   Family Medical Costs and Voluntary Health Insurance: A Nation-
wide Survey. New York: McGraw-Hill.

Anderson, Odin W.
1968   The Uneasy Equilibrium. New Haven: College and University Press.
1972   Health Care: Can There Be Equity? The United States, Sweden,
and England. New York: Wiley.

Anderson, Odin W. *and* Ronald Andersen
1972   "Patterns of use of health services." Pp. 386–406 in Howard E.
Freeman, Sol Levine, *and* Leo G. Reeder (eds.), Handbook of Medical Sociology. Englewood Cliffs, New Jersey: Prentice-Hall.

Baker, Frank
1970   "General systems theory, research, and medical care." Pp. 4–5
in Alan Sheldon, Frank Baker, *and* Curtis McLaughlin (eds.), Systems and Medical Care. Cambridge, Massachusetts: M.I.T. Press.

Bice, Thomas W. *and* Kerr L. White
1971   "Cross-national comparative research on the utilization of medical
services." Medical Care 9 (May–June): 253–271.

Bice, Thomas W., Robert L. Eichhorn, *and* Peter D. Fox
1972   "Socioeconomic status and use of physician services: A reconsidera-
tion." Medical Care 10 (May–June): 261–271.

Coleman, James S.
1971   "Problems of Conceptualization and Measurement in Studying Policy Impacts." Paper presented at the Conference on the Impacts of
Public Policies, St. Thomas, U. S. Virgin Islands (December 3–5).

Commission on Chronic Illness in the United States
1957   Prevention of Chronic Illness, Volume 1. Cambridge, Massachusetts:
Harvard University Press.

Cooper, Barbara S. *and* Nancy L. Worthington
1972   "National health expenditures, calendar years 1929–1970." Research and Statistics Notes (January 14): Note No. 1.

Falk, I. S., Margaret C. Klem, *and* Nathan Sinai
1933   The Incidence of Illness and the Receipt and Costs of Medical Care among Representative Families: Experiences in Twelve Consecutive Months in 1928–1931. Chicago: University of Chicago Press.

Field, Mark G.
1971   "Stability and change in the medical system: Medicine in the industrial society." Pp. 30–61 in Bernard Barber and Alex Inkeles (eds.), Stability and Social Change. Boston: Little, Brown.

Fox, Peter D.
1972   "Access to medical care for the poor: The federal perspective." Medical Care 10 (May–June): 272–277.

Goldsmith, S. B.
1972   "The status of health status indicators." Health Service Reports 87 (March): 212–220.

Greenlick, M. R., Arnold Hurtado, Claude R. Pope, Ernest W. Saward, *and* Samuel S. Yoshioka
1968   "Determinants of medical care utilization." Health Services Research 3 (Winter): 296-315.

Kriesberg, Louis
1963   "The relationship between socioeconomic rank and behavior." Social Problems 10 (Spring): 349.

Lerner, Monroe *and* Odin W. Anderson
1963   Health Progress in the United States, 1900–1960. Chicago: University of Chicago Press.

Lohr, William
1972   "An Historical View of the Research Done on the Behavioral and Organizational Factors Related to Utilization of Health Services." Unpublished paper (January). Rockville, Maryland: National Center for Health Services Research and Development.

McKinlay, John B.
1972   "Some approaches and problems in the study of the use of services—An overview." Journal of Health and Social Behavior 13 (June): 115–152.

Maclachlan, J. M.
1958   "Cultural factors in health and disease." Pp. 94–105 in E. G. Jaco (ed.), Patients, Physicians, and Illness. Glencoe, Illinois: Free Press.

Milbank Memorial Fund
1972   Current Program Policy and Organization: 5, 9. New York.

Moore, Wilbert E.
1969   "Social structure and behavior." Pp. 283–322 in Gardner Lindzey
       and Elliot Aronson (eds.), The Handbook of Social Psychology,
       Volume 4, 2nd edition. Reading, Massachusetts: Addison-Wesley.

Moriyama, I. W.
1968   "Problems in the measurement of health status." Pp. 573–600 in
       E. B. Sheldon and W.E. Moore (eds.), Indicators of Social Change.
       New York: Russell Sage Foundation.

National Center for Health Statistics
1965a Volume of Physician Visits by Place of Visit and Type of Service,
       Series 10, No. 18.

1965b Hospitalization in the Last Year of Life, Series 22, No. 1.

1968   Infant Loss in the Netherlands, Series 3, No. 11.

Newman, John F.
1971   The Utilization of Dental Services. Ph.D. dissertation. Emory
       University.

Newman, John F. and Odin W. Anderson
1972   Patterns of Dental Service Utilization in the United States: A
       Nationwide Social Survey, Research Series No. 30. Chicago:
       Center for Health Administration Studies, University of Chicago.

Richardson, William C.
1969   "Poverty, illness, and use of health services in the United States."
       Hospitals XLIII (July 1): 34–40.

1971   Ambulatory Use of Physicians' Services in Response to Illness Epi-
       sodes in a Low-Income Neighborhood, Research Series No. 29.
       Chicago: Center for Health Administration Studies, University of
       Chicago.

Rosenstock, I. M.
1966   "Why people use health services." Milbank Memorial Fund Quar-
       terly 44 (October-Part 2): 94–124.

Sheldon, Alan, Frank Baker, and Curtis McLaughlin (eds.)
1970   Systems and Medical Care. Cambridge, Massachusetts: M.I.T. Press.

Solon, J. A., James J. Feeney, Sally H. Jones, Ruth D. Rigg, and Cecil
       G. Sheps
1967   "Delineating episodes of medical care." American Journal of Pub-
       lic Health 57 (March): 401–408.

Suchman, E. A.
1965 "Health orientation and medical care." American Journal of Public Health 55 (November): 94–105.

Taylor, James C.
1971 Technology and Planned Organizational Change. Ann Arbor, Michigan: Institute for Social Research, University of Michigan.

U. S. Bureau of the Census
1965 Historical Statistics of the United States, Colonial Times to 1957; Continuation to 1962 and Revisions. Washington: U. S. Government Printing Office.
1971 Statistical Abstract of the United States, 1971. 92nd edition. Washington.

Warner, Homer R.
1972 "Problems and Priorities for Health Care Technology in the 1980s." Paper presented at the Conference on Technology and Health Care Systems in the 1980s, sponsored by the National Center for Health Services Research and Development, San Francisco (January 21).

Weinerman, E. Richard
1971 "Research on comparative health service systems." Medical Care 9 (May–June): 272–290.

Wirick, G. C.
1966 "A multiple equation model of demand for health care." Health Services Research 1 (Winter): 301–346.

Social-Psychological
Factors Affecting Health
Service Utilization

JOHB B. MCKINLAY
AND DIANA B. DUTTON

Perception of Need for Care

In studying the determinants of utilization of health services, re-searchers have generally reported what may seem to be an obvious conclusion: that need for care—an illness condition of some sort—is the primary cause of the decision to seek medical care (Ander-sen, 1968; Mechanic, 1969; Bice, 1971; Richardson, 1970). Yet the simplicity of the notion is deceptive.

What the "need" is—what factors are associated with the per-ception of medical need, how they are distributed among different population groups, and how they affect decision-making in the seeking of care are questions which do not have simple answers. Suchman (1965b) describes the decision to seek medical care as a progression of stages, beginning with the recognition of symptoms, leading to the definition of oneself as ill, followed by a possible de-cision to seek medical care. Each stage occurs within and is shaped by an aggregate context of social, cultural, economic, and situation-al circumstances, as well as an individual context of particular psy-

In *Consumer Incentives for Health Care*, edited by Selma J. Mushkin. New York: PRODIST, 1974.

chological attitudes and beliefs. In this paper we will discuss some of the social-psychological factors that bear on various stages in the decision to seek medical care.

Factors Influencing the Perception of Health and Recognition of Symptoms

A review of the literature does much to undermine the notion of "objective" illness. It is now apparent that illness is in large part "a matter of social definition which varyingly reflects cultural and individual differences in orientation toward the biological organism" (Twaddle, 1969:106). Most simply, illness is a subjective reaction to a physical state (Hochbaum, 1958; Kirscht, 1971), but it is the subjective reaction, and not the physical state, which is the measure of a person's "illness."

Investigators have noted the wide variety in popular conceptions of illness and symptoms (Lerner, 1969; Zola, 1966; Apple, 1960; Baumann, 1961; Robinson, 1971). Zola (1966) refers to the many factors that contribute to the shaping of definitions of health and illness and also to the sensitizing of people to certain physiological symptoms that are perceived as symptoms of illness or are accepted as the normal order of things. He suggests, for example, that if the symptom is very prevalent or if it is closely congruent with dominant or major value-orientations of the culture, then it is unlikely to be perceived as a sign of something wrong. Andersen et al. (1968) suggest that variation in the reporting of symptoms is related to demographic differences, in addition to cultural and societal differences in the interpretation of symptoms as disease. Even within a single culture, diseases are perceived in many ways. Content analysis of peoples' beliefs and perceptions about various diseases has revealed systematic differences among people with varying social, economic, and demographic characteristics (Jenkins, 1966).

Even what people mean by "good health" seems to vary. Analyzing responses to open-ended questions on perceptions of health and good physical condition, Baumann (1961) found three distinct orientations in the way "good health" was defined: (1) a general feeling of well-being; (2) the absence of general or specific illness symptoms; and (3) the ability to perform normal social roles. The symptom-oriented response was slightly more prevalent among more highly educated individuals, and the general-feeling orientation was more prevalent among those with less education. The third orientation, however, performance of social roles, was evenly distributed among all social classes.

Many studies have found that interference with the ability to perform normal social roles is the most common way for people to define a physical condition as "illness" or a physical sign as an "illness symptom" (Apple, 1960; diCicco and Apple, 1958). Furthermore, there are reported class differences in the use of inability to perform normal social roles as a criterion of self-defined "sickness." Gordon (1966), for example, gave a group of respondents twelve different descriptions of ill health and asked if each should be called sickness. Unfavorable prognosis was the most common factor considered to indicate sickness and did not seem to vary by social class.

Inability to work was found to be a more important determinant of what was viewed as sickness for upper income persons than for those with lower incomes. Thus, the more highly valued the activities of the "well role," the more likely that interference with them through adoption of the "sick role" is resisted (Twaddle, 1969; Zola, 1964; Robinson, 1971). Correspondingly, when the well role is unsatisfactory for some reason or when the individual feels a sense of failure in fulfilling that role, the sick role can provide a refuge from the well role (Twaddle, 1969; Cole and LeJeune, 1972). Illness can thus be used to legitimize a sense of failure to fulfill socially prescribed roles.

The point to be stressed is that adoption of the sick role, since it represents a rejection of well-role activities, will be very much affected by what those activities are and what valuation is placed on them. As Twaddle (1969:114) puts it, "Parsons suggested that exemption from normal activities depends on the severity of the illness, [but] it seems equally true that the respondents' assessment of severity depends on exemption from normal roles."

Factors Influencing the Differential Experience
of Illness Symptoms

It is not only the ways in which health and disease are perceived that are influenced by cultural and social characteristics but also apparently the *actual experiencing* of physiological symptoms. Wide divergencies between people's perceptions of their own diseases and the clinical diagnoses have been noted (Richardson, 1970; Zola, 1964; Kirscht, 1971; Maddox, 1964; Suchman et al., 1958; Friedsam and Martin, 1963). Two studies comparing physicians' evaluations with respondents' evaluations of their own health found that roughly forty percent did not agree.

There are clearly many factors related to the distortion of people's perceptions of their own health; unfortunately most of them are unknown. Kasl and Cobb (1966:256) discuss the effects of age and sex on the perception of symptoms, concluding that "men and older subjects are more optimistic about their health than women and younger subjects [although] one study found no age or sex differences." They go on to say that the conclusions are based on tendencies to underrate or overrate health conditions, and "since under-reporting varies with the nature of symptoms and since many symptoms are age or sex-related, or both, more refined analyses than are presently available need to be made."

In a comparison of matched groups of men and women, Hinkle et al. (1960) found significant differences in both the nature and number of illnesses reported by both groups. The women reported more illnesses that, although minor, were perceived as disabling, while the men were diagnosed as actually having more serious illnesses. Hinkle et al. (1960:1335) attributed the differences in perception of illness severity to "culturally and socially determined attitudes."

In addition to age and sex, other factors that have been found to be associated with differential response to disease symptoms are such social characteristics as religion, marital status, and living situation (Hessler et al., 1971)—and cultural differences among ethnic groups. Zborowski (1958) reported that ethnic values affect the reactions to physical pain—the "meaning" attached to it and the emotional content in its expression. Croog (1961) noted that in a group of army inductees, Jews at all education levels reported the greatest number of symptoms, reflecting greater concern with or sensitivity to illness symptoms.

Zola (1966) also reported that there are ethnic differences in reaction to symptoms. In a study of 196 hospital patients of Italian Catholic, Irish Catholic, and Anglo-Saxon Protestant backgrounds, he found that even with the same diagnosed disorder there were differences among those ethnic groups in the ways symptoms are perceived and experienced. The Irish tended to deny that they experienced pain in connection with their illness and typically described their problem in terms of specific dysfunctions while the Italians more often spoke of a diffuse difficulty, sometimes spreading and generalizing complaints into the area of interpersonal behavior.

Stress

Research on the relationship between psychological stress, physiological symptoms, and behavioral response has identified at least three potential roles for stress: (1) Severe or prolonged stress actually causes physiological illness. (2) Stress heightens symptom sensitivity, producing an increased awareness of illness symptoms that might otherwise have been ignored. (3) Stress increases the likelihood that some corrective action will be taken in response to a perceived symptom of illness—e.g., professional medical care will be sought. In fact, the evidence in support of all three roles is convincing. Stress has been reported to be associated, apparently physiologically, with the onset of a number of chronic diseases (see Sparer, 1956; Conference of the Society . . . , 1959; Travis, 1961; Holmes et al., 1951; Rahe, 1964), although it is not clear in some studies that new physiological symptoms have been distinguished from heightened sensitivity to symptoms already existing (Kasl and Cobb, 1966). For our purposes, it will not be important to distinguish the actual physiological effects of stress from its effects in heightening sensitivity, as both result in the perception of increased illness.

There is ample evidence that stress does increase the likelihood of perceiving illness, whether through increased mental or physical susceptibility. In a study of about 7,000 mothers in California, Berkman (1969) found that the stress resulting from being a spouseless mother was significantly related to the frequency of self-reported chronic conditions and functional disabilities, controlling for a number of other associated economic, environmental, and personality stresses. Similarly, Mechanic (1964) found that mothers under temporary psychological stress tended to report more illness symptomatology for both themselves and their children. In a study of 194 Underwater Demolition Team trainees, measures of stressful life changes were found to be significantly correlated with the development of severe illness (Rahe et al., 1972). Even the degree of "consonance" with respect to cultural and social characteristics among residents in a housing project was found to be related to the amount of physical and mental stress experienced (Hessler et al., 1971). Mechanic and Volkhart (1961) and Stoeckle et al. (1963) have reviewed a number of studies concerning the role of psychological stress that support the correlation between stress and increased prevalence, or at least awareness, of illness.

A close relationship between psychological stress and physiological disorders is also indicated in studies suggesting that certain individuals are particularly susceptible to both forms of distress. The work of Engel (1967) on "pain prone" individuals and a study by Fabrega and colleagues (1969) on the medical and behavioral features of low-income medical "problem patients" are illustrative of that relationship. The latter study found that patients identified as "problem patients" by a panel of doctors, according to such criteria as emotionalism, lack of cooperation, and vagueness in communication, were more likely to rate themselves as more physically "sick" than other patients (although their actual hospitalization rates were comparable) and were also more likely to introduce social problems into the medical consultation.

Finally, there is evidence that it may be not only difficult in practice to distinguish between the first two roles posited for stress, but that actually they may be interrelated. In other words, stress may first result in heightened (or imagined) sensitivities to illness symptoms but may then take a real physiological toll of health status. A study by Rosengren (1964) of two hundred maternity patients of various social classes concluded that lower class women and also women with class-inconsistent cultural values, role conflict, and recent social mobility tended to regard themselves as more "sick" during pregnancy than did women of middle or upper-middle class status. In fact, it turned out that those women who believed themselves to be sicker actually did have more difficult pregnancies. Though poorer general health status and lower quality care may have been partly responsible, it seems likely that the women's attitudes also affected their physiological states (McKinlay, 1972b).

Another example of the interaction between psychological and physiological states comes from a study by Epstein et al. (1957) of a homogeneous group of clothing workers in New York City. Rates of manifest arteriosclerosis were found to be twice as high among Jewish men as among Italian men and were associated with such factors as serum cholesterol levels, blood pressure, and body weight among the Italians but not among the Jewish men. Although real physiological differences existed, it is not clear whether their origins were physiological and psychological. The tendency of different ethnic groups to have different psychological reactions to physiological symptoms may result in real differences in physical symptom patterns.

In the context of influencing the concept of stress, the perception of physiological symptoms and utilization decisions is characterized by anxiety, discomfort, and emotional tension (Janis, 1958). Although the effects, in terms of increased sensitivity to physiological symptoms, of many forms of stress seem to be similar, sources of stress are numerous and varied. They include major changes in life situation (Rahe et al., 1972), overcrowding, inconsistency or ambiguity in tasks or roles, changes in customary activities (McGrath, 1970), low status (Meile and Haese, 1969), status inconsistency (Jackson, 1962; Jackson and Burke, 1965), social or marital incompatibility (Hochstim, 1968), and socio-environmental (Coe et al., 1969; Hochstim, 1968).

Two sources of stress that have been studied in detail are status inconsistency and lower class status. The findings suggestst that both are (independently) associated with higher than average stress symptoms. The degree of "status integration" is seemingly related to patterns of chronic illness in a number of empirical tests although alternative explanations of the relationship are possible (Dodge and Martin, 1970). Jackson and Burke (1965) found that the number and seriousness of stress symptoms experienced are related to the number and type of status inconsistencies as measured by occupation, education, and racial ethnic group.

An index of "psychophysiological disorder," based on twenty-two questions concerning both physical and mental disorders, has been used to study the relationship between mental stress, physical disorders, and social class. Crandell and Dohrenwend (1967) conclude from responses to those questions that "there is a distinct tendency on the part of lower-class groups to express psychological distress in physiological terms."

Meile (1972) claims, however, that this tendency represents not only a transference between psychological and physiological symptoms but the additional presence for lower class groups of real psychological burdens. Controlling for sex and education, he concludes that "structural variables may not only affect the type of expression of psychological disorder, but they may in fact be 'causally' linked to the presence or absence of the disorder."

Meile and Haese (1969) investigated the relationship between status inconsistency and status itself and found that lower class status, as measured by an average of socioeconomic status indicators, is more closely associated with mental and physical stress symptoms than is status inconsistency. They suggest that, as in the Crandell and Dohrenwend (1967) study, the association may be due to the presence of greater real sources of stress for the poor.

Additional evidence that lower class status is associated with greater experience of stress comes from studies contrasting the stress experiences of people living in poverty areas to those of people comparable in other respects but living in better-off neighborhoods. Two such studies concluded that the conditions of the poverty neighborhood itself constitute a source of stress for residents that is related to greater than average experience of illness, injury, and psychological disruption (Coe et al., 1969; Hochstim, 1968).

Salience of Health

A matter of some debate has been the question of possible differences in the "salience" of health and illness to different social groups. In particular, there has been a continuing argument about whether persons categorized as lower social class were more or less "concerned" about their health and its maintenance than are others. Koos launched the argument in 1954 by reporting that health is more salient to the upper classes, that lower class persons are more likely to "put up" with a variety of symptoms and not to seek medical care for them. It is important to note that this is not a single but a double claim, which deals with both the attitudinal as well as the behavioral response of persons to symptoms of illness. In fact, the claims should be evaluated separately, as different factors may influence each. Thus, one claim may be true and not the other. We shall first examine evidence regarding differences in the salience of health as measured by attitudes concerning health and illness.

Zborowski (1958) reported that more highly educated persons appear to be more conscious of their health and more aware of pain as a symptom of disease. That reaction is interpreted, however, as differential response to illness fostered by education and socialization rather than as an internal attitudinal difference. In the same year, in the field of mental health, Hollingshead and Redlich (1958) purported to document the relationship between social class and tolerance of symptoms of ill health. More recent evidence, however, clearly challenges the view that lower socioeconomic groups are less concerned about health or more tolerant of symptoms of ill health. Suchman (1965a) found little difference among socioeconomic groups in the interpretation of symptoms as indicating illness or in the amount of concern expressed about symptoms. Mc-Broom (1970) found no evidence that lower status persons tend to overreact to or overreport symptoms of illness, and little relation between socioeconomic status and perceived illness level. Mechanic

(1969) concluded on the basis of available research that there is little evidence of significant differences in response to pain and discomfort among various socioeconomic groups.

There is in fact some evidence that lower class persons *are more concerned* than upper class persons about their health. Crandell and Dohrenwend's findings concerning the tendency of lower class persons to translate psychological distress into physiological form suggest that the physical health of the body is of enough concern to them to serve as a vehicle for the expression of both mental and physical ills. Kadushin (1967) cites several studies, based on responses to check-listed items measuring concern with health or anxiety about physical symptoms, which suggest that lower class persons are more likely than upper class persons to worry about their health (Bradburn and Caplovitz, 1965; Crandell and Dohrenwend, 1967). These studies are particularly convincing since they avoid the pitfall of open-ended responses to questions that tend to elicit fewer responses from lower class persons, regardless of the questions being asked. As noted earlier, Rosengren (1964) found in his study of maternity patients that lower class women tended to regard themselves as more "sick" during pregnancy than women of middle and upper classes.

The suspicion may arise that the apparently greater concern of the poor for their health may be primarily because their health is worse. It is certainly true that the impact of illness is more burdensome for the poor, and it may be that past experiences, either personal or those of friends, have heightened the fear of repeated illness and have thus increased their concern about their health status. But it does not seem to be greater prevalence of present illness that accounts for their greater concern. Data from the National Health Survey suggest that, given comparable states of health, the poor are more concerned about their health. Self-administered medical history questionnaires given to a sample of adults were compared with the results of their medical examinations for hypertension and heart disease, and it was found that, at the lower income and lower educational levels, the self-reported disease prevalences were slightly exaggerated (National Center for Health Statistics, 1967). That is, lower income individuals tended to perceive themselves as sicker than they actually were as measured by clinical examination.

Use of Health Services

Since the perception and experiencing of illness symptoms affect a person's response to those symptoms, and since one possible response is the decision to seek medical care, all the factors discussed thus far bear at least indirectly on the decision to seek medical care. They affect the symptom-response (what might be termed the "pre-patient" or "pre-action") phase of the utilization-decision process. But many of them bear directly on utilization decisions as well. Stress seems to play a role both in increasing symptom sensitivity and in increasing the likelihood that the individual will seek professional medical care (Stoeckle et al., 1963). And it has been shown that seeking care is usually preceded by defining oneself as "ill" (Antonovsky, 1972). The connection between perceptions of illness and the decision to seek care is as tenuous, however, as the subjectivity of the notion of illness might suggest. Among a group of people who all perceived themselves as ill, it was found that the number or severity of illness symptoms was not significantly related to whether or not care had been sought (Ludwig and Gibson, 1969). Instead, situational factors and faith in the medical-care system were found to be most closely related to whether or not a doctor had been consulted.

In the same way that the perception and experiencing of symptoms are influenced by both external factors (social, cultural, economic, etc.) and internal (psychological) factors, so the subsequent decision to seek medical care, given certain perceived symptoms, is influenced by those factors. The role of external factors in influencing use of services is especially important. Many studies have shown that the availability, acceptability, and financial accessibility of services are critical factors in accounting for much variation in utilization behavior. In addition, the effects of demographic, social, and cultural factors have been found to be related to patterns of utilization (McKinlay, 1972a).

Tendency to Use Services

Little effort appears to have been made to distinguish the effects of psychological factors on the *decision* to seek care from their effects on the *perception* of symptoms, and this could be fruitfully pursued in future research. What work has been reported in the area has been primarily concerned with the measurement and/or explanation of a psychological state of "readiness" or "tendency" to use services. Typically, respondents have been asked if they would seek care if they noticed a given symptom of illness; their responses are then combined into an index, which is viewed as measuring the tendency or readiness to seek care. Some studies have treated the concept as an exogenous variable—a characteristic of people that is taken as given and is used in helping to predict utilization. More interesting are studies that have attempted to determine the characteristics to which such a tendency might be related and why.

The concept of readiness to initiate physician care was first employed by Koos in 1956 in the form of a collection of responses to the question of whether a doctor should be consulted for each of a list of common illness symptoms. In a subsequent study Hochbaum (1958) presented a model that specified three components of the state of psychological readiness to initiate care, especially preventive care—perceived seriousness of the disease, perceived vulnerability to the disease, and perceived efficacy of medical treatment. He contended that it was the presence of these beliefs that accounted for observed use patterns. Evidence has accumulated to support his claim, at least for discretionary use (preventive or patient-initiated therapeutic visits).

While Hochbaum's particular model dealt with psychological factors relevant to initiating the use of preventive services, most other studies of the tendency to use services have focused on psychological factors influencing use of therapeutic services, usually in response to the recognition of some sign of illness. Zola (1964) designates five "triggers" that may precipitate the decision to seek care. They are, briefly, interpersonal crisis, interference with valued social activity, sanctioning by others, threat to major activity, and nature and familiarity of symptoms. All are viewed as influencing both the perception of and the response to symptoms. Mechanic and Volkhart (1961), in contrast, emphasize that perception and response should be treated separately. They find that stress (in Zola's terms, interpersonal crisis) is related primarily to symptom sensitivity and perception, while a different psychological process —which they term "tendency to adopt the sick role"—which is a summary index based on the merged responses to several general symptom questions, and is thought to intervene between the perception of need for care and actual use of services.

Other findings on the role of "tendency to use services" have been somewhat mixed. Bice (1971) found that a measure of tendency to use services was important in explaining the use of preventive services but not in explaining any of his measures of symptomatic or therapeutic use. This is consistent with the original focus of the readiness concept in explaining use of preventive services. Kalimo (1969) and Antonovsky (1972) reported that measures of tendency to use physicians' services are positively correlated with total (preventive and therapeutic) utilization. In Andersen's model (1968) of families' use of health services, an index of "attitude toward physician use" was found to have only a slight positive relation to a measure of total physician use.

That the various findings differ somewhat is not surprising in view of the variation in the different tendency measures. Bice (1971) and Antonovsky (1972), for example, based their tendency measures on questions concerning psychosocial needs and problems (difficulty in getting along with other people, status, coping with failure, etc.), Kalimo's index (1969) was based on the perceived benefits and barriers to the use of medical services, and Andersen merged responses to questions about seeking physician's care for a number of physical symptoms of illness. The approaches taken by Hochbaum (1958) and Zola (1964) in their analyses of the psychological factors associated with readiness to seek care illustrates an even more fundamental difference in method. It is clear that there is no consensus on what psychological factors are involved in the tendency to use services or even on the best way to approach the formulation or measurement of such a concept.

Investigators have also been concerned with the relationship between some measure of tendency to use services and social class. To the extent that this psychological tendency is unevenly distributed among various social classes, it might account for use patterns that otherwise might be attributed to other characteristics of the groups. Koos (1954) and Rosenstock (1969) found, based on responses to check lists of medical danger signals, that persons classified as of upper socioeconomic status seemed more inclined to seek medical care for a given set of symptoms. Similarly, Hetherington and Hopkins (1969) reported that respondents of higher occupational status were more likely to judge that a list of symptoms warranted seeking medical care. The inclination to seek care was also related to a number of other social and demographic characteristics.

Other studies have failed to find a significant relationship between tendency to use services and social class (Feldman, 1966). Bice's (1971) measure of tendency to consult a doctor for a psychosocial problem was not related to either economic class or to education. Apple (1960) found that, in a sample of mostly middle class respondents, there was little variation in responses to a list of somatic symptoms by age, sex, occupation, or education, but the reason may have been the rather restricted range of educational and occupational groups included in the study.

In a study of the utilization behavior of older adults, Battistella (1968a) found that persons of lower socioeconomic status seemed to be more, rather than less, inclined to seek care in the presence of illness symptoms; they reported having delayed less than persons of upper status after they had recognized symptoms of disease. Battistella suggests that one explanation may be that the sick role offers lower status persons relief from the anxieties and strains of their normal social roles. No attempt, however, was made to determine if symptoms were recognized at comparable stages of seriousness by the two groups—a major weakness of the study that makes the findings somewhat inconclusive. On a larger scale, Andersen and colleagues (1968) found that social and economic factors seemed to account at least in part for international differences in utilization rates, although not for differences in the perception of symptoms.

It is difficult to draw a coherent picture from these widely different studies and the varied findings concerning the concept of tendency to use services. To some extent, variability is inherent in the nature of the phenomenon. Steele and McBroom warn that "health behavior"—use of preventive health services—is a multidimensional concept. Use of different types of preventive services varies among different groups and is differentially affected by various socioeconomic and situational characteristics (Steele and McBroom, 1972). Thus, one might expect that attempts to study psychological factors related to inclination or readiness to use different services would produce diverse results.

But much of the variety in the studies and findings results from inconsistencies in conceptualization and measurement and from further inconsistencies in the study contexts in which the concept is tested. One inconsistency is the type of utilization behavior the tendency measure is supposed to predict. Battistella (1968a) makes the important point that the appropriate measure of utilization in studying the role of psychological readiness or tendency to use services is the initial visit per illness episode, since the patient has maximum control over the decision to make the initial visit and much less control over the number and frequency of all subsequent visits. Thus, it is not surprising that studies find little if any relationship between tendency measures and total utilization frequencies; yet that is the relationship most frequently tested.

Perhaps the most fundamental weakness of research in the area is its failure to place the tendency concept in its proper context—as one of many factors affecting, or likely to affect, utilization. Battistella (1968b) has again correctly pointed out that whatever has been measured by the various indices of "subjective inclination to use health services" is relatively insignificant in relation to other factors affecting use, such as the accessibility and availability of physicians' services. Though there may in fact be real differences in such subjective tendencies, in general their effects have not been measured above and beyond the effects of other factors that are known to affect utilization patterns, such as availability of care, cultural and ethnic preferences, and age and sex effects. Characteristic of most studies is the analysis of single associations between measures of tendency and actual use or measures of socioeconomic status; the interrelation between even tendency, use, and social class is rarely examined. Bice's study (1971) is one exception. As a result, the effects of differences in subjective tendencies are probably largely lost among or at least confounded by the more predominant influences of all the other factors affecting use decisions, the effects of which are not controlled. A similar criticism is relevant to much of the work on the role of other psychological factors in utilization decisions, although it seems to be somewhat less critical to the analysis of factors affecting the symptom-response (pre-action) phase of the utilization decision-making process.

To some extent, the simultaneous interdependence of variables is rarely examined because to do so requires a fairly large data base that is often unavailable. But it also seems that the importance of the interdependencies has not been sufficiently appreciated, and the forms of multivariate analyses that would allow both an examination of and compensation for interrelations have only begun to be exploited. Advances in methodology may herald new substantive findings, or at least allow old disputes about the relative effects of variables that have been traditionally analyzed on a one-to-one basis to be laid to rest.

Influence of Stigma and the Labeling Process

A number of conditions and/or states are regarded, at least in Western societies, as stigmatizing those who possess them. Notable examples are alcoholism, venereal disease, mental illness, the menopause, obesity, drug dependence, and an unwanted pregnancy. One would suspect a priori that the possession of some stigmatizing characteristic may, in various ways, influence the use of services. Despite the fairly widespread recognition of its influence, however, stigma has received scant attention in this particular context. Little empirical research has been conducted on its nature, but there is a body of more theoretical social-psychological literature that does explore the dimensions of the question. Some of this work as it may relate to utilization behavior is considered below.

The most insightful work on the concept of stigma appears in the writings of Erving Goffman (1959) who began with an interest in "impression management." For him "impression management" denotes the efforts that people make to create and sustain desired images about themselves and thus to control the conduct of others, especially their responsive treatment, by controlling the types of information they receive. More recently, Goffman (1961) has focused specifically on the behavior of people with a stigma or "undesired differentness," and he identifies three main types: (1) physical disfigurement; (2) aberrations of character and/or personality; and (3) social categorizations, such as race, nationality, and religion. In short, "an individual who might have been received easily in ordinary social intercourse possesses a trait that can obtrude itself upon attention and turn those of us whom he meets away from him, breaking the claim that his other attributes have on us." Goffman argues that the type of impression management involved is largely a function of whether the stigma is visible or invisible, known about or not. If it is visible (e.g., facial deformities, polio paralysis), the person is *discredited*, knows or assumes that others are aware of the differentness, and the primary interactional task is the *management of tension*. If it is not immediately visible (e.g., an unwanted pregnancy, alcoholism, or the menopause) the person is only *discreditable* and his or her primary interactional task is the *management of information* about the condition.

From such a perspective, it is clear that the subjective meanings of their "undesirable differentness" for the stigmatized are of central importance. For those with some *permanent* stigma, a viable self-identity must be sustained; for the individual *acquiring* a stigmatized condition or entering a stigmatized state, a new self-identity must be created. They are no longer what they had presumed themselves to be and must devote considerable attention to achieving what is vaguely termed "acceptance" by the normal person. Goffman (1959, 1961, 1963), among others, describes at some length the protective or defensive strategies that constitute the impression-management repertoire of the stigmatized. Such tactics as "passing," "covering," and working out "lines" and "codes" of conduct help the "undesirably different" to cope with their discrediting or discreditable attribute and protect them from mortifying situations.

It seems that the stigmatized are involved in a tortuous dilemma of self-contradiction. They are clearly denied *real* acceptance in most social encounters, but they also, perhaps more importantly, act in such a way as to confirm the negative evaluation of their condition or state and remain stigmatized in their own eyes. The paradox of the situation is that, no matter how vast their repertoire of impression-management strategies or how successfully those strategies are deployed to manage tension or informaton, the stigmatized remain wedded to the same identity norms as normal persons—the very norms that disqualify them. Consequently, they are both *other*- and *self*-stigmatized.

One important influence of stigma on the utilization of health care relates to the involved person's *self-identity* and probably exerts an early influence in his help-seeking. Denial of the presence of some stigmatized condition (for example, conditions of a cosmetic nature like skin blemishes) may be viewed as an attempt to protect or delay some change in a person's own self-concept. Such denial is facilitated by the development of counterideologies or of self-rationalizations that the condition is, among other things, unimportant; that others' evaluations are misinformed; or that the condition is only temporary and will pass with time (Voysey, 1972a, b; Davis, 1961; Garfinkel, 1967; Glaser and Strauss, 1965). The self-rationalizations and the reluctance to alter behavior can be viewed as protective of those affected, or their significant others.

The alterations in behavior and ideology associated with self-identity should be distinguished from other behavior that relates to alterations in *social identity* (how *other* people and agencies react once disclosure occurs). Since many health and welfare agencies appear to shape the nature of a person's social identity through the isolation and confirmation of stigmatizing conditions, various types of utilization behavior (especially the delay and misuse of certain services) may be viewed as attempts to retain, for as long as possible, control of social identity.

Goffman (1963) has described a situation in which certain individuals are obliged to share some of the discredit of the stigmatized person to whom they are related. The relationship through the social structure leads the wider society to treat both the stigmatized person and his relations, in some respects, as one (Birnbaum, 1970). In such a situation the stigma flows from the initially discredited to his affiliates.

One can conceive of situations where stigma can initially reside in both mandated officials (e.g., the social worker, the policeman, the psychiatrist) and service organizations (abortion clinics, detoxification centers, welfare departments, and, perhaps, emergency rooms) and discredit those clients with whom they have contact. The stigma then flows *from the already discredited official or agency* to clients with whom they interact. It can of course be argued that the services—disease clinics, for example—receive a courtesy stigma because they interact with individuals and groups who are *already* stigmatized. The precise direction and sequence are, however, somewhat irrelevant as far as understanding utilization behavior is concerned, partly depending on the origins of particular organizations and the typical problems that they handled at their inception. Health and welfare facilities often have a reputation that precedes their current client membership, a prevailing ideology concerning their activities and clients and an existing set of typifications and degradation procedures that are learned by new personnel—all perpetuated by the agency and generally existing before current clients became members.

In addition, the stigma incurred by a multiservice health or welfare agency from one group of clients may be passed on to other clients with different problems or conditions who use the same agency. In Great Britain, for example, the agency that distributes unemployment benefits is also responsible for the employment services; to locate a new job a person has to risk the stigma of being labeled unemployed. If there is any doubt concerning whether or not health and welfare agencies are stigmatized, we can look at the almost perennial attempts that they make to change their public image by changing their name.

So far we have explored the possible importance of stigma in the decision to utilize a service and the possible utility of the concept in understanding utilization behavior in relation to specific agencies. The underuse or misuse of services can be viewed as an attempt to *avoid the application of a "label"* as a result of the recognition by others of some stigma. There is now a voluminous literature on the process by which professionals and organizations have a mandate to apply labels to behavior or conditions and the long-term consequences labeling often has for the perpetuation of the so-called "problem." The labeling perspective (often loosely termed the symbolic interaction, interactionist or societal reaction approach) has assumed prominence within sociology and social psychology and offers a valuable conceptualization of the development of deviant or illness careers that apparently become permanent.

In essence, labeling theory focuses on the ways "primary deviants" become "secondary deviants" and stresses the importance of the impact of societal reaction on the afflicted person rather than his individual characteristics. Primary illness or deviance may arise from many sources. The extent and nature of any societal reaction to an illness condition or stigma are functions of its visibility, the power vested in the social position of the afflcted person, and the normative parameters or tolerance for deviance and/or illness that exist within the community. Primary illness (heavy drinking, "idiosyncratic" behavior, etc.) that is visible and exceeds the community tolerance level may bring the actors to the attention of mandated labelers, such as psychiatrists, clinical psychologists, social workers, the police, and various "helping" organizations.

If the mandated agencies see fit to "officially" classify the actor as a type of ill person (or deviant), a labeling process is hypothesized to occur that eventuates in (1) a change in the person's self-identity and (2) a change in his social identity among significant others as well as in the wider community. Behavior that results from the revised identities is termed "secondary deviance." According to the labeling theorists, secondary deviance is substantially similar to the original primary deviance but has as its source the actor's revised self-identity, as well as the revised social identity he has in the community. We have already described how stigma may be related to both aspects of identity.

Previous research and theoretical literature have concentrated on the negative results of labeling, particularly in cases of mental illness, in terms of delayed help seeking and selective health-service utilization. Several writers have noted that the labeling process might in some cases have a positive effect on future behavior. Fear of stigma or of the application of some derogatory label may also serve to increase utilization or to terminate "at risk" behavior, depending on the nature and severity of the stigma involved, the contextual situation in which it presents itself and the availability of services. The labeling of certain conditions may pressure deviants to conform to group norms, relinquish earlier stigmatized life styles (promiscuity, obesity, alcoholism, etc.), and perhaps even reverse behavior in an attempt to delabel or relabel themselves.

It is clear from the preceding discussion that there is considerable uncertainty over whether and how stigma influences utilization behavior. Empirical investigations will do much to expand our knowledge of the various effects of labeling, and such research may show that its nature and force are a function of, among other things, the type of stigma, the social position of the stigmatized, whether the labeled person is a primary or secondary deviant, who the mandated labeler is, which organizations support the label, and whether the labeled behavior has ceased.

There is clear evidence that communities label and exclude through institutionalization a disproportionate number of "cultural marginals"—people classified as of lower social status and those more isolated from stable group ties who do not possess the power to resist (Gibbs, 1962; Leiffer, 1966–67; Linsky, 1970). Such differential labeling and exclusion by mandated professionals and organizations can be viewed as a form of social control and, given the increasing tendency towards the medicalization of everything (Zola, 1972) and the general permanence of labels, should be viewed with considerable alarm.

From such a perspective, underutilization becomes not a social problem to which resources are directed in order to eliminate it but, rather, healthy behavior to perhaps be encouraged. This notion, of course, questions the decision rule guarding the behavior of professionals operating with a medical model of illness; namely, when in doubt, diagnose, label, and treat—all in the interest of prevention. The labeling theorists, aware of the process described above, argue for the application of the converse decision rule; namely, when in doubt deny, in the interest of preventing the stabilization and exclusion of individuals for what may turn out to be only a transitory, unremarkable episode (Scheff, 1964; Scheff and Sundstrom, 1970).

Alienation

For several decades now social scientists—working mainly within a political context—have been concerned with the development and consequences of what is loosely termed the "mass society." The theory of mass society holds that the destruction of the old community has separated the individual from binding social ties and that his isolation produces a sense of powerlessness that can be both personally devastating and destructive of the democratic processes. The theory consists of an historically oriented account of contemporary social structure, a set of statements about the present and emerging alienating effects of that structure, and derived predictions about some possible behavioral consequences. It is clear that there is still debate over the mass-society thesis and the plausibility of some of its assumptions and implications. Some subscribe to the view that, far from functioning as mediating forces allowing individual expression and control, complex organizations are simply agencies for further alienation. C. Wright Mills espoused this view when he wrote:

> [that voluntary organizations] have lost their grip on the individual. As more people are drawn into the political arena, these associations become mass in scale, and as the power of the individual becomes more dependent upon such mass associations, they are less accessible to the individual's influence (1956:307).

While the debate on the mass-society thesis proceeds, some evidence has emerged that lends support to the view that membership in a work-based organization is associated with a relatively strong sense of control over events and that the greater powerlessness of the unorganized worker is not simply a function of his socioeconomic status. Although findings of this study appear relatively conclusive, attention is drawn to the obvious problem of causal imputation. Does participation in various kinds of complex organizations reduce alienation, or do only the nonalienated participate in organizations, whose essential purpose is to exercise control over certain spheres of life? If the former interpretation is correct, then it becomes clear that the estrangement of the poor from formal organizations (underutilization) can be regarded as a serious disadvantage and that the trend toward increasing bureaucratization—not only in health and welfare but also in the economic, occupational, and educational spheres—must result in further systematic exclusion and alienation of those in poverty from the main stream of social life. These statements are perhaps a little extreme, but their plausibility is often argued by social and political theorists. Their viability, of course, depends partly on the plausibility of the masssociety thesis and as yet, in our view, insufficient empirical evidence has been gathered with which to make a judgment.

There is an impressive body of evidence showing that the nature and extent of involvement in society (measured by participation in voluntary associations) are closely related to socioeconomic status; the lower one's social class, the less likely one is to belong to various types of organizations (Curtis, 1959; Babchuck and Edwards, 1965; Babchuck and Booth, 1969). Although voluntary association memberships showed a small but noteworthy overall increase between the mid-1950s and the early 1960s, involving particularly blacks and thus reducing previous subgroup differences, strong socioeconomic differentials still remain (Hyman and Wright, 1971). Such findings are manifestly important when the problem of the underutilization of health services is being considered, since they show that behavior to be not idiosyncratically specific to health but consistent with behavior in a number of related spheres of social life (e.g., education, leisure, religion, economics, politics). Such a perspective allows us to note several shortcomings of a purely social-psychological approach. First, it enables us to see how the emergence of particular behaviors may be realistic adjustments to one's social position and diminished life chances. Second, it facilitates the inference of so-called "pathologic" behavior in related spheres of life other than health. If certain individuals, groups, or social categories cling to certain health beliefs and action, it may be not only because they are traditional and familiar but also because they are linked to other important elements of their subculture. To effect a change in one area of a subcultural system (say, increased utilization of health services) may result in unanticipated changes in other areas in awkward dislocations (Paul, 1958).

Estrangement from major social organizations and the consequences for individual functioning have, of course, received considerable attention from social scientists over the past several decades. The concept that best captures the phenomenon that has been discussed and that also has been developed to a point of operational utility is "alienation." This concept has, of course, engaged the attention of thinkers since the time of Hegel (1955) and Marx (1963) (Fromm, 1955; Durkheim, 1933; Seeman, 1959; Nisbet, 1966; Blauner, 1964); and today is widespread. It has been usefully applied to the study of, among other things, educational achievement, ghetto life, work, reformatories, the behavior of interns, voting behavior, and public opinion on fluoridation. On the few occasions when it has been applied to utilization behavior, it has yielded promising results. Alienation has recently been challenged, however, on the grounds that it is the popular catchword of our age and is becoming a device to rationalize service inactivity (Feuer, 1963; Lee, 1972).

An early study by Seeman and Evans (1961, 1962) explored the relevance of alienation to health behavior with particular reference to hospital settings. They clearly demonstrated, in a group matched for background characteristics, that patients who felt more powerless were less able to learn about their disease (tuberculosis). They argue that it is a "sense of personal control which makes knowledge concerning one's affairs motivationally relevant" and conclude that an aspect of alienation (powerlessness) "serves as the hypothetical intervening variable between the individual's social circumstances (i.e., his social structural place) and his social learning."

A more recent investigation by Morris and his colleagues (1966a) related two components of alienation (powerlessness and social isolation) to well-child supervision. They found in a study of 246 black and white mothers of low socioeconomic status with ten-month old children, that the more powerless and socially isolated had received less preventive care for their children. Moreover, mothers who were more powerless were less in agreement with the statements of professionals about the purposes and potentialities of well-child supervision.

Another often neglected study analyzed the relationship between alienation as measured with Dean's (1961) alienation scale and polio immunization participation (Gray et al., 1967; Moody and Gray, 1972). The results are consistent with earlier studies and show that highly alienated mothers had their children immunized less frequently than did mothers showing less alienation and that the relationship held regardless of the subjects' socioeconomic status, age, education, and friends' expectations. We believe that the notion of alienation has been developed to a point of operational utility where it could, if systematically employed, contribute to the explanation of utilization behavior.

What Goes on Between Consumers and Health-Care Agencies

The preceding discussion of the various influences of alienation knowledge, perception, symptom recognition, stigma, stress, and satisfaction summarizes only a sample of the central issues in the social-psychological literature on utilization behavior that has appeared in the last few decades. We believe it fairly accurately reflects the predominant emphasis of past work—concern with important factors in the process of seeking care. In other words, attention has been principally directed at variables that exert some influence up to the point of utilizing some service, and not at what goes on between all those involved when a service organization is actually being utilized. In the light of recent developments in organization theory, it is clear that what goes on between clients and agencies may be as highly related to utilization behavior as the personal characteristics that so many have previously highlighted.

A growing body of knowledge of organizational structure and processes, as well as developments in theories of organizations, has made us aware that organizational factors encourage officials to develop particular orientations towards clients, with the result that service to them is measurably affected (Adams and McDonald, 1968; Janowitz and Delany, 1957–58; Blau, 1960–61; Walsh and Elling, 1968; Ben-David, 1958; Wilensky, 1964). In particular, it has been proposed that, in order to maintain itself, client-centered bureaucracy tends to neglect those in greatest need of its services —those the organization was, in fact, primarily established to assist —or who present difficult problems (Sjoberg et al., 1963; Zald, 1965; Cloward and Epstein, 1965; Beck, 1967; Scott, 1967; Levin and Taube, 1970; Lindenberg, 1958; Bredemeier, 1964; Hunt et al., 1958; Hollingshead and Redlich, 1958; Clark, 1960; Fisher, 1969). In a recent paper, Levin and Taube (1970) argue that, given client-centered bureaucracy's investment in its own success, it has little reason to accommodate itself to the orientation of those whom it perceives as impairing its capacity to achieve that success. It is clear that services to clients from lower socioeconomic categories are nearly always found to be limited by organizational factors (Miller, 1964; McKinlay, 1968; Walsh and Eling, 1968; Cloward and Epstein, 1965; Scott, 1967).

Numerous studies investigating certain aspects of lower working-class life have suggested that members of that particular social category do not have the requisite expertise for performing effectively in various types of bureaucratic settings. Summaries of these and other studies, not directly related to utilization, are available (Boum and Rossi, 1969; Rosenblatt and Suchman, 1964a, 1964b; Jefferys, 1957; Osofsky, 1968; Zola, 1964; Shostak and Gomberg, 1964; Gans, 1962; Cohen and Hodges, 1962; Miller, 1964; Young and Willmott, 1960; Schatzman and Strauss, 1955; Hausknecht, 1964; Bernstein, 1959, 1967).

Through increasing knowledge of working-class behavior and experience with ill-fated health and welfare programs, intervention studies, eradication programs, etc.—principally with the poor—the difficulties of changing the knowledge, attitudes, and practice of any group in relation to health, illness, and other social problems have been recognized. Workers have commented on the ever-widening gap between modern medical care, as it is being increasingly provided, and certain groups of the population who continue to cling to what are regarded as traditional beliefs. Consequently, recognition has been increasingly given to the need for services themselves to be tailored to meet the particular needs of clients. It is perhaps noteworthy that the suggestion has almost always followed recognition of the failure of some initial attempt to change knowledge, attitudes, and practice.

Another factor, related to those already discussed but worthy of separate consideration, concerns our knowledge of the systematic uniqueness of the values, beliefs, definitions of situations, and life styles of the poor. Far from being random and idiosyncratic, their knowledge, attitudes, and practice can be viewed as responses that are consistent with, and understandable in relation to, problems associated directly with their social structural position. More than any other, the notion that has fathered that particular view is the concept of a "subculture" or a "culture of poverty," which—like many other concepts currently in vogue—is not without its ideological, analytical, and empirical limitations (Jaffe and Polgar, 1968). Despite its limitations, the concept has focused attention on the fact that behavior from this perspective appears to be patterned and systematically interrelated rather than idiosyncratic.

Recognition of the interrelatedness has led to the view that attempts to change aspects of lower working-class life, without also alleviating or altering the social structural problems to which certain types of behavior are adjustments, may do more harm than good. We have already alluded to the suggestion by Schneiderman (1965) that the underutilization of certain types of services by various subgroups of society may, in some senses, be regarded as healthy behavior. It is suggested that the general factors outlined here helped promote a concentration on organizational and client-agency interaction factors in the use of services and reoriented efforts away from the personal pathologies of underutilizers.

Social scientists studying formal organizations have produced considerable evidence suggesting that not all subgroups of society have an equal facility with and the requisite expertise for performing effectively in various types of formal organizational situations. As yet, however, only a relatively small amount of the material has been employed in the study of services—their organization, provision, and rates of utilization. It is now clear that the middle class have a considerable advantage over the poor in the field of medical care and social welfare as long as services are presented in an almost exclusively bureaucratic fashion. Some of the reasons that experts have given for their relatively advantaged position are listed below.

(a) The basic assumptions underlying the structure of health services (rationality, future orientation, etc.) are often reported as being consonant with the values and life styles of the middle class.

(b) Professional health-care personnel are generally middle class in origin and thus there is minimal status sensitivity during an encounter between them and middle class recipients, and they are best able to understand middle class problems.

(c) Middle class socialization patterns provide individuals with a role repertoire that enables them easily to adopt the role of listener, understand and tolerate the object orientation of officials, and maintain considerable role distance during an encounter.

(d) Socialization, combined with middle class educational advantages, provides a general middle class facility with form-filling and fosters the ability to verbalize feelings, attitudes, and need.

(e) Middle class education and socialization also fosters greater receptivity to health-education campaigns, which, it is often claimed, tend to be biased in their favor.

Health and welfare services then, it is claimed, tend to be based on a middle class rationale, require middle class knowledge and sophistication, generally recruit staff from the middle class, and to many, are open only in middle class hours!

The nature of the interaction between clients and agencies probably varies among different types of organizations (for voluntary organizations, for example, and for universities and churches), as well as among comparable organizations that appear to undertake different activities (a prison, compared with a hospital for the criminally insane). Not only have there been few discussions of the interaction of clients with officials and organizations, but the methodology for such studies remains inadequately developed, although some work in the area is now underway.

Particularly promising is the work of Danet and her colleagues, who have attempted to isolate and describe the attempts by external participants (clients) to influence bureaucratic decisions in their favor (Katz and Danet, 1966). They focus on the kinds of reasons or "persuasive appeals" that clients offer to substantiate their requests to officials in formal organizations, and they identify five sets of organizational circumstances in which "persuasive appeals" may occur.

They are, first, appeals to reciprocity, in both positive and negative forms (inducements and threats). This type of appeal takes the form: "if you grant the request, I will reward you," or, "if you don't, I will deprive you." Second, there are appeals based on pure persuasion as in "you will reward yourself." Third, there are appeals to altruism—"if you grant the request, you will reward me." All three persuasive strategies appeal to someone's profit, while depending on some aspect of the personal exchange relationship of the two parties involved, and compliance is, in principle, voluntary.

The two remaining types of appeals listed are normative in character, and compliance is supposedly obligatory. Danet distinguishes between appeals to the norm of reciprocity and appeals to impersonal norms. While appeals to simple reciprocity say, "I will reward you" (future tense), appeals to the norm of reciprocity say, "you owe it to me now because I have rewarded you in the past." Although the latter type of appeal also involves an exchange relationship between the parties, compliance is presumably experienced as obligatory. In the case of appeals to impersonal norms, which is the fifth basic type of persuasive appeal, compliance is also obligatory but independent of past interaction or any personal acquaintance between the two parties. ("You owe it to me because some abstract principle you have internalized obliges you to do so.")

In one study, Katz and Danet (1966) investigate the relationship between the background characteristics of clients and variations in their use of the different types of appeals, as well as the relationship between different appeals and different organizations. Four hypothetical situations, in which a client seeks services from an official, were presented to a heterogeneous sample of Israeli army reservists. The men were all asked to state what they thought should be said in each case, in order to get the official to grant the request. The authors were particularly interested in the variability of persuasive appeals, and in whether some clients discriminated more than others in what they said to different organizations, as well as in whether certain organizations were distinguishably similar or different judging from the variability in types of appeals addressed to them.

The arguments or persuasive appeals suggested by the reservists were found to vary with both their personal background and the type of organization involved. In general, it seems from the evidence presented that the nature of the organization did influence the types of persuasive appeals of clients in trying to get what they wanted. It is perhaps noteworthy that the content of the appeals appeared to be influenced more by the normative basis on which the organization rested (the prime beneficiary whom it was serving) than on the client's ability to offer his resources in exchange for the services offered by the organization.

In a subsequent report Danet (1971), employing a promising methodological technique, examined the patterns of variation in the language of persuasive appeals to the Israeli customs authorities. Persuasive appeals were chosen as the focus of the study on the grounds that they would reflect client orientations to bureaucracy. It was found that there were no appeals to reciprocity or attempts at pure persuasion. The clients neither offered inducements, nor did they threaten customs officials. Moreover, of the three basic types of appeal that were common, appeals to impersonal norms ("the customs owes me rights") were least frequent.

It was found that only fifteen percent of all appeals were to normative obligations, compared with twenty-three percent to the norm of reciprocity and a high forty-one percent to altruism. The proportion of appeals to altruism is perhaps an indication of the weakness of external clients in that particular organizational situation. Since appeals to impersonal norms were low, it was suggested that the clients lacked both bargaining power, which would be best expressed by appeals to impersonal norms. Danet further suggests that even in a powerful commonweal organization, the properly socialized client feels equal to the official before the law in some ultimate sense, while those less socialized define themselves as more subservient and make their appeals in a style that the socialized would regard as degrading and perhaps obsequious.

Some recent attempts have been made to study the strategies designed to gain or maintain personal power, using the techniques of laboratory experimentation. Jones (1964), perhaps more than any other, has developed a promising approach to what he terms "strategic behaviors." He notes that all interpersonal relationships involve some mutual dependence and that each party to a social interchange has potential influence over cetain rewards available to and costs incurred by some other. If the dependence of one on the other are not only mutual but approximately equal, then there is a balance of power in which each can either enforce a minimal set of rewards through his capacity to act or fail to enact the responses sought by the other. When the power in a two-person relationship is asymmetrical, Jones suggests that a repertoire of strategic alternatives is open to the dependent person that guarantees him a certain minimum of rewards but does so at the expense of confirming or strengthening the power asymmetry that defines his dependence.

An example suggested is compliance—the use of overt obedience to avoid punishment and secure available rewards. Other strategies, however, may be effective in modifying the asymmetry itself so that the dependent person's power is in the long run increased. Ingratiation is regarded by Jones as power-enhancing or dependence-reducing. He suggests that, by making himself attractive, the more dependent person reduces the value of his own sanctioning responses and at the same time makes it more difficult for the powerful person to apply the full range of sanctions that were initially part of his repertory.

In our view then, much can be gained in the understanding of health-service utilization by looking at the interaction between clients and agencies, and we have noted some promising beginnings. A concern with such issues will complement much of the work to which earlier sections of this paper are devoted and consequently lead to a more complete picture of the use of services.

Lacking the requisite expertise in and feeling estranged from bureaucratic settings, the lower class often opts for a more person-oriented, individualistic type of medical care. Studies have pointed to the tendency of people of low socioeconomic status to choose the more personal, continuous, and noncoercive care of local general practitioners, corner drugstores, and semiprofessionals. It is plausible to regard a closely knit lay referral system as a direct reaction against increasingly formal and confusing health services. That reaction, of course, while functioning to insulate the lower class from impersonalization and frustration, further widens and reinforces their alienation from the very care to which they are entitled.

Current trends suggest, however, that the days of even the insulative reaction patterns are numbered. For various reasons, lower class persons will probably find it increasingly difficult to retain the traditional, simple, and essentially individualistic medical-care arrangements to which they are accustomed.

The rationalization of services can be seen in both the trend toward group practice and the interest in the development of health centers. Can that mean that even the traditionally inviolable doctor-patient relationship is being eroded—is eventually to be replaced? The rationalization of pharmaceutical services and the establishment of clinics are events that will likely exacerbate lower class alienation. Bureaucratization in the field of health and welfare is, of course, not developing in a vacuum. It is occurring alongside and is probably being reinforced by a more general trend toward impersonality in the political, occupational, educational, and economic spheres.

Suggestions aimed at minimizing lower class frustration with bureaucratic settings have been presented during the past few years. Some researchers, apparently assuming the sanctity of bureaucracy, have suggested that special programs should be established to educate the lower class in the skills and knowledge required for effective functioning in a formally organized society. Such campaigns, however, appear to require the establishment of more and more bureaucracy. The problems arising out of bureaucracy are, if you like, to be solved by bureaucracy. Researchers and administrators seldom consider the possibility of different and more effective forms of organization.

Few attempts have been made to study the doctor-patient relationship in a variety of organizational settings. Research so far has largely concerned itself only with doctor-patient communication in outpatient departments and health clinics. Almost without exception the studies report a breakdown of communication with lower class patients. How does the doctor-patient relationship vary in different settings? Why is the traditional surgery situation for general practitioners often thought to be conducive to good communication? How do outpatient departments, child health and welfare, family planning, and antenatal clinics inhibit personal relationships? These questions have yet to be answered. It is possible that comparative studies of situational influences on the doctor-patient relationship may uncover techniques for enhancing such individuality and for reducing the confusion that members of some subgroups experience in formal organizations.

Clearly a more flexible, innovative, and even daringly experimental approach to medical-care organization and delivery is urgently needed. We also need more than a simple variation on the bureaucratic theme. Fresh attempts must be made to devise entirely new forms of delivery that take account of and overcome many of the problems outlined in the preceding sections. Perhaps we are seeing the beginning of a more innovative approach with the development of such phenomena as storefront clinics, outreach programs, crisis intervention units, and hotlines. At the same time there appears to be some emphasis on broadening the scope of traditional health personnel to include paraprofessionals, indigenous workers, and other entirely new categories of personnel. There is a suggestion that such services are more understandable and culturally acceptable to the poor in particular because they are more akin to their own life styles.

Some commentators may suggest that the proposed more innovative approach, by taking account of particular needs, involves the provision of special facilities for "different" groups. On the surface that may seem to involve a radical departure from traditional health-service philosophy—namely, relinquishing the principle of universality. One can, however, after highlighting the social class differentials in utilization under the present unitary bureaucratic structure, maintain that greater selectivity in provision may result in greater universality in use.

Some Doubts about "Patient Satisfaction"

In recent years attention has been devoted to the influence of patient satisfaction on utilization behavior. It is assumed that people expressing satisfaction with some type or aspect of medical care will be more likely to utilize medical facilities, follow regimens, comply with advice, etc. Such an assumption appears unwarranted since researchers have pointed out that few studies have been able to establish any sort of correlation between expressed attitudes and subsequent behavior (Festinger, 1964; Kegeles, 1967). Despite this and other known limitations, such studies, for a variety of questionable reasons, continue to engage the attention of medical-care researchers.

There is, of course, a range of different techniques for measuring attitudes and satisfaction. Some researchers make vigorous efforts to measure satisfaction in an objective and structured fashion (Hulka et al., 1971). Others, adopting less structured approaches, have listed several major factors associated with patient satisfaction (waiting time, time spent with the physician, ease of communication, exactness of diagnosis, etc.) and have requested responses regarding satisfaction or dissatisfaction with each of them. Another approach is simply to ask respondents what they like or dislike most about utilizing a particular health facility; a more recent, imaginative technique is to offer subjects several hypothetical situations or short vignettes and require them to state feelings and attitudes.

Many researchers employ some combination of structured and unstructured techniques. Subjects may, for example, be interviewed about their expectations before utilizing a service; then, by content analysis of the recorded happenings, an effort is made to determine the influence of expectations on satisfaction (Francis et al., 1969; Reader et al., 1967; Deisher et al., 1965).

When reviewing the plethora of studies of patient satisfaction and considering the wide variation in methods employed, we note a surprising consistency in findings. The expressed satisfaction with physicians and medical care is phenomenally high for all social categories and, where there is variation, it presented as varying levels of positive attitudes rather than as really negative sentiment. One of the very lowest levels of satisfaction appears to be the seventy-six percent reported in a study of doctor-patient communication (Francis et al., 1969), but the usual figure is around the ninety-eight percent found in a study of mothers' opinions of their pediatric care (Deisher et al., 1965).

The high expressions of satisfaction found in many studies may be a function of who sponsors the research, the subject content of the inquiry (nearly always associated with pediatrics), and where the interviews are conducted. It has often been reported that respondents tend to reply in a stereotyped, socially acceptable manner, and hesitations are often noted. One group of researchers concedes that those conducting the survey had some feeling that the respondents were generally reluctant to express any dissatisfactions they might have had because of the nature of the doctor-patient relationship (Deisher et al., 1965).

With such constraints, it is surprising that researchers continue to elicit responses through interviews and/or written questionnaires at the very place that respondents are expected to comment on and even continue to utilize. Respondents in several earlier investigations of patient attitudes and satisfactions clearly reported positively (and therefore produce the phenomenally high rates of satisfaction) for fear of possible recriminations. A comparable situation in criminology would be a study by prison guards of the satisfaction of long-term prisoners with the treatment received from the guards.

Information concerning satisfaction with care elicited from respondents when they are not actually utilizing a facility may also show a higher degree of satisfaction. When not actually receiving a service, respondents may tend to overlook matters that trouble them when they are using it; satisfaction is expressed rather with its availability. The person making only occasional visits to health facilities can tolerate irritations or inefficiencies that may accompany such infrequent visits without becoming dissatisfied with the system of care. Or the costs of potentially dissatisfying aspects of care may, for the patient, be outweighed by the long-term benefits of the treatment. Kosa and his colleagues (1967) noted that the "errors of recall are not simple functions of forgetfulness but tend to follow a complex, psychologically motivated selectivity." They felt that a person "when furnishing information, feels impelled to apply a selective censorship, separating the reportable events and suppressing the others."

Some of the most insightful work on attitudes and beliefs associated with medical care comes from Kegeles, who has expressed open skepticism with earlier work and has advanced several ideas worthy of serious attention. He writes:

> . . . as to attitude surveys as means of gathering information, people will generally answer questions posed them by interviewers in surveys. This will happen whether they have ever thought of the question or not. There seems to be a growing body of data which indicates that such expressed attitudes have no functional significance unless they fit into the cognitive organization of the person (Kegeles, 1967:921).

Kegeles points out that Converse (1963) has already labeled such statements "non-attitudes"—which seemingly bear no relationship to the behavior of the persons or to anything else and argues that, "without demonstration that such attitudes have relevance for behavior, they provide merely interesting and perhaps useful hypotheses for further testing." Kegeles also suggests that there are few indications of the persistence or reality of the beliefs and attitudes studied and that the best prediction of subsequent behavior is previous behavior.

These criticisms of attitude and satisfaction studies are clearly not exhaustive but relate principally to utilization behavior. Many other researchers have considered a number of the more technical methodological problems with attitude studies per se. Certain questionable ideological factors appear to perpetuate those studies, despite their dubious status on other methodological grounds.

Studies of patient satisfaction often appear to be value-laden and biased in their allocation of responsibility for dissatisfaction. When almost everyone, according to researchers, is satisfied with his medical care, it becomes easy to allocate culpability to some seemingly negligible minority, especially since it has been repeatedly claimed that dissatisfaction is more often present among the aged, the less educated, and lower socioeconomic groups. Hulka and her colleagues (1971) in a recent paper claim that the "use of the medical care system and knowledge of how to use it, as evidenced by having a regular doctor and hospital insurance, are associated with increased total satisfaction." What appears to be implied in such a statement is that those people unfortunate enough not to have a regular doctor or health insurance do not know how to use the system correctly and have brought upon themselves any dissatisfaction they might experience. The same implication is present in some of the work of Suchman, who suggests that if an individual maintains an informed, objective, professional, and independent approach to illness and health care, then he will be likely to express satisfaction with it.

Such research appears to justify the status quo and provides a rationale for either inactivity or lack of progress. According to this view, it is not that the service is inequitable or inefficient but that the nature and characteristics of the recipients obstruct effective delivery and undermine purposeful social policy. It follows that such a perspective and the findings of the studies which it employs, tend to support the existence of demonstrably ineffective programs. Accompanying the federal and private funding in the health field has been the formal or informal requirement that service agencies who receive funds must occasionally justify their continuance. Evaluation studies, with patient satisfaction as a principal component, have been conducted as one of their primary aims

For some time behavioral scientists (especially sociologists and psychologists), who have been interested in utilization behavior, have ascribed culpability for underutilization (or overutilization) to particular individuals or groups—usually the poor—employing such labels as distrustful, disreputable, irresponsible, alienated, parochial, dissatisfied, etc. By adopting such a perspective, we have attempted to deemphasize social structural or organizational determinants of utilization and have disproportionately highlighted the characterological features of clients. We believe that social scientists, among others, guided in part by the availability of funds, have acted as midwives during the birth of much of the present day punitive welfare legislation. While most of them have not actually designed and administered the legislation, they have, through certain findings and concepts, facilitated its delivery. Coser (1969) has noted that researchers espouse a status quo ideology and fail to consider the unanticipated consequences of their liberal theorizing. We have already alluded to studies, mainly in the area of deviance, which show how the process of labeling an offender, and making him conscious of himself as a deviant may evoke the very behavior that is thought to be undesirable (Becker, 1963; Kitsuse, 1964; Scheff, 1966; Lemert, 1951). It surely must be time for researchers to reappraise the effects of their involvement and their perennial invention of new words and concepts. Becker (1967), for example, has described how officials develop ways both of denying the institution's failure to perform as it should and of explaining those failures that cannot be hidden. He also reminds us that researchers who favor officialdom are almost always spared the accusation of bias. Perhaps we should, along with Becker, consider whose side we are on, the various consequences of our research involvements, and the extent to which we are prepared to comply in the coverup of the real sources of dissatisfaction.

There is one outstanding issue that relates to the extent to which so-called patient satisfaction (leaving aside all its methodological and ideological questionability) should be an ingredient in the evaluation of the quality of medical care. We do not deprecate the importance of lay consumer attitudes, nor do we believe that

John B. McKinlay and Diana B. Dutton

they must be confined to such relatively minor aspects of care as working time, tone and manner of the physician, and clinic surroundings. We must, however, be mindful of the many limitations of attitudinal research and the real possibility that consumers may be misguidedly satisfied with what is actually medical care of poor quality or dissatisfied with what is actually care of good quality.

References

Adams, P. L. *and* N. F. McDonald
    1968   "The clinical cooling out of poor people." American Journal of Orthopsychiatry 38 (April): 457–463.

Andersen, R.
    1968   A Behavioral Model of Families' Use of Health Services. Chicago: University of Chicago, Center for Health Administration Studies.

Andersen, R., O. W. Anderson, *and* B. Smedby
    1968   "Perceptions of and response to symptoms of illness in Sweden and the United States." Medical Care 6: 18–30.

Andersen, R., L. M. Gunter, *and* E. Kennedy
    1963   "Evaluations of clinical, cultural and psychosomatic influences in the teaching and management of diabetic patients." American Journal of Medical Science 76:682–690.

Antonovsky, A.
    1972   "A model to explain visits to the doctor: With special reference to the case of Israel." Journal of Health and Human Behavior 13 (December): 446–454.

Apple, D.
    1960   "How laymen define illness." Journal of Health and Human Behavior 1 (Fall): 219–225.

Babchuck, N. *and* A. Booth
    1969   "Voluntary association membership: A longitudinal analysis." American Social Review 34 (February): 31–45.

Babchuck, N. *and* A. Edwards
    1965   "Voluntary associations and the integration hypothesis." Sociological Inquiry 35 (Spring): 149–162.

Battistella, R. M.
1968a "Factors associated with delay in the initiation of physicians' care among late adulthood persons." American Journal of Public Health 61 (July): 1348–1361.
1968b "Limitations in use of the concept of psychological readiness to initiate health care." Medical Care 6: 308–319.

Baumann, B. O.
1961 "Diversities in conceptions of health and physical fitness." Journal of Health and Human Behavior 2: 39–46.

Beck, B.
1967 "Welfare as a moral category." Social Problems 14 (Winter): 258–277.

Becker, H.
1963 Outsiders: Studies in the Sociology of Deviance. New York: The Free Press.
1967 "Whose side are we on?" Social Problems 14 (Winter): 239–247.

Ben-David, J.
1958 "The professional role of the physician in bureaucratized medicine." Human Relations 11 (August): 255–274.

Bergner, L. *and* A. Yerby
1968 "Low income and barriers to use of health services." New England Journal of Medicine 278 (10): 541–546.

Berkman, P.
1969 "Spouseless motherhood, psychological stress and physical morbidity." Journal of Health and Social Behavior 10 (4): 323–334.

Bernstein, B.
1959 "A public language: Some sociological implications of a linguistic form." British Journal of Sociology 10 (December): 311–326.
1967 "Social class and linquistic development." Pp. 288–314 in Halsey, A. H., J. Floud, *and* C. A. Anderson (eds.), Education, Economy and Society. New York: The Free Press.

Bice, T. W.
1971 Medical Care for the Disadvantaged. Baltimore: Johns Hopkins University, Department of Medical Care and Hospitals.

Birnbaum, A.
1970   "On managing and courtesy stigma." Journal of Health and Social Behavior 11 (June): 196–206.

Blau, P. M.
1969-61   "Orientation towards clients in a public welfare agency." Administration Science Quarterly 5: 341–361.

Blauner, R.
1964   Alienation and Freedom. Chicago: University of Chicago Press.

Blum, Z. D. *and* H. Rossi
1969   "Social class research and images of the poor: A bibliographic review." Pp. 343–397 in Moynihan, D. P. (ed.), On Understanding Poverty. New York: Basic Books.

Bradburn, N. H. *and* D. Caplovitz
1965   Reports on Happiness. Chicago: Aldine Publishing Co.

Bredemeier, H. C.
1964   "The socially handicapped and the agencies: A market analysis." Pp. 205–235 in Riessman, F., J. Cohen, *and* A. Pearl (eds.), Mental Health of the Poor. New York: The Free Press.

Clark, B.
1960   "The 'cooling out' function in higher education." American Journal of Sociology 65 (May): 569–576.

Cloward, R. *and* I. Epstein
1965   "Private social welfare's disengagement from the poor. The case of family adjustment agencies." Pp. 623–644 in Zald, M. N. (ed.), Social Welfare Institutions. New York: John Wiley and Sons.

Coe, R. M., J. M. Goering, *and* M. Cummins
1969   Health Status of Low Income Families in an Urban Area. Final Report for the Bi-State Regional Medical Program. St. Louis: Medical Care Research Center.

Cohen, A. K. *and* H. M. Hodges
1962   "Characteristics of the lower blue-collar class." Social Problems 10 (Spring): 303–335.

Cole, S. *and* R. Lejeune
1972   "Illness and the legitimation of failure." American Sociological Review 37 (June): 347–356.

Conference of the Society for Psychosomatic Research, Royal College of
  Physicians
  1959   The Nature of Stress Disorder. Springfield, Ill.: C. C.
            Thomas.
Converse, P.
  1963   Attitudes and Non-Attitudes; Continuation of a Dialogue.
            Washington, D.C.: International Congress of Psychiatry.
Coser, L. A.
  1969   "Some unanticipated conservative consequences of liberal
            theorizing." Social Problems 16 (Winter): 263–272.
Crandell, D. L. *and* B. P. Dohrenwend
  1967   "Some relations among psychiatric symptoms, organic ill-
            ness and social class." American Journal of Psychiatry 123:
            1527–1538.
Croog, S. H.
  1961   "Ethnic origins, educational level and responses to a health
            questionnaire." Human Organization 10 (Summer):
            65–69.
Cumming, J. *and* E. Cumming
  1965   "On the stigma of mental illness." Community Mental
            Health Journal 1: 135–143.
Curtis, R. F.
  1959   "Occupational mobility and membership in formal volun-
            tary associations: A note on research." American Sociologi-
            cal Review 34 (December): 846–848.
Danet, B.
  1971   "The language of persuasion in bureaucracy: 'Modern' and
            'traditional' appeals to the Israel customs authorities."
            American Sociological Review 36 (October): 847–859.
Davis, F.
  1961   "Deviance disavowal: The management of strained interac-
            tion by the visibly handicapped." Social Problems 9
            (June): 120–132.
Dean, D. G.
  1961   "Alienation: Its meaning and measurement." American So-
            ciological Review 26 (October): 753–758.
Deasey, L. E.
  1956   "Socio-economic status and participation in the poliomylitis
            vaccine trial." American Sociological Review 21 (April):
            185.

Deisher, R. W., et al.
  1965   "Mothers' opinions of their pediatric care." Pediatrics 35
          (January): 82–90.
diCicco, L. *and* D. Apple
  1958   "Health needs and opinions of older adults." Public Health
          Reports 73: 479–481.
Dodge, D. *and* W. T. Martin
  1970   Social Stress and Chronic Illness: Mortality Patterns in In-
          dustrial Society. Notre Dame, Indiana: University of Notre
          Dame Press.
Durkheim, E.
  1933   Suicide. Glencoe, Illinois: The Free Press.
Engel, C. L.
  1967   "Psychogenic pain." Journal of Occupational Medicine 3:
          249–257.
Epstein, F. H., E. P. Boas, *and* R. Simpson
  1957   "The epidemiology of arteriosclerosis among a random
          sample of clothing workers of different ethnic origins in
          New York City: I and II." Journal of Chronic Diseases 5:
          300–341.
Fabrega, H., R. Moore, *and* J. Strawn
  1969   "Low income, medical problem patients: Some medical and
          behavioral features." Journal of Health and Social Behavior
          10 (4): 334–343.
Feldman, J. J.
  1966   The Dissemination of Health Information. Chicago: Aldine
          Publishing Co.
Festinger, L.
  1964   "Behavioral support for opinion change." Public Opinion
          Quarterly 28 (Fall): 404–417.
Feuer, L.
  1963   "What is alienation? The career of a concept." New Politics
          1 (Spring): 116–134.
Fisher, B. M.
  1969   "Claims and credibility: A discussion of occupational iden-
          tity and the agent-client relationship." Social Problems 16
          (Spring): 423–433.
Francis, V., B. M. Korsch, *and* M. Morris
  1969   "Gaps in doctor-patient communication: Patients' responses

to medical advice." New England Journal of Medicine 280: 535–540.

Friedsam, H. J. *and* H. W. Martin
1963   "A comparison of self and physicians' health ratings in an older population." Journal of Health and Human Behavior 4: 179–183.

Fromm, E.
1955   The Sane Society. New York: Rinehart and Company.

Gans, H. J.
1962   The Urban Villagers. New York: The Free Press.

Garfinkel, H.
1967   Studies in Ethnomethodology. Engelwood Cliffs: Prentice-Hall.

Gibbs, J. P.
1962   "Rates of mental hospitalization: A study of societal reaction to deviant behavior." American Sociological Review 27 (December): 782–792.

Glaser, B. G. *and* A. L. Strauss
1965   Awareness of Dying. Chicago: Aldine Publishing Co.

Goffman, E.
1959   The Presentation of Self in Everyday Life. New York: Doubleday.
1961   Asylums. Chicago: Aldine Publishing Co.
1963   Stigma. Engelwood Cliffs: Prentice-Hall.

Gordon, G.
1966   Role Theory and Illness: A Sociological Perspective. New Haven, Conn.: College and University Press.

Gray, R. M., J. P. Kesler, *and* P. M. Moody
1967   "Alienation and immunization participation." Rocky Mountain Social Science Journal 4 (April): 161–168.

Hausknecht, M.
1964   "The blue-collar joiner." Pp. 402–431 in Shostak, A. B. *and* W. Gomberg (eds.), Blue Collar World. Englewood Cliffs: Prentice-Hall.

Hegel, G. F. W.
1955   The Phenomenology of Mind, 2nd ed., rev. New York: Macmillan and Co.

Hessler, R. M., P. Kubish, P. Kong Ming New, P. L. Ellison, *and* F. H. Taylor

John B. McKinlay and Diana B. Dutton

1971   "Demographic context, social interaction and perceived health status: Excedrin headache #1." Journal of Health and Social Behavior 12 (3): 191–199.

Hetherington, R. W. and C. E. Hopkins
1969   "Symptom sensitivity: Its social and cultural correlates." Health Services Research 4 (1): 63–75.

Hinkle, L., R. Redmont, N. Plummer, and H. Wolff
1960   "An examination of the relation between symptoms, disability and serious illness in two homogeneous groups of men and women." American Journal of Public Health 50: 1327–1336.

Hochbaum, G. M.
1958   Public Participation in Medical Screening Programs: A Socio-Psychological Study. Washington, D. C.: Government Printing Office.

Hochstim, J. R.
1968   "Poverty area under the microscope." American Journal of Public Health 58 (10): 1815–1827.

Hollingshead, A. B. and F. C. Redlich
1958   Social Class and Mental Illness. New York: John Wiley and Sons.

Holmes, T. H.
1951   "Psychosocial and psychophysiological studies of tuberculosis." Psychosomatic Medicine 19: 134–143.

Hulka, B., S. Thompson, J. Cassel, and S. Zyzanski
1971   "Satisfaction with medical care in a low-income population." Journal of Chronic Disease 24: 661–673.

Hunt, R. G., O. Gurrslin, and J. L. Roach
1958   "Social status and psychiatric service in a child guidance clinic." American Sociological Review 23 (February): 81–83.

Hyman, H. and C. R. Wright
1971   "Trends in voluntary association memberships of American adults: Replication based on secondary analysis of national sample surveys." American Sociological Review 36 (April): 191–206.

Jackson, E. F.
1962   "Status inconsistency and symptoms of stress." American Sociological Review 27 (August): 469–480.

Jackson, E. F. *and* Peter J. Burke
  1965   "Status and symptoms of stress: Additive and Interaction
          effects." American Sociological Review 30 (August):
          556–564.
Jaffe, F. S. *and* S. Polgar
  1968   "Family planning and public policy: Is the 'culture of pov-
          erty' the new cop-out?" Journal of Marriage and the Fami-
          ly 30 (May): 228–235.
Janis, I. L.
  1958   Psychological Stress. New York: John Wiley and Sons.
Janowitz, M. *and* W. Delany
  1957–58 "The bureaucrat and the public: A study of informa-
          tional perspectives." Administrative Science Quarterly
          2: 141–162.
Jeffreys, M.
  1957   "Social class and health promotion." The Health Education
          Journal 15 (May): 109–117.
Jenkins, C. D.
  1966   "The semantic differential for health: A Technique for
          measuring beliefs about diseases." Public Health Reports 81
          (6): 549–558.
Jones, E. E.
  1964   Ingratiation. New York: Appleton-Century-Crofts.
Kadushin, C.
  1967   "Social class and ill health: The need for further research.
          A reply to Antonovsky." Sociological Inquiry 37: 323–332.
Kalimo, E.
  1969   Determinants of Medical Care Utilization. Helsinki: Re-
          search Institute for Social Services, National Pensions Insti-
          tute.
Kasl, S. *and* S. Cobb
  1966   "Health behavior and sick role behavior." Archives of En-
          vironmental Health 2: 246–266.
Katz, E. *and* B. Danet
  1966   "Petitions and persuasive appeals: A study of official-client
          relations." American Sociological Review 31 (December):
          811–822.
Kegeles, S. S.
  1967   "Attitudes and behavior of the public regarding cervical cy-

John B. McKinlay and Diana B. Dutton

tology: Current findings and new directions for research." Journal of Chronic Diseases 20 (December): 911–922.

Kegeles, S. S., J. P. Kirscht, D. P. Haefner, *and* I. M. Rosenstock
1965   "Survey of beliefs about cancer detection and taking papanicoloau tests." Public Health Reports 80: 815–824.

Kirscht, J. P.
1971   "Social and psychological problems of surveys on health and illness." Social Science and Medicine 5: 519–526.

Kirscht, J. P., D. P. Haefner, S. S. Kegeles, *and* I. M. Rosenstock
1966   "A national study of health beliefs." Journal of Health and Human Behavior 7: 248–254.

Kitsuse, J.
1962   "Societal relations to deviant behavior: Problems of theory and method." Social Problems 9 (Winter): 247–256.

Koos, E. L.
1954   The Health of Regionville: What the People Thought and Did About It. New York: Columbia University Press.

Kosa, J., J. J. Alpert, *and* R. J Haggerty
1967   "On the reliability of family health information: A comparative study of mothers' reports on illness and related behavior." Social Science Medicine 1 (July): 165–181.

Kutner, B. *and* G. Gordon
1961   "Seeking care for cancer." Journal of Health and Human Behavior 2: 128–145.

Lee, A. M.
1972   "An obituary for 'alienation.'" Social Problems 20 (Summer): 121–127.

Leiffer, R.
1966–67 "Involuntary psychiatric hospitalization and social control." International Journal of Social Psychiatry 13: 53–58.

Lemert, E. M.
1951   Social Pathology. New York: McGraw-Hill.

Lerner, M.
1969   "Social differences in physical health." Pp. 69–112 in Kosa, J., A. Antonovsky, *and* I. Zola (eds.), Poverty and Health. Cambridge: Harvard University Press.

Leventhal, H., I. M. Rosenstock, *and* G. M. Hochbaum
1960   The Impact of Asian Influenza on Coming Life: A Study

in Five Cities. Washington, D. C.: Government Printing Office.

Levin, J. *and* G. Taube
1970   "Bureaucracy and the socially handicapped: A study of lower-status tenants in public housing." Sociology and Social Research 54 (February): 209–219.

Lindenberg, R. E.
1958   "Hard to reach: Client or casework agency." Social Work 3 (October): 23–29.

Linsky, A. S.
1970   "Who shall be excluded: The influence of personal attributes in community reaction to the mentally ill." Social Psychiatry 5: 166–171.

Ludwig, E. *and* G. Gibson
1969   "Self perception of sickness and the seeking of medical care." Journal of Health and Social Behavior 10: 125–133.

Maddox, G. L.
1964   "Self-assessment of Health Status: A longitudinal study of selected elderly subjects." Journal of Chronic Diseases 17: 449–460.

Marx, K.
1963   Early Writings. London: C. A. Watts and Co.

McBroom, W. H.
1970   "Illness, illness behavior and socio-economic status." Journal of Health and Social Behavior 11 (December): 319–326.

McGrath, J. E. (ed.)
1970   Social and Psychological Factors in Stress. New York: Holt, Rinehart and Winston, Inc.

McKinlay, J. B.
1968   "Better maternity care for whom. . . ?" Medical Officer 3147 (November 15): 275–276.

1972a   "Some approaches and problems in the study of the use of services: An overview." Journal of Health and Social Behavior 13 (June): 115–152.

1972b   "The sick role—illness and pregnancy." Social Science and Medicine 6: 561–572.

Mechanic, D.
1964   "The influence of mothers on their children's attitudes and behavior." Pediatrics 33: 444–453.

John B. McKinlay and Diana B. Dutton

1969   "Illness and cure." Pp. 191–214 in Kosa, J., A. Antonovsky, *and* I. Zola (eds.), Poverty and Health. Cambridge: Harvard University Press.

Mechanic, D. *and* E. H. Volkhart

1961   "Stress, illness, behavior, and the sick role." American Sociological Review 26: 51–58.

Meile, Richard L.

1972   "The 22-item index of psychophysiological disorder: Psychological or organic symptoms?" Social Science Medicine 6: 125–135.

Meile, R. J. *and* P. N. Haese

1969   "Social status, status incongruence and symptoms of stress." Journal of Health and Social Behavior 10 (3): 237–244.

Miller, S. M.

1964   "The American lower classes: A typological approach." Sociology and Social Research 48 (Spring): 1–22.

Mills, C. W.

1956   The Power Elite. New York: Oxford University Press.

Moody, P. M. *and* R. M. Gray

1972   "Social class, social integration, and the use of preventive health services." Pp. 250–261 in Jaco, E. G. (ed.), Patients, Physicians and Illness. New York: The Free Press.

Morris, N., M. H. Hatch, *and* S. S. Chipman

1966a   "Alienation as a deterrent to well-child supervision." American Journal of Public Health 56 (November): 187–192.

1966b   "Deterrents to well-child supervision." American Journal of Public Health 56 (August): 1232–1241.

National Center for Health Statistics

1967   Three Views of Hypertension and Heart Disease. Washington, D.C.: Government Printing Office.

Nisbet, R. A.

1966   The Sociological Tradition. New York: Basic Books.

Osofsky, H. J.

1968   "After office hours: Some social psychological issues improving obstetric care for the poor." Obstetrics and Gynaecology 31 (March): 437–443.

Paul, B.

1958   "The role of beliefs and customs of sanitation programs." American Journal of Public Health 48 (November): 1502–1506.

Pratt, L.
1971   "The relationship of SES to health." American Journal of
        Public Health 61: 281–291.
Rahe, R. H.
1964   "Social stress and illness onset." Journal of Psychosomatic
        Research 8: 35–44.
Rahe, R. H., R. J. Biersner, D. H. Ryman, *and* R. J. Arthur
1972   "Psychosocial predictors of illness behavior and failure in
        stressful training." Journal of Health and Social Behavior 3
        (December): 393–397.
Reader, G. G., L. Pratt, *and* M. C. Mudd
1967   "What patients expect from their doctors." Modern Hospi-
        tal 89 (July): 88–94.
Richardson, W. C.
1970   "Measuring the urban poor's use of physician services in re-
        sponse to illness episodes.' Medical Care 8: 132–142.
Robinson, D.
1971   The Process of Becoming Ill. London: Routledge and Ke-
        gan Paul.
Rosenblatt, D. A. *and* E. A. Suchman
1964a   "Blue-collar attitudes and information toward health and
        illness." Pp. 324–333 in Shostak, A. B. *and* W. Gomberg
        (eds.), Blue Collar World. Englewood Cliffs, N.J.: Pren-
        tice-Hall.
1964b   "The underutilization of medical care services by blue col-
        larites." Pp. 341–349 in Shostak, A. B. *and* W. Gomberg
        (eds.), Blue Collar World. Englewood Cliffs, N.J.: Pren-
        tice-Hall.
Rosengren, W. R.
1964   "Social class and becoming ill." Pp. 362–370 in Shostak, A.
        B. *and* W. Gomberg (eds.), Blue Collar World. Englewood
        Cliffs, N.J.: Prentice-Hall.
Rosenstock, I. M.
1966   "Why people use health services." Milbank Memorial Fund
        Quarterly 44 (3, Part 2): 94–127.
1969   "Prevention of illness and maintenance of health." Pp.
        168–190 in Kosa, J., A. Antonovsky *and* I. Zola (eds.),
        Poverty and Health. Cambridge: Harvard University Press.
Rosenstock, I. M., D. P. Haefner, S. S. Kegeles, *and* J. P. Kirscht
1966   "Public knowledge, opinion and action concerning three

public health issues: Radioactive fallout, insect and plant sprays and fatty foods." Journal of Health and Human Behavior 7 (2): 91–98.

Samora, J., L. Saunders, *and* R. F. Larson
1961   "Medical vocabulary knowledge among hospital patients." Journal of Health and Human Behavior 2: 83–92.

Schatzman, L. *and* A. Strauss
1955   "Social class and modes of communication." American Journal of Sociology 60 (January): 329–338.

Scheff, T. J.
1964   "Preferred errors in diagnosis." Medical Care 2 (July/September): 166–172.
1966   "Typification in the diagnostic practices of rehabilitation agencies." Pp. 139–147 in Sussman, M. B. (ed.), Sociology and Rehabilitation. Washington, D.C.: American Sociological Association.

Scheff, T. J. *and* E. Sundstrom
1970   "The stability of deviant behavior over time: A reassessment." Journal of Health and Social Behavior 11: 37–43.

Schneiderman, L.
1965   "Social class, diagnosis and treatment." American Journal of Orthopsychiatry 35 (January): 99–105.

Schonfeld, J. et al.
1963   "Medical attitudes and practices of parents toward a mass tubercular testing program." American Journal of Public Health 53: 14–18.

Scott, R. A.
1967   "The selection of clients by social welfare agencies: The case of the blind." Social Problems 14 (Winter): 248–257.

Seeman, M.
1959   "On the meaning of alienation." American Sociological Review 24 (December): 783–791.

Seeman, M. *and* J. W. Evans
1961   "Stratification and hospital care I: The Performance of the medical intern." American Sociological Review 26 (February): 67–80.
1962   "Alienation and learning in a hospital setting." American Sociological Review 27 (December): 772–782.

Shostak, A. B. *and* W. Gomberg (eds.)
1964   Blue Collar World. Englewood Cliffs, N.J.: Prentice-Hall.

Sjoberg, G., R. A. Bryner, *and* B. Farris
    1963   "Bureaucracy and the lower class." Sociology and Social Research 50 (April): 325–337.

Sparer, P. (ed.)
    1956   Personality, Stress and Tuberculosis. New York: International University Press.

Steele, J. L. *and* W. H. McBroom
    1972   "Conceptual and empirical dimensions of health behavior." Journal of Health and Social Behavior 13 (December): 382–392.

Stoeckle, J. D., I. K. Zola, *and* G. E. Davidson
    1963   "On going to see the doctor, the contributions of the patient to the decision to seek medical aid: A selected review." Journal of Chronic Diseases 16: 975–989.

Suchman, E. A.
    1964   "Sociological variations among ethnic groups." American Journal of Sociology 70: 319–331.
    1965a   "Social factors in medical deprivation." American Journal of Public Health 55 (11): 1725–1733.
    1965b   "Stages of illness and medical care." Journal of Health and Human Behavior 6: 114–128.

Suchman, E. A., B. S. Phillips, *and* G. F. Streib
    1958   "An analysis of the validity of health questionaires." Social Forces 36: 223–232.

Taglacozzo, D. M. *and* I. Taglacozzo
    1970   "Knowledge of illness as a predictor of patient behavior.' Journal of Chronic Diseases 22: 765–775.

Travis, G.
    1961   Chronic Disease and Disability. Berkeley: University of California Press.

Twaddle, A. C.
    1969   "Decisions and sick role variations: An exploration." Journal of Health and Social Behavior 10 (2): 105–115.

Voysey, M.
    1972a   "Impression management by parents with disabled children." Journal of Health and Social Behavior 13 (March): 80–89.
    1972b   "Official agents and the legitimation of suffering." The Sociological Review 20 (November): 533–551.

Walsh, J. L. *and* R. H. Elling
    1968   "Professionalism and the poor: Structural effects and professional behavior." Journal of Health and Social Behavior 9 (March): 16–28.

Watts, D.
    1966   "Factors related to the acceptance of modern medicine." American Journal of Public Health 56 (8): 1205–1212.

Wilensky, H. L.
    1964   "The professionalization of everyone?" American Journal of Sociology 70 (September): 137–158.

Williams, T. F. et al.
    1965   "The clinical picture of diabetic control, studied in four settings." Paper presented before the Association of Public Health Administrators Meeting, Chicago, Illinois.

Young, M. *and* P. Willmott
    1960   Family and Class in a London Suburb. London: Routledge and Kegan Paul.

Zald, M. N. (ed.)
    1965   Social Welfare Institutions. New York: John Wiley and Sons.

Zborowski, M.
    1958   "Cultural components in response to pain." Pp. 256–268 in Jaco, E. G. (ed.), Patients, Physicians, and Illness. Glencoe, Illinois: The Free Press.

Zola, I. K.
    1963a   "Problems of communication, doctors, and patient care: The interplay of patient, physician, and clinic organization." Journal of Medical Education 38: 829–838.
    1963b   "Socio-cultural factors in the seeking of medical aid: A progress report." Trans-Cultural Psychiatric Research 14:62–65.
    1964   "Illness behavior of the working class: Implications and recommendations." Pp. 350–361 in Shostak, A. B. *and* W. Gomberg (eds.), Blue Collar World. Englewood Cliffs: Prentice-Hall.
    1966   "Culture and symptoms—an analysis of patients' presenting complaints." American Sociological Review 31: 615–630.
    1972   "Medicine as an institution of social control." The Sociological Review 20: 487–504.

Factors Associated with Patient Evaluation of Health Care

LAWRENCE S. LINN

The purpose of this paper is to study the relationships among patient characteristics, characteristics of a health care encounter, and patients' evaluation of that encounter. On the basis of 1739 patient-provider encounters in eleven ambulatory care settings, three relatively independent correlates of patient satisfaction were found: age; community satisfaction; and the nature and degree of continuity of care which characterized the visit. Patients' sex, marital status, religion, and the number and kind of services provided were not related to the evaluations patients made. Greatest differences in patient satisfaction were from setting to setting, and these differences probably can be attributed to the types of patients which they recruit or service (i.e., age, level of community satisfaction) and setting policy and procedures regarding continuity of care.

In spite of the fact that many social scientists and most physicians have questioned the validity and significance of evaluations patients make of their medical experiences, several recent studies have demonstrated their importance. Alpert et al. (1970) has noted that changing attitudes and satisfactions with medical care are not only worthwhile goals in themselves, but have some very practical consequences. One of those consequences has been reported by Francis, Korsch, and Morris (1969) who found that patients highly satisfied with their last visit to the doctor were significantly more likely to follow the doctor's orders than patients who were dissatisfied. In terms of the validity of patient assessments of care, Kisch and Reeder (1969) found that the client's appraisal of physician performance was highly correlated with professional criteria for assessing competent professional performance. Finally, Reeder (1972) has pointed out how the growth of consumerism in American society has begun to affect the traditional doctor-patient relationship. Patients as "consumers" in the medical care system are becoming increasingly powerful to the extent that their needs and satisfactions can no longer be neglected by either physician "providers" or by social scientists.

Published studies of patient satisfaction seem to fall into three general categories: (1) studies of satisfaction among group health plan members or satisfaction with group health insurance coverage; (2) satisfaction with physicians in general or with specified doctor visits in particular, and (3) satisfaction with new non-physician providers of health care.

The first group of studies shows much similarity in findings greatest satisfaction being with the technical standards of health care and less satisfaction with the doctor-patient relationship itself (Weinerman, 1964). Anderson and Sheatsley (1959) and Freidson (1961) both found that patients seeing solo practitioners on a fee-for-service basis elicited more satisfaction than patients seeing physician members of group practice. Similar to the earliest report of patient satisfaction (Koos, 1955), complaints with physicians in group practice involved the lack of personal interest, insufficient explanation of the patient's condition by the doctor, complaints about house calls, and waiting time. However, more recent studies of this type have found very high levels of satisfaction among members. Bashshur et al. (1967) found that 78 percent of the union workers studied liked their plan, and Gerst et al. (1969) found that 77 percent of the government employees studied were satisfied with their coverage. In examining factors associated with the levels of satisfaction expressed, Bashshur found that the patient's education, income, and race were not related. However, satisfaction was higher among the married than among singles and among those with longer employment. Gerst also found that singles were significantly less satisfied than married members, but also found that higher income and educational levels were directly related with higher levels of satisfaction. Older people and males were somewhat more satisfied than their counterparts but not significantly so.

Similar to the first group of studies, the studies of attitudes toward doctors or doctor visits also show high percentages of patients satisfied with the care they receive. Francis et al. (1969) found that 76 percent of the outpatient visits studied resulted in high patient satisfaction. Deisher et al. (1965) in a questionnaire survey of mothers' opinions found that 95–98 percent were very satisfied with the pediatric care their children were receiving in terms of doctor interest, examination time, and the doctor's willingness to receive phone calls. Mothers were less satisfied with fees, house calls, and waiting time, but less than 5 percent indicated high dissatisfaction with any of these aspects. Alpert et al. (1970) in a study of three groups of low-income families who utilized an emergency clinic between 1964 and 1968 measured satisfaction with last doctor visit using both general and specific questions. All groups expressed high levels of satisfaction with the doctor giving enough time and being easy to talk to (75 – 78 percent). The only major source of dissatisfaction involved waiting. Finally, Hulka et al. (1971) studied satisfaction with medical care in a low-income population on three dimensions: professional competence, personal qualities, and cost-convenience. Although all three were found to correlate significantly with each other, satisfaction with personal qualities of doctors was greatest and satisfaction with cost-convenience the least. No differences in satisfaction levels were found in relationship to age, race, sex, census tract, marital status, time in the community, or health status. However, for their low-income sample it was found that as family size increased, satisfaction decreased, and as education and occupational status increased, satisfaction increased.

Finally, the third and most recent group of studies have examined patients' satisfaction with and acceptance of new health practitioners such as physician assistants and nurse practitioners. Spitzer (1974), for example, reports that there have been very few instances of rejection of nurse-practitioner services by patients. Ninety-six percent of the patients who saw a nurse practitioner were satisfied with the health services they received as compared with 97 percent who saw a physician. Similarly, Day et al. (1970) reported that 95 percent of their sample of mothers expressed satisfaction with their contact with a pediatric nurse practitioner. Finally, Nelson et al. (1974) report that patient acceptance of physician assistants they studied was extremely high, with 89 percent assessing the Medex studied as "very competent," 83 percent as "sure of himself," and 86 percent as "very professional in his manner." In looking at the effects of age, sex, and social class on the attitudes patients expressed, Nelson found that younger patients consistently perceived the Medex to be less technically competent than did older patients, but Nelson reported no other significant differences between patient characteristics and evaluations of competency.

From this brief review, several basic points become evident: (1) a number of techniques have been used to measure satisfaction with health care (single items, attitude scales, open-ended items, etc.); (2) a number of different populations have been studied (i.e., patient populations, union members, clinic utilizers, low-income residents); and (3) a number of different objects of satisfaction have been evaluated (i.e., last doctor visit, doctors in general, health plans, health insurance, new health professions). Yet, in spite of these diversities, several uniformities are apparent:

(1) All studies found high levels of patient satisfaction.

(2) There is a lack of consistent findings between social or cultural factors and patient satisfactions.

(3) Specific characteristics of the medical encounter have not been identified or examined in relationship to levels of satisfaction expressed by patients.

The Purpose of the Present Study

Since the recent growth of consumerism in the health care field may have had some impact on the perceptions, attitudes, and feelings of patients, there seems to be a need to evaluate the current status of satisfaction among patients within different kinds of ambulatory health care settings. Therefore, the purpose of the present investigation will be twofold:

(1) to ascertain levels of patient satisfaction employing multiple criteria that are meaningful and important to patients and yet acceptable to providers of health care.

(2) to analyze the relationships among patient characteristics, characteristics of the health care encounter, and patient satisfaction with that encounter.

As such, patient satisfaction is conceptualized as an outcome variable, being a product of the social, cultural, and psychological character of the patient on the one hand and certain aspects of the delivery of care on the other. Of course, in the larger perspective, patient satisfaction is probably an intervening variable, being antecedent to such outcomes as patient compliance, recovery, or wellness.

Method

The Sample and Design

The data presented in this report were collected in eleven Southern California ambulatory health care settings: two solo-practitioner general practices; two university student health centers; two health department community health clinics; one large private group practice; two outpatient clinics affiliated with small hospitals; one large county outpatient clinic; and one large clinic of a prepaid HMO. The settings were not randomly selected but chosen because of entree in connection with the training and preceptorship of a nurse practitioner program at UCLA. Thus, although the settings are probably typical of family or general ambulatory care settings in Southern California, caution must be exercised in making generalizations.

In each of the settings, all patient visits were studied during a period of one five-day work week. As the patients arrived at each setting, they were greeted by a member of the UCLA research team who explained the study and asked them to complete an anonymous questionnaire in either English or Spanish.[1] At this time, a number-coded encounter form which was to be completed by all health care providers (physicians, nurses, nurse practitioners) was attached to the patient's chart and the number entered on the top of the patient's questionnaire. Patients were asked to read over their questionnaires and to complete and return them to the UCLA representative after they had received treatment. This system permitted an analysis of who provided care, what was provided, and how the care was evaluated by the patient. Thus, the encounter form allowed us to determine the type or types of providers. However, since some patients were examined or treated by both a nurse and a physician, there were separate sets of questions to evaluate the services of each on the patient questionnaire. Rates of response varied from 80−99 percent, with few patient refusals. Non-responses were generally in large settings where patients could leave without turning in their questionnaire or where some providers failed to complete encounter forms. The total number of complete patient-provider encounters which is the basis of this report is 1,739.

[1]The directions on the questionnaire were as follows: The people who have just given you medical care are interested in how they can do a better job. In order to help them find out, we at U.C.L.A. are asking you to fill out this survey about the care you just received. Your answers will be kept private so that you can feel free to answer the questions in a straightforward and honest way. Be sure to answer all of the questions on this page and the back page (page 4). You should answer questions on page 2 *only* if you saw a physician as part of your visit. Answer questions on page 3 if a nurse treated you today. If both a nurse and a doctor treated you today, answer all questions on pages 2 and 3. Finally, pay no attention to the numbers along the right-hand side of the page. They are for the computer.

Thank you very much for your help, and if you have any problems with the questions, ask for help.

Measurements: Patient Encounter Form

Although a number of different kinds of information were ascertained about each provider-patient encounter, the following three categories of characteristics will be discussed: (a) general characteristics of the visit, (b) services performed or provided, and (c) the disposition. The general characteristics of the visit include the provider's estimate of time spent with the patient, whether or not the patient had been seen before in the setting, whether or not he had seen the provider in a previous visit, and if he had, whether or not that visit concerned the same health problem. The services performed or provided include a general or limited history, a general or limited physical examination, lab tests, X rays, drug therapy, therapeutic listening or counseling, or advice concerning exercise, diet, or habits. Finally, the disposition of the visit involved whether or not follow-up was planned and, if so, whether the patient was to return at any time or at a specific time.

Measurements: Patient Characteristics

Seven patient characteristics were ascertained in the pencil-and-paper questionnaire: age, sex, race, marital status, educational background, religion in which the patient was raised, and, finally, the level of satisfaction with the community in which he was currently living.

Measurements: Patient Evaluations of Care (Satisfaction)

The first measure of patient evaluation of care to be analyzed in this report is a General Evaluation Index and is based upon responses to the following six items (scoring value in parenthesis):

1. Do you feel that the medical attention you received today is better than what most people get, about the same, or not as good? (3,2,1)

2. Regarding today's visit, do you feel that there were any tests or procedures used on you which were *not* necessary? (1,2)

3. Regarding today's visit, do you feel that *more* tests or procedures were necessary to understand your problem? (1,2)

4. Would you say that the medical care you received today was better than usual visits, about the same, or not as good? (3,2,1)

5. How well do you feel you understand your present medical condition? (Check one)

I understand very well	(4)
I think I understand	(3)
I am not sure I understand	(2)
I don't understand very well	(1)

6. Which of the following statements *best describe* your feelings about the person(s) who gave you medical care today? (Check one)

I would prefer to see the same person(s) again	(3)
It wouldn't make much difference whether or not I saw the same person on my next visit	(2)
I would prefer to see someone else	(1)

On the basis of the sum of his responses to these six questions, each patient in the sample was assigned a quartile rank of 1 to 4, with 4 indicating the highest positive evaluation of care and 1 the lowest. Because of the skewed distribution of scores, the following classification resulted: Quartile 1 (Scores 8 – 13) 16 percent; Quartile 2 (Score of 14) 20 percent; Quartile 3 (Score of 15) 33 percent; and Quartile 4 (Scores 16 – 17) 31 percent.

The second measure of patient care to be discussed in this report is an Index of Satisfaction with Physician Care and is based upon responses to the following four items:

1. Would you say that the doctor spent more than enough time with you today, enough time, or not enough time? (3,2,1)

2. Do you feel that the doctor understood what was bothering you? (Check one)

understood very well	(4)
understood somewhat	(3)
didn't understand very well	(2)
didn't understand at all	(1)

3. How much interest and concern did the doctor show for you? Was the doctor: (Check one)

extremely concerned	(6)
very concerned	(5)
somewhat concerned	(4)
somewhat unconcerned	(3)
very unconcerned	(2)
extremely unconcerned	(1)

4. In general, how satisfied were you with today's contact with the doctor? (Check one)

extremely satisfied	(6)
very satisfied	(5)
somewhat satisfied	(4)

somewhat dissatisfied	(3)
very dissatisfied	(2)
extremely dissatisfied	(1)

Again, each patient in the sample was assigned a quartile ranking on the basis of the sum of his responses to the four items above. A rank of 1 indicated the lowest level of satisfaction; a rank of 4 the highest. In this process, the following distribution resulted: Quartile 1 (Scores 6 − 14) 21 percent; Quartile 2 (Score of 15) 13 percent; Quartile 3 (Score of 16) 32 percent; and Quartile 4 (Scores 17 − 19) 34 percent.

The items in each index were chosen because they were thought to measure directly satisfaction with the care received or to reflect positive or negative aspects of a health care encounter. However, since no provision was made to weight the items within each index equally, the simple summation process employed has some systematic bias, giving greater weight to items with more answer categories.

Finally, it should be noted that because of the design of the patient questionnaire, the General Evaluation Index referred to attitudes regarding the entire visit; the Index of Satisfaction with Physicians referred only to encounters with a physician.[2] However, in examining the relationship between the two indices, a strong statistically significant correlation was found ($r = .57$ $p > 001$). Therefore, the analysis presented in this report should not be interpreted as advocating two distinct satisfaction dimensions. They were not combined into a single index because of the possible differences which may arise in their relationship to the independent variables under examination.

Results

Consistent with previous findings, patients generally evaluated the care they had received in a highly positive way. For example, with regard to patients' general evaluation, 97 percent felt the medical attention they received was about the same or better than what most people get, 98 percent felt their visit was about the same or better than usual visits, 98 percent did not feel that they were subjected to unnecessary tests, and 86 percent did not feel that more tests were necessary. Two thirds of the sample felt they un-

[2] In some settings, non-physicians also render care, and the relationship between type of provider and evaluation of care will be discussed elsewhere (Linn, 1975).

derstood their medical condition very well, 25 percent thought they did, but for 10 percent, lack of understanding was certainly an issue. Finally, 80 percent of the patients indicated that they would prefer to see the same providers of care again, 18 percent indicated apathy, and 2 percent preferred to see someone else.

With regard to satisfaction with physician care rendered, generally only 3 − 5 percent of patients indicated any clear dissatisfaction on the four questions. However, one needs to make a value judgment regarding whether the response of "somewhat concerned" (as opposed to alternative choices of very or extremely) represents an acceptable level of response for patients to make regarding their attitudes toward the interest and concern shown by the doctor. Similarly one also might argue that because of the importance of doctor-patient encounters, a response of "somewhat satisfied" really is not very good.

When the two indices constructed from these items were examined across the 11 medical settings studied, significant differences among patients were clearly observed. For example, the range of patients highly satisfied (third and fourth quartile scores) on the General Evaluation Index was 44 − 87 percent; the range on the Index of Satisfaction with physicians was 52 − 84 percent.[3]

Patient Characteristics and Satisfaction

In this regard, the religion in which patients were raised, their sex, and their marital status were not found to be significantly related to either measure of patient satisfaction. However, as can be seen in Table 1, the oldest patients were the most likely group to be satisfied on both measures. The least satisfied group of patients were the young adults, ages 18 − 24.

The second major finding in Table 1 indicates that patients who were more satisfied with living in their community were significantly more satisfied with their medical care. This most interesting finding suggests that perhaps patients who express dissatisfaction with care are more likely to express dissatisfaction with other aspects of their life than more "satisfied" patients do. Perhaps dissatisfied patients are dissatisfied people, and one significant factor in determining patient satisfaction is the general psychological predisposition or personality of the patient.

Finally, with regard to the findings concerning educational background and race, Table 1 indicates no significant relationship

[3]Because of the skewed distribution of scores, the third and fourth quartiles together constituted 64 percent of the scores on the General Evaluation Index, and 66 percent on the Index of Satisfaction with Physicians.

TABLE 1

Patient Characteristics and Satisfaction with Medical Care

Patient Characteristics	High General Satisfaction			High Satisfaction with Physician		
	%	N	Total	%	N	Total
Age						
≥ 17 years	66	160	243	63	175	278
18-20	55	85	156	55	73	132
21-24	50	97	193	67	121	182
25-29	68	95	139	61	76	124
30-39	64	88	138	64	101	159
40-49	72	70	97	69	88	128
50-59	65	67	103	70	87	125
60 >	78	79	101	81	99	122
	$X^2 \, p < 001$			$X^2 \, p < 01$		
Race						
White	63	543	856	64	559	886
Black	68	67	98	75	80	106
Spanish	65	120	185	71	160	228
	X^2 NS			$X^2 \, p < 001$		
Educational Background						
Some grade school	65	46	71	77	66	86
Completed grade school	74	46	62	79	66	84
Some high school	60	120	201	71	153	218
Completed high school	61	156	256	59	169	286
Some vocational school	61	25	41	59	28	48
Completed vocational school	70	26	37	63	29	49
Some college	61	253	413	62	239	384
Completed college	64	94	147	64	82	128
	X^2 NS			$X^2 \, p < 05$		
Community Satisfaction						
Extremely satisfied	71	152	215	77	176	229
Very satisfied	64	307	478	68	337	494
Somewhat satisfied	57	209	366	61	239	394
Somewhat, very, or extremely dissatisfied	61	119	194	54	112	206
	$X^2 \, p < 05$			$X^2 \, p < 001$		

between the two variables and patients' general evaluation of care. However, patients with less formal education (some high school or less) were significantly more likely to be highly satisfied on the Index of Satisfaction with Physicians than patients with more education. Similarly, black and Spanish-speaking patients were more satisfied with the care the physicians rendered than white patients. Although these findings may only reflect the local situation in Los Angeles County, racial minorities and less educated people do not seem to be overly dissatisfied with the way in which physicians treat them; rather, they hold more favorable opinions than the white and educated majorities.

Patient Satisfaction and Characteristics
of the Medical Encounter

Traditional studies of patient satisfaction generally examine the relationship between patient characteristics and evaluations of care. However, since satisfaction might not be determined by patient contingencies alone but may be affected by either services provided or policies within the health care setting, the present study is also concerned with the relationship between satisfaction and characteristics of the encounter being evaluated.

General characteristics   Table 2 shows that there was no significant difference in satisfaction levels between new and old patients. However, patients who had been seen by their provider of care on a previous visit were significantly more satisfied with their care in general and with the doctor in particular than patients who saw a new provider. Similarly, patients who had been seen before by the same person for the same problem were significantly more likely to be satisfied than patients who saw a familiar provider but for a new

TABLE 2

Patient Satisfaction and the General Characteristics of the Patient Visit

General Characteristics of Doctor Visit	High General Satisfaction			High Satisfaction with Physician		
	%	N	Total	%	N	Total
First Visit to Setting						
Yes	62	69	111	66	71	107
No	63	652	1032	65	726	1117
	x^2 NS			x^2 NS		
First Visit to Provider						
Yes	57	192	338	60	193	321
No	67	485	720	68	535	789
	$x^2\ p < 001$			$x^2\ p < 01$		
First Visit to Familiar Provider for Present Problem						
Yes	67	145	218	60	149	248
No	69	360	520	71	397	560
	x^2 NS			$x^2\ p < 02$		
Duration of Visit with Provider						
5 min. or less	67	209	311	63	210	334
6-10 min.	63	259	414	63	289	462
11-15 min.	63	131	209	69	160	231
16 min. or more	59	90	152	70	111	159
	$x^2\ p < 05$			x^2 NS		

problem. Thus, although there is no difference in attitude between new and returning patients, among the latter group there seems to be strong evidence that they favor continuity of care. Highest levels of physician satisfaction were expressed by patients who had previously seen the same person for the same problem.

Finally, the findings in Table 2 concerning estimated time spent with the patient indicate that patients who had shorter visits with the provider (five minutes or less) were significantly *more* satisfied on the General Evaluation Index than patients who had longer visits (16 minutes or more). However, although not statistically significant, the trends regarding satisfaction with the physician and duration of visit indicate the opposite. Thus, although greater time spent by the doctor with the patient results in greater patient satisfaction with that doctor, it nevertheless results in less overall satisfaction with the medical visit.

Services rendered The provider of care was asked to check those services that were provided to each patient from the following list: (1) a general or limited history; (2) a general or limited physical exam; (3) lab tests; (4) X rays; (5) drugs given or prescribed; (6) therapeutic listening; or (7) advice or counseling. In looking at the relationship between the provision of each service and both measures of patient satisfaction, only advice or counseling was found to be significantly related. More specifically, 71 percent of the patients who received advice or counseling had high scores on the General Evaluation Index as compared with 60 percent who did not receive any advice ($p < 01$). However, there was no significant difference between advice and satisfaction with the physician. Generally, then, almost none of the specific services provided to patients seemed to have any effect on their overall assessments of care.

Regarding this finding, it may be that what is really important is not specific services but the *number* that are provided to patients. However, when the number of services was examined in relationship to both measures of patient satisfaction, no statistically significant differences were found. Thus, in the present study, there seems to be little or no relationship between patients' satisfaction and either the number or kind of services provided to them.

Disposition of the visit The final aspect of the patient-practitioner encounter under examination is the disposition of the visit. Providers were given a list of possible dispositions and asked to check all that applied to their decision. In looking at the relationship between patient satisfaction and the three most frequently checked dispositions (no follow-up, return at specific time, or return any time), it was found that patients who were given a scheduled return appointment were significantly more satisfied with their care in general and their interactions with physicians than patients who had no return appointment scheduled. Similarly, the trends on the Index of Physician Satisfaction suggested that patients who were told to return any time or for whom no follow-up was planned were less satisfied than patients with other dispositions.

The finding that patients are significantly more satisfied if they see the same doctor for the same problem and if a return visit is scheduled suggests a strong positive argument for continuity of care. To illustrate this finding more explicitly and for more precise analysis, each of the patient encounters has therefore been classified into one of the following six categories:

(1) familiar provider, familiar problem, return visit scheduled

(2) familiar provider, familiar problem, no return visit scheduled

(3) familiar provider, new problem, return visit scheduled

(4) familiar provider, new problem, no return visit scheduled

(5) new provider, return visit scheduled

(6) new provider, no return visit scheduled

In looking at the relationship between this classification and patient evaluations, Table 3 shows a statistically significant as-

TABLE 3

Patient Satisfaction and Continuity of Care

Continuity	High General Satisfaction			High Satisfaction with Physician		
	%	N	Total	%	N	Total
Same M.D., same problem, return visit	69	273	394	71	300	420
Same M.D., same problem, no return visit	69	87	126	69	97	140
Same M.D., new problem, return visit	71	61	86	63	64	101
Same M.D., new problem, no return visit	58	56	96	56	62	111
New M.D., return visit	61	90	147	65	89	137
New M.D., no return visit	52	98	187	56	101	180
	($p < 01$)			($p < 01$)		

sociation with both measures as well as some very interesting patterns. For example, patient evaluations are more favorable when patients see the same practitioner for the same (or familiar) problem, regardless of whether or not a return appointment is scheduled. However, among patients with new problems, the importance of the return visit for patient satisfaction emerges, with patients having return visits scheduled being more satisfied. Similarly, among patients whose visits were to new providers, satisfaction was greater when a return appointment was scheduled.

Patient Factors vs. Contingencies of the Visit

In brief review, three main factors were found to be significantly related to the evaluations patients made of their medical care: (1) age, (2) level of satisfaction with living in their community, and (3) the nature and degree of continuity of care which characterized their visit. In looking at these factors two at a time in relationship to both measures of satisfaction, with few exceptions the original relationships were sustained. Therefore, age, community satisfaction, and continuity of care seem to be three relatively independent correlates of patient satisfaction (or dissatisfaction) as well as the three most important correlates considered in this report.

Discussion and Summary

To review, the present study has confirmed the findings of previous studies: that patients are generally very satisfied with their medical care. When index scores were examined in relationship to other factors, the greatest differences occurred between settings. In order to account for these differences, characteristics of both patients and visits were examined with the following results:

(1) Neither measure of satisfaction was significantly related to patients' sex, marital status, or the religion in which they were raised.

(2) Patients with less education or from minority groups (black and Spanish-speaking) were significantly more likely to evaluate their physicians more positively than patients who were white or with more education. However, education and race were not significantly related to patients' scores on the General Evaluation Index.

(3) Generally, patients over 60 years and under 18 (often mothers' evaluations of their infants' or children's care) were significantly more satisfied with their medical encounters than patients in other age groups. Young adults (18−21 or 21−25) were

the least likely age group to be satisfied. Such differences probably reflect the different social and psychological needs of the age group.

(4) Patients who were more satisfied with living in their community were significantly more likely to be satisfied with their medical visit as well as their interactions with doctors than patients who were less satisfied with their community life. This finding represents a reconfirmation of a previously unpublished finding from a large household survey (Linn and Reeder, 1973) which found a relationship between satisfaction with last doctor visit and satisfaction with community life, facilities, and services. The interpretation of this finding in the present report is that the high correlation between evaluations of medical care and community life probably reflects a more general tendency to view one's world either positively or negatively. As such, perhaps dissatisfied patients are dissatisfied people, and that one major determinant of patient satisfaction is the cognitive style or personality of the patient.

(5) There was no significant difference in evaluations of care between new and old patients. However, among old patients, those who got to see the same provider were significantly more satisfied than those who saw someone new. Similarly, satisfaction with the physician was greatest among patients who saw the same doctor for a problem they had seen him about on a previous visit. Finally, patients were significantly more satisfied with their visits and doctors if a return appointment was scheduled. Together, these findings provide strong evidence that patients like continuity of care. Looked at in another way, it appears that patients are most satisfied when they are allowed to develop an expected, consistent, and structured relationship with a provider of care.

(6) With little exception, both the number and kind of services provided during the visit has little effect on patient evaluations of care or providers.

(7) When age, community satisfaction, and the nature and degree of continuity of care are examined in relationship to satisfaction, two variables at a time, the results indicate that the three factors are relatively independent sources of satisfaction.

Returning then to the question of why the greatest differences in satisfaction levels occurred between settings, additional examination of the data suggest that it is because of differences in patient characteristics and setting policies which characterize them. For example, the settings with the highest patient satisfaction levels generally provided greater continuity of care, had more patients with favorable community attitudes, and had more patients very young or very old. Similarly, settings with low levels of satisfaction had more patients who were young adults, scheduled few return visits, did not emphasize seeing the same provider each visit, and so on.[4]

Finally, the implications of these findings are that although in general patient satisfaction is already high, it probably will not be increased by providing more services to patients. Similarly, the experiences, needs, and attitudes related to certain age groups cannot easily be altered by health care providers, nor can the personality characteristics of certain patients be changed. However, policies within the health care system can be changed to favor continuity of care, so that patients can develop a continuing relationship with the same provider.

[4]Although it is probable that some differences in continuity of care may be related to differences in patients' medical problems, the data from apparently similar kinds of primary care settings in the present study suggests an alternative hypothesis: that in primary care settings, whether or not patients are asked to return at a specific time and whether or not they will see the same provider on their return is more likely to be a function of physician or setting policy than an attribute of the presenting complaint. This, of course, is something which needs to be pursued further.

Lawrence S. Linn, PH.D.
Primex Project
University of California, Los Angeles
924 Westwood Boulevard, Suite 520
Los Angeles, California 90024

The research reported here was supported by a grant from the National Center for Health Services Research and Development, U.S. Department of Health, Education, and Welfare No. HS90085. The author is indebted to Dr. Charles E. Lewis for his cooperation and support.

References

Alpert, J.J., J. Kosa, L.J. Haggerty, L.S. Robertson, and Mageret C. Heagarty
    1970   "Attitudes and satisfactions of low-income families receiving comprehensive pediatric care." American Journal of Public Health 60, 3 (March): 499 – 506.

Anderson, D.W., and P.B. Sheatsley
    1959   Comprehensive Medical Insurance—A Study of Costs, Use, and Attitudes Under Two Plans. Research Series 9. Chicago, Illinois: Health Information Foundation.

Bashshur, R.L.
1967   "Consumer satisfaction with group practice, the cha case." American
        Journal of Public Health 57, 11 (November): 1991 – 1999.

Day, Lewis R., R. Egli, and Henry K. Silver
1970   "Acceptance of pediatric nurse practitioners." American Journal of
        Diseases of Children 119 (March): 204 – 208.

Deisher, R.W., W.L. Engel, R. Spielholz, and Susan J. Standfast
1965   "Mothers' opinions of their pediatric care." Pediatrics 35 (January):
        82 – 90.

Francis, V., B.H. Korsch, and Marie J. Morris
1969   "Gaps in doctor-patient communication patients' response to medical
        advice." New England Journal of Medicine 280, 10 (March):
        535 – 540.

Freidson, E.
1961   Patients' View of Medical Practice. New York: Russell Sage Founda-
        tion.

Gerst, A., L. Rogson, and Robert Hetherington
1969   "Patterns of satisfaction with health plan coverage: a conceptual ap-
        proach." Inquiry 6, 3: 37 – 51.

Hulka, B.S., S.J. Zyzanski, J.C. Cassel, and Shirley J. Thompson
1971   "Satisfaction with medical care in a low income population." Journal
        of Chronic Diseases 24: 661 – 673.

Kisch, A.I., and L.G. Reeder
1969   "Client evaluation of physician performance." Journal of Health and
        Social Behavior 10, 1 (March): 51 – 58.

Koos, E.L.
1955   "Metropolis what city people think of their medical services."
        American Journal of Public Health 45, 12 (December): 1551 – 1557.

Linn, Lawrence S.
1975   "Patient acceptance of the family nurse practitioner." Medical Care
        (forthcoming).

Linn, Lawrence S., and Leo G. Reeder
1972   Satisfaction with last doctor visit in a general population sample. Un-
        published monograph.

Nelson, Eugene, A.R. Jacobs, and Kenneth G. Johnson
1974   "Patients' acceptance of physician's assistants." JAMA 228, 1 (April
        1): 63 – 67.

Reeder, L.G.
1972   "The patient-client as a consumer: some observations on the changing professional-client relationship." Journal of Health and Social Behavior 13 (December): 406–412.

Spitzer, Walter O.
1974   "A strategy for evaluation of new health professionals." Paper presented at Conference of New Health Manpower, sponsored by Association of Teachers of Preventative Medicine, NIH, Bethesda, Maryland (May).

Weinerman, E.R.
1964   "Patients' perceptions of group medical care." American Journal of Public Health 54, 6 (June): 880–889.

II Professional Behavior

The Social Control
of Organizations
in the Health Care Area

M. DAVID ERMANN

Available data suggest that the influence and autonomy of health care professionals have been declining. Of course, professional impact remains higher in health care than perhaps any other economic sphere, but the locus of much health care decision making has been shifting from independent professionals to employed personnel of large-scale governmental, hospital, insurance, and research organizations. The question therefore arises as to what shall replace this previous reliance upon individual professional ethics to assure the society that its newly powerful health care organizations are functioning in a desirable manner. In other words, what are to be the preferred mechanisms for socially controlling health care organizations.

This paper traces three dominant belief patterns about how the characteristics of health care organizations and their environments produce desired control. It proposes that belief patterns have emphasized (1) the non-profit motives of many health care organizations; (2) the system of interrelationships that surround health care organizations; and (3) the vast differences among health care consumers. Choices from among these models continue to depend less upon knowledge of organizational functioning than upon political dispositions and social fancy.

In 1928-29, expenditures for physicians' services were the largest category of medical cost in the United States, accounting for 28 percent of all health expenditures. Hospitals, which were second with 18 percent of total expenditures, were workshops of physicians and were dominated by them. Following expenditures for hospitals were expenditures for drugs (17 percent), dental services (13 percent), and "other professional services" (7 percent) (Cooper and Worthington, 1973:12). The bulk of care thus was dispensed in settings controlled by professionals, and the cost and quality of care were in large measure determined by the decisions of these individuals. Much has changed since then.

By 1971-72, expenditures for hospitals had grown to be the largest category of medical cost, more than doubling in relative share to 39 percent of total health expenditures. The relative share of physicians meanwhile had declined to 19 percent, after which came drugs (9 percent), research (7 percent), and dental services (6 percent). Organizations thus had increased their importance in the arrangements by which Americans received medical care, with three organizationally dominated areas (hospitals, drugs, and research) accounting for more than one-half of all expenditures. Furthermore, the immense power of physicians and other professionals in these organizations had been somewhat weakened while the power of administration had increased, particularly in hospitals (Perrow, 1961; White, 1971). Health care organizations and their administrative structures were becoming the focus of planning, decision making, sanctioning, and much else in health care.

Because of this ongoing shift, there developed a need to change assumptions about motivations and controls in the health care field. The tradition of professional motivation to serve clients could less and less be relied upon as a way to assure laymen that medical institutions function "properly." Patient-oriented professionals do not control medical organizations; organizationally oriented employees do. Unfortunately, however, little is understood about circumstances that would encourage the elites of health care organizations to provide quality care at reasonable prices.

Social Control of Medical Organizations

The health care field is not unique in its failure to understand the control of organizational activities. Public inability to control corporate political contributions and CIA domestic spying, as well as the nearly universal failure of federal regulatory agencies, are just a few illustrations that available technology for external control of organizational actions is weak in many areas. Little is known about how organizations can be controlled. In a controversial area such as health care, this lack of knowledge leaves a costly vacuum where strategies for control reflect little more than the political and social predispositions of their advocates (see Reinhardt, 1973). But, as illustrated by experiences with Blue Cross, Medicare, and Comprehensive Health Planning, the usefulness of these predispositions has not been affirmed by experience. Control has been difficult to obtain, and health care organizations have proven more complicated and intractable than expected, with narrow organizational interests regularly undermining outsider preferences. For instance, while it may be rational for a hospital to abandon an emergency room or purchase open-heart surgery facilities, this may not be desired by concerned outsiders. Hospitals nevertheless continue to buy unneeded technology and companies continue to sell it.

These behaviors are sociologically defined as deviant; they are contrary to the standards and expectations defined by important groups in society. However, incomplete knowledge about the relationship between these deviant organizational behaviors and the societal responses to them results in fostering behaviors that are neither intended nor immediately obvious (Ermann and Lundman, 1975). This tendency prompted Somers (1969:ix) in her excellent book on hospital regulation, to observe succinctly that hospitals so far have "defied conventional public regulation"; despite past failures, or perhaps because of them, the search for organizational knowledge and regulatory technology has continued.

Models of Behavior and Control of Medical Organizations

This paper analyzes changing models of organizational behavior and control in the health care field. It argues that these models, in their times, have been used by the public and by elites (1) to describe the internal dynamics of medical organizations, and (2) to prescribe the conditions that should exist to encourage medical organizations to perform in socially desired ways. Though the models are not mutually exclusive in theory, an emphasis on one has tended to be accompanied by relegation of the others. The models, like the conceptual scheme used here to describe them, are of necessity crude because of the recent importance of large medical organizations and the resulting newness of the need to control them. When applied, these models have enjoyed little success—partly as a result of problems of their unstated and therefore untested nature which we will here try to remedy.

Available data suggest three partly overlapping stages of American beliefs about how medical organizations operate. The first model stressed that the non-profit status of most hospitals and some other medical care organizations makes them substantially immune from corruption of their health care goals. Conversely, it assumed that the profit motive in medicine has a powerful corrupting influence. The second model emphasized systemic ties of hospitals to a wide range of organizations in their environments. It implied that connections, exchanges, and coordination involving health organizations are the most important constraints on their performance. The third and most recent model, just now emerging, emphasizes the impact of the immediate environment of medical organizations. It proposes that the idiosyncratic differences among health care recipients are or should be the major determinants of the performance of medical care organizations.

These three models have remarkably different implications for choices regarding how hospitals and other medical organizations are to be controlled. Each will be analyzed in detail in the following sections.

The Non-Profit Motivation Model

The non-profit motivation model, which has had the longest history and probably the most influence of any model, emphasized distinctions between profit-making and non-profit organizations. It placed great emphasis on the altruistic goals of formally non-profit organizations (Lentz, 1956) and on the parallel unworthiness of those that seek "to make profit from the suffering of others." Because this model accepted the official service goals of non-profit organizations, and because it has been influential, attempts to control non-profit medical organizations until recently have been minimal. Why, it was asked, should we regulate organizations whose only goals are public service? The description below shows that the answer to this question in the case of voluntary hospitals and Blue Cross often was that they need not be regulated.

Voluntary hospitals for a long time escaped common law and legislated controls, such as a financial penalty for poor performance, applied to most other organizations. For example, malpractice suits, despite their notoriety, are a recent and incomplete phenomenon for hospitals. Beginning with a case in 1876 (Somers, 1969:29) voluntary hospitals have been protected from liability under a doctrine of "charitable immunity." (In that 1876 case the court ruled that a patient whose fractured thighbone allegedly was incompetently treated by an intern could not receive damages from the non-profit Massachusetts General Hospital, even if he proved his allegations, because hospital funds were held in trust solely to maintain the hospital.) Despite a trend in the past thirty years toward reduction in hospital immunity, Zald and Hair (1972:62) characterize 1967 rulings in seven states as still conveying "full immunity" and in eight as "qualified immunity" for voluntary hospitals.[1]

Voluntary hospitals continue to be exempted from control in other areas as well. They have been exempted from most labor legislation, including legislation controlling working conditions and minimum wages until recently. They are specifically excluded from six of the 14 state laws patterned on the federal government's National Labor Relations Act (Metzger, 1970:83), and were until mid-1974 excluded from the federal law as well. The origins of this federal exclusion vividly illustrate the non-profit model as applied to hospitals. In 1947, the Taft-Hartley Amendments to the Wagner Act excluded employees of non-profit hospitals from NLRB protection as a result of the efforts of Senator Tydings, who, in making his proposal (U.S. House of Representatives, 1973:2), explained that the exclusion was:

> designed merely to help a great number of hospitals which are having very difficult times. They are eleemosynary institutions, *no profit is involved in their operations;* and I understand from the Hospital Association that this amendment would be very helpful in their efforts to serve those who have not the means to pay for hospital service. [Emphasis added.]

There was little opposition voiced to this exclusion of protection of workers solely because a hospital was non-profit.

Non-profit status as a basis for regulation has not been limited to hospitals. The American Hospital Association, shortly after creating Blue Cross as a non-profit insurance organization, sought and received for Blue Cross special regulatory treatment despite its basic similarity to profit-making insurance programs. Among the items sought were exemption from state insurance laws and from reserve requirements applied to commercial insurers. Law (1974:9) found that all states but three now have "special enabling legislation for hospital service organizations, and in 20 states such corporations are exempt from taxation." She also found (Law, 1974:17) that most states do not even require Blue Cross to file proposed increases with their insurance departments. Here again

---

[1] For 1967-68, Somers (1969:29-31) characterized two states (Massachusetts and South Carolina) still offering total immunity and 20 with "liability limited in one way or another."

medically related organizations were given special treatment—and subjected to relatively loose control—because they were deemed to be non-profit.

By comparison, the level of control of proprietary hospitals and commercial insurance companies has been high, partly because of low legitimacy of commercialism in these areas. Proprietary hospitals always have been subject to malpractice suits, labor legislation, and regular taxation. Commercial insurance companies have been regulated by state insurance commissioners for more than 100 years (Kulp and Hall, 1968:958-959). They were not given special treatment for their involvements in health care.

The level of regulation of these medical businesses appears to change in concert with regulatory trends in the society. When the regulatory movement in the general economy is in a laissez-faire direction and controls on businesses are being loosened, health-related businesses also have their controls lessened. At other times medical businesses join non-medical businesses in being closely regulated.

American public opinion appears to be in a period of increasing distrust of commercial organizations, growing desires to control them, and decreasing support for laissez-faire economics—and these attitudes are carrying over into the medical field. Recent studies of nursing care facilities and their failures, for example, have focused on the need to control the medical practices, as well as the high profits, of commercial nursing homes. A Senate report (U.S. Senate, 1974:225) on "Profits and the Nursing Home: Incentives in Favor of Poor Care" quoted a Dr. Butler expressing this focus quite clearly:

> After 15 years of research and practice, I come now to believe that the profit motive must be eliminated from our care systems including medicine and institutional care and its alternatives. There are many fine and well-intentioned nursing home owners. They are not all miscreants...But the conflict between profit and service is too great to overcome.
>
> Only in the United States and Canada (to my knowledge) is there "commercialization..."

The report itself, as well as its title, placed its authors with Dr. Butler among the critics of profit-making nursing homes.

The non-profit motivation model, in sum, presumes differential need to control health care organizations based on a single criterion—whether they officially seek a profit. Those organizations holding official non-profit goals tend to be less controlled than profit-making organizations engaged in similar activity. In health care sectors where non-profit organizations account for much activity (e.g., hospitals and insurance), emphasizing this dimension has resulted in low levels of societal control.

The Systemic Model

The systemic model has been replacing the profit motivation model in American regulatory imagery. Unlike its predecessor, the systemic model as applied to health and other fields does not focus on internal (profit-related) motives; rather, it focuses on external relations with other organizations.

This systemic approach when applied to health problems emphasizes that all hospitals (whether voluntary or proprietary) buy from commercial pharmaceutical firms, that non-profit Blue Cross is disbursing agent for the government's Medicare program to proprietary hospitals, and that university-based research centers rely on federal funding. The systemic approach is unconcerned with adjectives like "profit-making," "voluntary," or "governmental." It emphasizes instead how organizations interconnect (Levine and White, 1961). Its current popularity is evident in the widely used phrases like "health care delivery systems" and the "chaos" of the "health care non-system." The word "system" in particular is emphasized.

Fortune magazine, in an issue ushering in the present decade devoted primarily to "Our Ailing Medical System," made this model as uncomplicated and explicit as possible. Its editorial (Fortune, 1970:79) explained that "most Americans are badly served by the obsolete, overstrained Medical system that has grown around them helter-skelter." Its first article offered (Fortune, 1970:2) prescriptions based on the systemic model:

> ...What is needed is a drastic restructuring of the medical system. The federal government, which is paying a sizable share of present medical costs, should encourage the establishment of more efficient systems of medical care, particularly group-practice plans....Also private insurance companies should begin challenging high medical costs more firmly...

Letters to the editor, even critical ones, published in subsequent months all accepted the underlying systemic assumptions.

A more thought-provoking article in *Modern Hospital* (1970), summarizing a five-day "off the record" meeting of 23 hospital-related leaders, used the systemic model with greater sophistication. It predicted a future with three power coalitions in the medical care field, each vying with the others. The coalitions would be (1) physicians, allied professionals, and medical managers, (2) consumers and their agents, Blue Cross, Blue Shield, and other third-party purchasers, and (3) government. The creation and interaction of these three groups, the article concluded, would determine the future course of American health care.

The popularity of the systemic model for understanding and controlling health organizations goes beyond these descriptions and predictions—it is reflected in current regulatory activities. Hospitals are being required to buy generically from pharmaceutical manufacturers, and Blue Cross is being pressured by Medicare to contain hospital costs. Use of the model is evident in some aspects of all national health insurance proposals, and in recent legislation such as the National Health Planning and Resources Development Act of 1974 (P.L. 93-641).

Three of the six most important national health insurance bills introduced into the recent Ninety-third Congress share wholeheartedly the assumptions of the systemic model. They postulate that health care is a system of interrelated parts, and that the parts' relations with one another should be altered. They differ about what relationships should be altered, which is not surprising given their divergent support, but they agree on the need for alterations. The Senate sponsor of the strongest and best known of them, the Kennedy-Griffiths bill supported by organized labor, made these assumptions perfectly clear in his introduction to the bill (Kennedy, 1973:1)

> ...The history of medicare and medicaid has taught us that attempts to offer health insurance on a piecemeal basis to segments of our population—without major efforts to expand and reform our health care system—result in increased inflation which robs Americans of much of the benefit of the new insurance....The answer to this problem is not to cut back on benefits, to raise insurance premiums even more, or to simply offer more insurance to more Americans. The answer is to reform our health care system and bring these costs under control.

Control of medical organizations under Kennedy-Griffiths rests with a unitary, inclusive program administered and coordinated by the federal government, with special boards and councils to make policies and administer them within the Department of Health, Education, and Welfare. Medicare, Medicaid, Maternal and Child Health, and other programs would terminate as separate programs. In sum, the "system" of health care "delivery" would have the relation of its parts reordered and rationalized.

One of the earliest and clearest examples of the systemic model is the Comprehensive Health Planning (CHP) Act, passed (O'Connor, 1974:391) in 1966 amid "great hopes for a rationalization of what has recently come to be called the American medical care 'non-system' [through the] application of sophisticated planning technology." The act created local and state agencies to plan for and coordinate activities in their (O'Connor, 1974:393) "medical catchment areas." As its title implied, it was to be comprehensive, including all segments of the health care industry, and (O'Connor, 1974:394) "looking at the system as an operating unit." However, achievement of desired coordination has been more difficult than its conceptualization. CHP is widely considered a failure. Its planning agencies have had little influence on the coordination of health care activities, apparently spinning their wheels and accomplishing little, and influencing few behaviors of other organizations in the health field.

The failure of CHP may be due more to the accuracy of the systemic model and its assumptions than to their inadequacy. The model correctly avoids superficial assumptions that non-profit organizations which fail to serve the public will change their behaviors readily in order to serve, and that profit-making organizations will change to protect or enhance profits. It emphasizes instead that organizations tend toward stability and autonomy because of the constraints of other organizations with which they interact. As a result, medical organizations often resist external forces trying to disrupt their existing patterns—to the immense frustration of critics. The following criticism of reforms (Alford, 1972:128) vividly summarizes the frustrations (and the assumptions) of the systemic model:

> ...The overwhelming fact about the various reforms of the health system that have been implemented or proposed—more money, more subsidy of insurance, more manpower, more demonstration projects, more clinics—is that they are absorbed into a system which is enormously resistant to change. The reforms which are suggested are sponsored by different elements in the health system and ad-

vantage one or another element, but they do not seriously damage any interest. This pluralistic balancing of costs and benefits successfully shields the funding, powers, and resources of the producing institutions from any basic structural change.

This disillusionment with the systemic approach is understandable when one considers American health-planning experiences to date, and basic American attitudes toward planning. American distrust of planning runs deep and strong. George Wallace had little difficulty finding audiences sympathetic to his attacks on pointy-headed bureaucrats who plan other people's lives; calls for reduced governmental planning gain support at all points of the political continuum on all types of issues.

Despite these misgivings (engendered by recent experiences and anti-planning biases), the systemic model has enjoyed popularity among health care professionals because it is consistent with many of the growing technical and scientific subcultures within American society. Management information systems, operations research, and inventory control are just a few instances of this approach in business. In the social sciences, econometric modeling and interorganization studies have gained popularity more recently. As can be seen by the statements from *Fortune* and Senator Kennedy, use of the systemic approach in other areas has provided powerful imagery for the systemic models of health care.

In sum, the systemic model's emphasis on interconnections is being challenged because it creates frustration and distrust. Frustration results from the accuracy of the model's emphasis on interconnections that inhibit change, as well as from the failure of legislation based on systemic approaches. Distrust by a large segment of American society results from the model's implication of large-scale government planning.

The Idiosyncratic Needs Model

More consonant with current American beliefs than the systemic model is a model that emphasizes the peculiar, idiosyncratic nature of the geographic, racial, class, age, and other categories of health care recipients. Focusing on differences between categories, this model deemphasizes the interconnections among (and profit-making traits of) health care providers. Instead, it implies that the differences between black urban ghettos, rural backwaters, and suburban sprawls are more important than similarities—so their health care organizations must be different and locally controlled. Preferably these organizations would be controlled by those being served, because centralized planning and controlling agencies, even when they attempt to be flexible, are seen as incapable of serving such a wide divergence of health care needs. With its emphasis on diversity and decentralization, this model, not surprisingly, is useful to a number of groups.

First, as used by those on the political left, differences in needs require local "community control" of health care so that the special interests of consumers, particularly the downtrodden, can be asserted and protected. *The American Health Empire* (Ehrenreich and Ehrenreich, 1971), a well-received critique of American health care, makes essentially this case when it argues that health care presently is controlled by and serves profitable commerical ventures and uncaring hospital leaderships. But health care could be consumer-controlled, the book suggests. The final chapter is entitled, "The Community Revolt: Rising Up Angry," and expresses belief in a community's ability to deal with a neighborhood health center it so far had been unable to control. "With literally a century of struggle behind it, the lower east side community is too old and too experienced to be discouraged by one short skirmish" (Ehrenreich and Ehrenreich, 1971: 279). The book illustrates that the idiosyncratic needs model, as implemented by the political left, assumes communities have relatively homogeneous needs which (1) differ from the needs of other communities, and (2) should and can be served.

In the same vein is the Office of Economic Opportunity (OEO) program of Neighborhood Health Centers begun in the mid-1960s. OEO's policy was to encourage "maximum feasible participation" by local poverty groups. According to the positive evaluation of one physician (Sheps, 1972:69), this use of the idiosyncratic needs model advocated "a much greater role, in fact a controlling role, for the consumer [as] an essential condition for future success in our *pluralistic* health system" [emphasis added].

Second, as used by the political right, the model directs more attention to individual differences and less to group differences. Consistent with classical economics, this use of the idiosyncratic model would permit each individual to purchase the services that his own peculiar configuration of needs dictates. The American

Medical Association's national health insurance proposal, "Medicredit," is in this category. It implies that the nation's most significant health care problem is paying health insurance premiums, and proposes little more than federally subsidized optional private insurance so that individual citizens can buy the particular configurations of health care they desire.

Finally, as used by health care administrators, the idiosyncratic model discards the bad old days when local differences were ignored in favor of formulas applicable to a wide range of cases (e.g., Hill-Burton had a small number of population-to-hospital ratios applied over a broad array of circumstances). Somers (1969:217) supports this trend in seeking "a practical, achievable, federal-state system, encompassing the essential aspects of regulation, and *flexible* enough to permit a *creative* mix of controls and incentives" [emphasis added]. This goal of a flexible system based on rational incentives underlies recent interest in using prospective reimbursement to encourage hospital administrators to make cost-conscious decisions reflecting local needs. It also is part of what Ellwood (1974:85) calls the "competitive HMO model" under which federal planners adopt "certain positive programs to aid in the development of HMOs and to further a competitive health market." It has been criticized (Navarro, 1973:228-237) because planner responsiveness to consumers would be undermined by the tendency toward monopoly that characterizes health care providers.

In sum, although no version of the idiosyncratic-needs model has been widely accepted, the model nonetheless is attractive to a diversity of political and professional groups because it has components they share. It advocates a decentralized control system, consumer choices, and the avoidance of "big brother," all of which makes it appealing in American culture. Consequently, it appears to be gaining attractiveness in the general society as "think small" becomes desirable, and as sentiment among citizens and leaders grows against bigness in government and commerce. (Even pornography is now legally definable by community idiosyncrasies.) In health, once the controversy over national health insurance is resolved, this "back to the roots" movement may enter with full force. This model may be attractive enough to dominate future health care control decisions.

The Sociological Imagination and the Social Control of Medical Organizations

This paper has attempted to clarify the alternative ways Americans have gone about modeling the increasingly apparent problems of controlling their powerful health care organizations. It has argued that American thought gradually has been abandoning profit as a prime explanatory variable in many areas and moving toward the idea of a system. Now, as nostalgia for simpler days is gaining strength, as large institutions generally are falling into disfavor, and as sexual, age, and ethnic groups are asserting their distinguishing traits, health beliefs and preferences are discouraging bureaucratic impersonality and efficiency in favor of the charms of group differences.

The changing health attitudes described here parallel Charles Reich's (1970) interesting but overstated description of the sequence of "world views" held by Americans. Reich's categories can be seen as the larger context for the sequence of views on controlling medical care organizations described here. "Consciousness I," the earliest of the world views, belonged to the small businessmen, farmers, and pioneers whose life experiences taught them that man's natural condition is to struggle. "One worked for oneself, not for society. But enough individual work made the wheels turn" (Reich, 1970:22). Some people were profit-motivated, others were not.

"Consciousness II," the replacement for "Consciousness I," belongs to those whose most compelling experiences were with the interdependences and interconnections of large organizations, and who came to believe that organized rationality is man's most necessary state. And, finally, Reich's "Consciousness III" is held by an emerging group who seek a stronger respect for people. "In place of the world seen as a jungle, with every man for himself (Consciousness I), or the world seen as a meritocracy leading to a great corporate hierarchy of rigidly drawn relations...(Consciousness II), the world [of Consciousness III] is community" (Reich, 1970:227).

Beliefs of health care leaders, like those of laymen, are influenced by societal trends and fancies. These changing social attitudes in general could have unfortunate consequences for health care organizations if applied indiscriminately in the health field. This writer believes that there may be unfortunate consequences if social trends lead to wholesale acceptance of the idiosyncratic model. While many of the most noticeable American medical care problems are visible at the community level, their roots lie deeper in the social structure. Attracting health personnel from affluent suburbs to urban ghettos and poor rural regions, for example, cannot be accomplished by the poor communities; a mechanism encompassing the relative surplus and shortage communities is needed. Medical care requires resources that are spread throughout the society, resources that cannot be mobilized locally but must be organized regionally or nationally.

Similarly, hospitals are in a national nexus of government programs, commercial manufacturers, insurance organizations, and professional associations. The growth of this system has outstripped Americans' understanding of necessary circumstances for health care organizations to provide reasonably priced high-quality care. As Mills (1959:3) noted, "the more aware [people] become, however vaguely, of ambitions and of the threats which transcend their immediate locales, the more trapped they seem to feel." The idiosyncratic model in health care may turn out to offer a false road to losing the sensation of being trapped and powerless.

It would be unfortunate to end this paper defending the systemic model, however, because the goal of this paper has not been to boost one model and disparage others. Convincing data for doing this are unavailable in any case. The goal, rather, has been to draw attention to the need to understand and make explicit the models proposed for controlling increasingly dominant organizations in American health care. Professional responsibility will not work because professionals, even when they happen to be client-oriented, do not control medical organizations. What is needed in the health care area is organizational control *knowledge* as the basis for developing organizational control technologies. Current technology, in the absence of knowledge, has become an offshoot of idiology and popular culture.

M. David Ermann, PH.D.
Department of Sociology
University of Delaware
Newark, Delaware 19711

I am indebted to Dan Ermann for his critical reading of an earlier draft of this paper.

References

Alford, Robert R.
    1972   "The political economy of health care: dynamics without change."
            Politics and Society 3 (Winter): 127-164.

Cooper, Barbara S., and Nancy L. Worthington
    1973   "Health care expenditures, 1929-1972." Social Security Bulletin
            36(January): 3-19.

Ehrenreich, Barbara, and John Ehrenrich
    1971   The American Health Empire. New York: Vintage Books.

Ellwood, Paul M., Jr.
    1974   "Models for organizing health services and implications of
            legislative proposals." Pp. 67-95 in Zola, Irving K., and John B.
            McKinlay (eds.), Organizational Issues in the Delivery of Health
            Services. New York: PRODIST.

Ermann, M. David, and Richard J. Lundman
    1975   "Organizational control of organizational deviance." Paper presen-
            ted at the 70th Annual Meeting of the American Sociological
            Association, San Francisco (August).

Fortune
    1970   "Our ailing medical system." Fortune 81(January).

Glaser, William A.
    1966   " 'Socialized medicine' in practice." The Public Interest 1 (Spring):
            90-106.

Kennedy, Edward
    1973   Pp. 1-4 in Congressional Record, Vol. 119, No. 17, January 31.

Kulp, C.A., and John W. Hall
    1968   Casualty Insurance (4th edition). New York: Ronald Press.

Law, Sylvia A.
    1974   Blue Cross: What Went Wrong? New Haven and London: Yale
            University Press.

Lentz, Edith
  1956   "The American voluntary hospital as an example of institutional change." Unpublished Ph.D. Dissertation. Cornell University, Ithaca, New York.

Levine, Sol, and Paul E. White
  1961   "Exchange as a conceptual framework for the study of interorganizational relationships." Administrative Science Quarterly 5(March):583-601.

Metzger, Norman
  1970   "Labor relations." Hospitals 44(March):80-84.

Mills, C. Wright
  1959   The Sociological Imagination. New York: Grove Press.

Modern Hospital
  1970   "Experts see new balance of health care forces." Modern Hospital 14(April): 39-40d.

Navarro, Vicente
  1973   "National health insurance and the strategy for change." Milbank Memorial Fund Quarterly/Health and Society 51 (Spring): 223-251.

O'Connor, John T.
  1974   "Comprehensive health planning: dreams and realities." Milbank Memorial Fund Quarterly/Health and Society 51(Spring): 223-251.

Perrow, Charles
  1961   "The analysis of goals in complex organizations." American Sociological Review 26(December):854-866.

Reich, Charles A.
  1970   The Greening of America. New York: Random House

Reinhardt, Uwe E.
  1973   "Proposed changes in the organization of health-care delivery: an overview and critique." Milbank Memorial Fund Quarterly/Health and Society 51(Spring): 169-222.

Sheps, Cecil G.
  1972   "The influence of consumer sponsorship on medical services." Milbank Memorial Fund Quarterly (October, Part 2): 41-69.

Somers, Anne R.
  1969   Hospital Regulation: The Dilemma of Public Policy. Princeton, New Jersey: Industrial Relations Section, Princeton University.

U.S. House of Representatives

1973   Extension of NLRA to Non-Profit Hospital Employees. Hearings before the Special Subcommittee on Labor of the Committee on Education and Labor. 93rd Congress, 1st Session (April 12 and 19).

U.S. Senate

1974   Nursing Home Care in the United States: Failure in Public Policy. (Supporting Paper No. 1: The Litany of Nursing Home Abuses and an Examination of the Roots of Controversy.) Prepared by the Subcommittee on Long-Term Care of the Special Committee on Aging. 93rd Congress, 2nd Session (December).

White, Rodney F.

1971   "The hospital administrator's emerging professional role." Pp. 51-69 in Arnold, Mary F., L. Vaughn Blankenship, and John M. Hess (eds.), Administering Health Systems: Issues and Perspectives. Chicago: Aldine-Atherton.

Zald, Mayer, and Feather Davis Hair

1972   "The social control of general hospitals." Pp. 51-82 in Georgopoulos, Basil S. (ed.), Organizational Research on Health Institutions. Ann Arbor, Michigan: Institute for Social Research, University of Michigan.

The Erosion of Professional Authority:
A Cross-Cultural Inquiry
in the Case of the Physician

MARIE R. HAUG

The extent to which the erosion of professional authority observed in the United States is also occurring in the United Kingdom and the U.S.S.R. is examined in the case of the primary care physician. Informal interviews with health practitioners in these diverse societies revealed that the model of the professions which bases physicians' autonomy and authority on the occupational characteristic of a monopoly of specialized knowledge is subject to some revision. Education of the patient emerged as a critical factor in eroding physician authority in both countries, while patient age affected authority relations differentially in the two societies. Despite variations in the level of bureaucratization of health care, the role of the physician, as gatekeeper to non-medical benefits, served to counteract the erosion trend in both. The legacy of deference to the upper classes in Great Britain and in the U.S.S.R., an ideology of health as a citizen's obligation plus the "mothering" ambience of a largely female personnel are varying societal characteristics which also affect physician authority.

Theoretical Issues

One of the phenomena which seems increasingly to characterize relationships between professionals and their clients in the United States is an unwillingness on the part of the client to accept without question the authority of the professional. The "revolt of the client" (Haug and Sussman, 1969), and the demand for accountability (Reiff, 1971) signify a growing public suspicion that neither the expertise nor the good will of the professional are to be taken on trust, at face value. While this trend can be observed in the United States, having been noted by writers with respect to medicine as well as other professional fields (Reeder, 1972; Eulau, 1973; Haug, 1975), its occurrence in other parts of the world with differing social, cultural and economic structures and various divisions of labor in the human services, has not yet been systematically studied. The research outlined in these pages represents a preliminary attempt to determine the nature and extent of this phenomenon in the case of the physician, in two different societies, the United Kingdom and the U.S.S.R. Utilizing a

M M F Q / Health and Society / *Winter 1976*

sociological perspective, the study explores the basis of primary care physician authority in the context of two types of socialized delivery system of medical care. The aim is to identify those societal characteristics as well as those individual characteristics of patients and physicians which affect the authority relationship in these diverse national contexts.

Most sociologists in the United States have modeled their definitions of profession on the historic trio of medicine, law, and the clergy, focusing on the command of an esoteric body of knowledge acquired through academic training, and a service orientation, which account both for professional freedom from lay control, i.e., autonomy in work performance, and socially sanctioned power over clients, i.e., authority in the practitioner-client relationship. According to this view, it is the professions' monopoly over knowledge not easily accessible to the public, coupled with a claim to a public service outlook, which legitimates the professional's authority in dealing with clients, and institutionalizes client obligations to trust the professional and comply with his prescriptions (Moore, 1970). Even those who have argued that profession is essentially a folk concept (Becker, 1962) concede that knowledge claims undergird professionals' work autonomy and client acceptance of their authority. In fact it has been suggested that the presence or absence of this power position is what distinguishes professions from non-professions (Freidson, 1970). The sick-role concept (Parsons, 1951), the most widely used sociological interpretation of the doctor-patient relationship, is a derivative of the theory of professions: it is the obligation of the sick to seek expert help in order to get well, and thus to defer to the physician's professional authority. The "competence" gap between doctor and patient justifies the asymmetrical power relationship and the patient's trust, confidence, and norm of obedience.

Implicit in the focus on professional autonomy is the likelihood of conflict with the authority structure of bureaucratic organizations, in which professional work is increasingly located. Indeed, the literature on this topic has been voluminous in recent years (Perrow, 1972). However, the strain between the two power bases may currently be more imagined than actual. In fact, professions often in practice forge a partnership with bureaucracy in organizational work settings, in order to buttress their relations with clients (Freidson, 1970). In this case, the bureaucratic rules and regulations are used to enforce professional decisions with respect to client actions, whether or not the client has accepted the value stricture that it is in his best interests to comply.

Given these multiple pressures on the client to conform, how does it happen that both the autonomy and authority of the professional are nevertheless being challenged, at least in this country? Explanations for the American phenomenon have been sought in the erosion of the professional's monopoly over knowledge, the sophistication attending rising educational levels of the general public, and new divisions of labor which redistribute expertise in the human service field. Changes in control over esoteric knowledge, as its storage and retrieval are computerized, present a potential threat to the eroding monopoly. Furthermore, aggregation of clients in bureaucratic settings may have the unanticipated consequence of stimulating a form of "client consciousness" of their common fate, leading to social movements which challenge professional power and demand accountability for practitioners' actions (Haug, 1973; 1974).

It is apparent that these developments apply to the physician in the United States. Popular knowledge of health issues is disseminated by the media; health organizations urge people to watch for signs of cancer or heart disease; Dr. Spock is only one of a range of do-it-yourself medical guides, of which a more recent example is *Our Bodies Our Selves* (Boston Women's Health Book Collective, 1973); patients with chronic conditions are trained for self-care; and the fact that the majority of the adult American public has completed more than 12 years of schooling (U.S. Bureau of the Census, 1972: 111) implies not only some basic education in nutrition and hygiene but also potential for skepticism about others' knowledge claims (Wilensky, 1964). The computerization of many aspects of medical services is already an established fact (Schwartz, 1970).

As for changes in the division of labor, these also are characteristic of the medical profession. The extent to which tasks of the physician are gradually being given to paraprofessionals or to those now claiming to be professionals in their own right is well documented (Lefkowitz and Ausmus, 1970). Babies are delivered by a midwife with specialized training, and the nurse-clinician handles many aspects of infant and child care; the intensive-care-unit nurse deals with postoperative crises, and the physician's assistant takes over tasks previously performed by a doctor. One prominent physician educator has suggested that by 1980 physician's assistants or technicians will be setting simple fractures and taking out appendixes (Geiger, 1972: 109).

A complexity which is most marked in medicine is the sexual division of labor. In the United States, the most powerful role, that of the physician, is largely in male hands, while most persons to whom former physician tasks have devolved, as a result of the change in the division of labor, are female. To the extent that societal values produce differences in acceptance of autonomy and authority on the basis of the sex of the authority figure, this confounds an estimate of the effect of the new occupational mix on patient responses to the claims of expertise.

Moreover, physicians are not immune to the loss of autonomy inherent in demands for accountability, and public rather than peer evaluation. The evidence for this development is more tenuous, and it may be related to factors in addition to schooling increments and the changing labor mix. Thus the well-documented increases in malpractice suits may spring at least in part from a general consumerism ideology. On the other hand, proposed legislation to monitor physician use of human subjects in medical research has political overtones. Organized patient movements for improvements in hospital ambulatory clinic care challenge physician control of service delivery at the institutional level, and offer a portent of future developments when patient care is dispensed in a bureaucratized setting. Each of these is in its own way a sign that the doctor's dictum is not necessarily taken as the last word.[1]

In sum, it is suggested here that profound change in authority relations is occurring in which knowledge is losing its role as a

[1] It might be argued that the voluminous literature on failures and factors in patient compliance (Marston, 1970; McKinlay, 1972) indicate that not following a physician's advice is a common phenomenon. Although this is undoubtedly the case (Freidson, 1961), compliance and non-compliance as such are not logically equivalent to acceptance-rejection of physician authority. Patients can accept medical authority, that is the right to advise and the obligation to obey, but still fail to fulfill that obligation by complying. Conversely, in terms of the bargaining-negotiating model of the medical encounter (Balint, 1957), it is possible that a patient complies with a regimen because he has bent the practitioner to his will, securing the diagnosis and treatment plan which he was desirous of having confirmed when entering the interaction.

power base as it becomes demonopolized, and that the medical profession may be viewed as a prototype of this trend.

Research Question and Method of Data Collection

But is this an emergent phenomenon peculiar to the United States? Is the professional authority model applicable cross-culturally? Specifically, is physician medical knowledge the explanation for this occupation's legitimated power over patients under varying societal conditions, or are there other factors which structure the doctor-patient relationship? Derivative questions address whether variations in patient acceptance of medical-practitioner authority occur by (a) various *individual* characteristics, for example, level of patient education; and (b) various *societal* characteristics, for example, bureaucratic structure.

Data relevant to these research questions have been collected through informal interviews conducted by the author with medical practitioners and knowledgeable informants in Great Britain and the U.S.S.R. during the winter and spring of 1974. The focus was on general practice, as offering the widest range of physician-public interactions. Great Britain and the U.S.S.R. were selected for study because they varied from each other and from the United States on a number of major parameters.

Although both offer a form of socialized medicine, in Great Britain primary care is still dispensed largely by solo practitioners or small group practices, while the Soviet system provides care in large centers or polyclinics. Educational levels and the sexual division of medical labor in Great Britain are more similar to the situation in the United States, while fewer average years of schooling and a predominantly female medical profession characterize the U.S.S.R. Finally, the British and American concepts of profession are virtually identical, whereas the Soviets have no comparable definition; in fact the Russian language does not even have a word for profession in our sense, using the term "intelligentsia" for a more general category.

There was no attempt at random sampling of interviewees. Instead a *purposive* sample was selected, taking into account geographic location and position in the health delivery system. In Britain key respondents were chosen on the advice of British social scientists knowledgeable about their country's health system, and practitioners of varying ideological stance. From this beginning a "snowballing" technique was used, in which respondents were selected from persons recommended by those already interviewed as having information germane to the study, including those with different perspectives. In all, 47 persons, including 15 physicians in general practice, were formally interviewed.

In the U.S.S.R., heads of medical facilities were selected on the basis of their availability for interview as determined by Intourist, the official tourist agency. Eleven physicians, in seven polyclinics from Leningrad to Tblisi, were among the 22 interviewed. In both Britain and the Soviet Union, respondents were secured from several geographic areas, and from academic medical figures as well as from active practitioners.

All interviews were reconstructed on tape immediately after the interview, using field notes and recollections. Although the interviews were informal and unstructured, they followed a general format which began with a question about the current characteristics of doctor-patient relationships from the interviewee's perspective, followed by inquiries about recent changes, if any, in the nature of that interaction. Questions about the effect of age, education, and occupation of the patients on the relationship were included, as well as probes about those persons considered easiest and most difficult to treat, and why.

In both the U.S.S.R. and Great Britain the data are chiefly from a medical practitioner's perspective, since no patients' organizations are such were found in the U.S.S.R., and only limited contact was possible in Great Britain with two existing groups, themselves circumscribed in scope. Despite this shortcoming, it was possible to gather indications of developments relevant to the research questions posed and thus with impact on theories of professions, and derivatively on doctor-patient relationships in the sick role.

Research Findings

Several themes emerged from these experiences. First, on a general level, physician authority is currently being challenged, and this phenomenon is by no means idiosyncratic to the United States. Moreover, from the physician's perspective, in both Great Britain and the U.S.S.R., professional authority in the physician-patient relationship varies with patient education, but patient age also is an important variable. In both countries, despite the differences in the bureaucratization of the medical care delivery systems, health practitioners have similar gatekeeper roles from which they derive power over patients not directly related to their medical expertise, since physicians control access to many non-medical benefits valued by the public. An unexpected finding is the overriding importance of historical developments, cultural traditions, and ideology in explaining the position accorded physicians in the division of labor and public acceptance of their authority. The specific impact of the discovery and the development of technological aids of various kinds is only one of these factors, along with the effects of war, social-class history, and the sex of the practitioner. Each of these themes suggest, from different perspectives, the changing role of knowledge monopoly, and the extent to which factors other than knowledge undergird professional power in general and physician authority in particular.

Individual Characteristics: The age variable

In Great Britain, several informants suggested that older patients are more willing to accept the physician's authority because they are grateful for the "free" medical care, remembering the period before World War II when the fee-for-service system existed and care was beyond the reach of many. As one Welsh physician commented, some of the elderly are very respectful and deferential, "excusing themselves for bothering the doctor, bringing gifts of boxes of chocolates at Christmas, or half a dozen eggs during the year."[2] On the other hand, another general practitioner, in a Midlands health center, had noted the disaffection of some older patients who "expected the doctor to drop in and have a cup of tea and a chat," as in an earlier, more leisurely time, and were upset when this did not occur. In general, however, British health workers considered the older patients more accepting of the physician's authority than the younger, who, many felt, tend to argue, question, and reject authority. The explanation offered, it should be noted, was not only a habit of deference among the

[2]Quotation marks represent statements reconstructed from notes and tapes, not always exact quotes, particularly in the U.S.S.R., where respondents were translated.

elderly, but the experiences of this age cohort from a period prior to the establishment of the National Health Service.

In the U.S.S.R. age was also viewed as a meaningful variable, but with a somewhat different focus. Some physicians felt, in the words of one informant, that "the aged, when they are ill, are eager to be cured and so carry out all instructions as carefully as possible, while with the young people it is just the opposite—they refuse to obey." Another theme was more dominant—that the elderly are more demanding, questioning, and unwilling to bow to the doctor's orders. Since they are not working, not busy, they come in more often for small matters, although usually all they need is reassurance. As one woman general practitioner put it, "The retired who have grandchildren to care for do not come as frequently, but if they are not working and have nothing to do, they read *Health,* a popular magazine, or medical columns in the paper, or listen to radio and TV, and come in asking for one pill or another, or insist that they have symptoms requiring medication, or just because they want a social visit with the doctor." Since the primary health care system in the U.S.S.R. is based on a network of regional or neighborhood "polyclinics," easily accessible, at least in the city, to would-be patients without charge, the structural arrangements facilitate "overutilization" coupled with challenges of the physician's advice.

Variation in acceptance of professional authority by client age cohort is congruent with a model of profession based on the occupational characteristic of knowledge monopoly to the extent that the age variable is related to educational level and thus to differential breakdown of that monopoly. Indeed, in the U.S.S.R. this relationship is made explicit. It is because the old have time and inclination to read and listen to health education materials that they develop knowledge claims of their own and challenge the word of the doctor.

Individual Characteristics: The education variable

Education of the client as a critical factor in eroding professional authority emerged clearly in both countries studied, although in Britain it was often expressed in social-class terms, whereas in the U.S.S.R. the differences were formulated in terms of schooling and health education, as well as non-manual versus manual categories. One eminent general practitioner in London pointed out that middle- and upper-class patients more critical than working-class patients. For them, he commented "the knowledge and skill of the general practitioner in terms of his present training is not too much unlike their own sophistication because they also have university degrees." A Midlands physician said he preferred local poor people, because they are "grateful for any help; but couldn't stand Londoners and middle-class types," who were full of questions and arguments. Indeed a thread ran through many of the British interviews, that patients were growing more knowledgeable, demanding more explanations, and in this sense, for some doctors, becoming more difficult, i.e., less willing to accept authority, a finding congruent with data reported by Mechanic (1970) from an earlier study of a larger sample.

In the Soviet Union, a similar theme was expressed by several polyclinic physicians. As one remarked, "it is much easier to treat manual workers as patients. The intelligentsia and the non-manual workers are educated. They read books, literature, listen to radio, watch TV; when they speak of an illness they give not only the symptoms but also the diagnosis. It is easier for the doctor if the patient does not try to tell the doctor what to do." On another occasion, during a group interview, a male doctor had said that it was necessary to explain everything to neurotic patients because they want to know everything. The researcher then probed about the effect of education and asked, apropos of the fact that the Soviet state had recently set compulsory education at 10 years, what would happen when all Soviet citizens had a university education. The head of the clinic, a woman physician, laughed, and said that "then all patients will be neurotic, there will be much work for the doctor, lots of arguments and different kinds of diseases to deal with."

There was, however, a striking difference between the U.S.S.R. and Great Britain on the education variable. In the U.S.S.R. there was heavy constant emphasis on teaching patients about health matters. Every polyclinic had posters and displays in hallways and waiting rooms about nutrition, hygiene, exercise, care of chronic conditions, infant development, and the like. Available in waiting rooms were varicolored illustrated folders on specific diseases and treatment, some with diagrams of various organs to explain the purposes of medical procedures. In several polyclinics the researcher noticed that physical therapy rooms had large wall displays with photographs of each piece of equipment along with statements of their purpose and benefits. In each facility visited there was an office responsible for fostering patient education, although much of the material was obviously centrally prepared. The medical staff was well aware of the dilemma involved in educating patients while at the same time preferring them to accept the physician's advice without question. Several explained that the education material focused on treatment, rather than symptoms, because if there was too much information about symptoms, the polyclinic might have an excess of patients with imaginary ailments. On the other hand, some others suggested that a few early symptoms were specified, and not too much about treatment, to encourage consultation with a physician.

There was one point on which doctors in both countries firmly agreed, and that was that patients should *not* have access to their own medical records. As one doctor in the U.S.S.R. put it, "patients should *not,* of course, know everything," echoing a general practitioner in Great Britain who responded emphatically in response to an inquiry about patients' seeing their files, "That's stupid...ignorance is bliss for most." The implication was clear that knowledge should not extend to the point where it would be painful tò a person. For the patient's own protection, the doctors agreed, there were some things that only they should know. The paradox in this view was understood by a Soviet cancer specialist, who wondered how patients could be persuaded to trust their doctors, and believe what they were told, when at the same time it is common knowledge that doctors may fail to tell cancer victims what their diagnosis is, or even lie about it.

Societal Characteristics: Doctors as bureaucratic gatekeepers

The gatekeeper role of the physician emerged as a reinforcement of medical power under the British National Health Service as well as the Soviet medical system. In Britain, general practitioners must sign "certificates" which validate illness claims and thus a person's right to paid sick leave if he is off work for more than three days. One informant noted that just before the 1974 miners' strike, surgeries and hospital casualty departments in Wales were flooded with patients—miners claiming they were sick in order to get social security payments during the strike. Many physicians are annoyed by certification duties because they view this as essentially non-medical dirty work, in which the task involves striking a bargain with the worker as to how much of the desired time off is reasonably justified. In some cases this bargaining job has been sloughed off on nurse or receptionist, but the doctor's signature is still needed on the form. The physician's work is also critical in getting a priority for an elderly patient in "council housing," the publicly supported dwellings for the aged and needy, or a telephone installed for an old or sick person living alone. In rural areas or smaller communities the doctor is still presumed to know people on his patient roster well enough to sign gun-license applications or provide character references for young job hunters.

The British general practitioner's control over access to values in the medical arena is also a buttress to his authority, and indeed one protection against encroachments from paraprofessionals. He provides the only entry through the public system to hospitals, and the consultants, or specialists, located there. He is the only channel to medications on prescription-only lists, such as the barbiturates and tranquilizers. Some practitioners indicated that a large part of their practice consisted of prescribing these drugs to individuals with personal and emotional problems. One unpublished study shows that more than half the British practitioners surveyed believe from one third to two thirds of their consultations have a psychogenic component, and four out of five estimate that 80 percent or more of their patients arrive at the surgery expecting a prescription.[3] One physician interviewed estimated that nearly half of his consultations involved psychosocial problems, anxiety, and depression, often of women patients, both young and middle aged, who would come in for tranquilizers. If the doctor tries to deny the prescription the patient will say, "I've got to have them. I can't cope. The children are getting on my nerves," and feeling the patient is in a state, the doctor gives the prescription.

In the U.S.S.R., the medical system is the gatekeeper not only for paid absences from work, but also for continuation on the job, as well as side benefits such as special vacation privileges. The general practitioner in the regional polyclinic certifies workers for sick leave and approves pay for illness. More than this, in order to stay on the job, whether in production industry or in a white-collar

---

[3]Personal communication from Martin Bridgestock, Medical Sociology Research Centre, Swansea, Wales.

enterprise, workers must receive an annual, or in some cases, a semi-annual, medical checkup. They must show their "card" at the enterprise to prove that they have complied with this requirement in order to continue employment. These examinations are often given at the "enterprise polyclinic," an all-purpose primary and chronic care medical center attached to large establishments such as factories, merchandising complexes, or universities. These enterprise polyclinics, as distinct from the regional polyclinics which are based on neighborhood subdivisions, also have the special gatekeeper role of deciding which workers will be able to take advantage of the health resorts, spas, and vacation facilities run by the enterprise union. Since space is limited, and the benefits of cut-rate prices at desirable vacation locations are much sought after, the physician's gatekeeper role and attendant authority is by no means inconsiderable. Notably in the U.S.S.R., as in Great Britain, sick-leave certificates and other similar gatekeeper functions are based on striking a bargain with the applicant, in order to maintain the patient's good will and cooperation for the future, and not solely on medical criteria or professional expertise.

Societal Characteristics: Technology and authority

Still another pervasive theme, but stressed mainly in the British data, is the modified role of the medical professional as a result of historical changes in conceptions of the nature of health and illness, following in part from the discovery of new drugs and therapies and the invention of medical technologies, tests, and diagnostic and treatment devices. As one general practitioner in London put it, "There has been a profound change in the last twenty years...The person sees himself as ill at an earlier stage and with fewer symptoms...It is an age in which people are not willing to tolerate anxiety or minor symptoms; they want alterations in their experience of life and they turn to the general practitioner," who has been forced to change his attitudes. "His apostolic function has been reduced. No longer can he say, 'I'm the doctor, do as I tell you.' Now there is a transaction, with the outcomes the result of a collusive effort." Another physician, in a Midlands medical center, also remarked that the concept of illness and medicine has changed, but focused on drug discoveries during and after World War II as explanation. Before that, "doctors had only a bedside manner, colored water, and aspirin." Now patients know about the new magic of pills and technical procedures, and demand that these services be made available by the doctor. In fact several informants noted that patient requests to be referred for diagnostic tests, as carried out in hospitals, were a way of rejecting the authority of the physician in favor of the authority of technology. And a nursing officer commented that godlike tests were replacing the godlike physician as a subject for obeisance and belief.

Only passing references to these developments appear in the Soviet data, and when they do, the perspective is different. Instead of tests substituting for the authority of the primary care physician they are viewed as reinforcing it. Several polyclinic chiefs announced with pride that their staff had a perfect record—all diagnoses made by the general practitioners without the benefit of the technical apparatus available in hospitals and specialty clinics, had been validated by the tests of the specialists. One chief pointed out that the way new doctors in the clinic gained authority was by having their diagnoses and treatment plans coincide with the recommendation of the hospital specialists.

Thus while new medicines and technologies were seen by practitioners in both countries as affecting doctor-patient relationships, the direction of the effect vis-à-vis professional authority was conceptualized in different ways. The findings suggest that various aspects of a physician's tasks differentially affect his authority image. Uncertain diagnosis diminishes, whereas verified diagnosis enhances, that image.

Societal Characteristics: History, culture, and ideology

Medical history is only one among the set of variables found to affect the phyician-client relationship; other historical, cultural, and ideological forces also shape, and perhaps even determine, the meaning of the professional category in the division of labor in these two countries.

In Great Britain, there were repeated references to these factors as of critical importance, particularly with respect to the general practitioner, whose *need* for clinical knowledge and whose *command* of psychosocial knowledge were both seen as limited. One prominent general practitioner said of his colleagues that perhaps the quip was true: they are overtrained for what they do and undertrained for what they are supposed to do. Their authority, then, comes from sources other than body of knowledge.

The most salient supportive factor is the aristocratic tradition, which still casts its aura over medicine. Despite the absorption of lower-class apothecaries and barbers into the occupation of physician and surgeon, the status of the upper-class incumbents remains dominant. As more than one informant pointed out, until fairly recently upper-class families expected the oldest son to take over the estate, the second son to enter the clergy, and the third son to become a physician. All went to a university, and this fact, more than the specific skills acquired, distinguished them from the common folk, who in the class system in Britain were expected to respect and defer to their betters. In some back-country sections of Scotland and Wales, patients still stand when they come in to see the doctor, and actually or symbolically "touch their forelocks." The giving of gifts at Christmas is another manifestation of this habit of deference.

Furthermore, part of the aristocratic tradition is the lord's obligation for public service, a carryover of the feudal value system in which the lord was presumed to have the best interests of his poor and ignorant serfs at heart. The claim that medicine has scientifically based curative power is a relatively new basis for physician authority, and is grafted onto the earlier and more internalized public belief that the doctor's social position merits faith and compliance. Thus as one informant declared, "Doctors are living on the trust engendered from the earlier model of the physician." And another noted that the doctor's ability to secure non-medical services, like better housing and a telephone, is a hangover from "the old days when their word counted for a lot because of their upper-class position rather than their medical status."

An interacting trend is the spreading ideology of collectivism and socialism in Britain. This orientation contains the notion of obedience, the value of deferring to the common good, and the belief that authority should flow to the experts who have the common good at heart. A curious anomaly is that this belief structure also puts physicians in the role of public servants, whose training is paid for by the public and whose services are a public right. Thus the general practitioner should always be available, night and day, to anyone who asks for his attention. The outcome of this mix of forces was verbalized by one of a group of radical medical students in this way: "There is a tension between the traditional deference of the working class toward the upper class, and their sense of conflict with them over many vital aspects of their lives. The place where the classes meet is localized to the medical arena. In other circumstances the classes do not meet.'' As a result of this cross-pressure, the average working person is not comfortable with the physician. He may not openly challenge the physician's authority, but neither may he comply with the medical recommendations after he gets home.

The historical, cultural, and ideological trends which emerged in the Soviet Union were also critical explanatory variables for physician power, but of quite a different sort. Three factors in particular merit attention: the impact of the death and destruction of World War II, the pervasiveness of medical oversight coupled with citizen obligation to attend to his health, and the special ambience attached to the fact that so many primary care physicians are women.

Although the Second World War severely damaged Britain, its land was not invaded, and the rate of civilian casualties was less than that endured in the U.S.S.R. Accordingly the war is still a very salient issue there, at an intensity difficult for the American visitor to comprehend. Mass graves and monuments to war heroes constantly remind the public of the suffering of the period, when there were 20 million dead. An example of the continued concern is the custom for brides in many cities to place their bridal bouquets on the tomb of the local World War II unknown soldier, immediately after the ceremony. During the war, the physicians were literally life savers, and their role in rescuing and treating victims under bombing and artillery fire is remembered by anyone over 40 today. The possibility of challenging a doctor's decision in such situations of danger and stress undoubtedly did not often arise, while the physicians' self-sacrificing attention to the needs of the injured was evident. Attitudes from that period have clearly carried over to the present. For example, respondents to a survey undertaken by one of the regional polyclinics for its district, showed that some of the physicians received high praise because they were "just like doctors in the war: very concerned, very active, very willing to help."[4]

[4]As an aside, the survey showed that complaints of the patients in the U.S.S.R. echoed those reported in the United Kingdom (Klein, 1972): lack of attentiveness, rudeness, hasty care. In both countries even these complaints were rare.

Another facet of the Soviet medical system difficult for Westerners to understand is the all-pervasiveness of health supervision. Children and students must be examined periodically in the schools, through the special maternal and child health clinics. They receive checkups before being allowed to go to summer camp. As for adults, no one who is working can escape. The need for periodic examinations in order to continue employment has already been alluded to. Tourist guides, because they meet all kinds of foreigners and their germs, are given annual innoculations; some of the young women try to get out of it to no avail; the physician comes to the office to do the job. According to several informants, there are medical stations in every area of major industrial establishments, satellites of the enterprise polyclinic, where physicians and "feldshers"—specially trained intermediate health personnel (Sidel, 1968)—are located. They get to know the workers well, check on their health, follow up those with chronic conditions, lecture on health matters, and monitor compliance with safety and sanitary rules. Women workers are given regular gynecological examinations whether they want them or not. One polyclinic doctor stated that in industry every employee has a "sports rating," and the "coffee break" is an "exercise break," with calisthenics for fifteen minutes. This physician noted that some managed to slip away and have a smoke in the washroom instead. Workers who are recalcitrant and refuse to follow the doctor's treatment recommendations, or insist on treatment for ailments which the doctor considers imaginary, will be put in the hospital as inpatients for a complete workup and specialist's examination.

Moreover the regional polyclinic structure permits close health supervision in the neighborhoods. One physician with long experience in one such polyclinic told the researcher about how well she knew her blocks of families. They called her "Aunt M——," she was invited to weddings and funerals, and made social visits as well as house calls. She felt that if she noticed someone not looking well, she would be able to urge him or her to get a medical examination, because everyone in her district trusted her, they knew her so well. Several polyclinics explained the system of patient follow-up. If someone with a chronic condition, for example, fails to keep a regular checkup appointment he is sent a letter or postcard. If this fails to work a nurse visits him, then visits his family, and as a last resort the manager of the enterprise where he works will be asked to get him to come in.

In this all-encompassing atmosphere, many polyclinic doctors interviewed seemed to find it hard to imagine any serious challenge of a physician's expertise, or to view the admitted examples of questioning physician authority as anything but examples of aberrant behavior. At an enterprise polyclinic, the chief of staff said, "The doctor doesn't tell the worker how to work and does not expect the worker to tell the doctor how to take care of his responsibility." The fact is, however, that patients do perceive differences in physician ability and sources of medical care. Thus one informant suggested that enterprise polyclinics were better than regional ones, because both union and management, as well as the establishment's political committee, were concerned with the quality of the medical care. These clinics were able, with union-negotiated funds, to provide better equipment and pay higher salaries, thus attracting more able staff. According to this informant, regional polyclinics catered largely to pensioners, an opinion not incongruent with research observations. Also there is a small private practice sector chiefly in the form of cooperatives of male specialists, in a few cities and in the South, and some of the intelligentsia prefer these services if they are seriously ill.

Public acceptance of the pervasiveness of the medical system is partly ideological. There is apparently a strong sense that maintaining one's own health is an obligation of citizenship. It is a person's public duty to keep well, and if ill, to get well. In this effort, cooperation with the health practitioners is part of the obligation. Indeed this ideology has been incorporated into law, on both a national and individual republic basis. One polyclinic director displayed copies of the legislation for the Ukrainian Republic, whose preamble states that the attitude of a person to his own health is a concern of the state. Thus in the U.S.S.R. the Parsonian conception of the sick role as including the obligation to get well (Parsons, 1951) has been institutionalized in the formal legal structure.[5]

Perhaps another basis for the acceptance of all-encompassing medical attention is social-psychological, and is related to the fact that most primary care physicians, and indeed most physicians, have been women, a statistic true at least since 1940. The constant

[5]For a further discussion of the Soviet health system, with a similar perspective, see James E. Muller et al. (1972).

oversight, the continued concern about health, the persistent follow-ups and reminders about taking care of oneself are reminiscent of a mothering role. This impression grew during the data collection, as polyclinic after polyclinic was visited, and the researcher was introduced to many women phusicians—in medical departments, minor surgery, orthopedics, and all the other sections of the medical center—and often they were indeed maternal in appearance and manner.

One non-medical informant actually verbalized the mother ambience by talking about an instance where he had a false reading of high blood pressure, and had quite an argument with the doctor who wanted him to change his entire life style. The doctor talked to him "like a grandmother about all the dangers of not caring for himself and was shocked at his cavalier attitude."

The evidence is scanty and impressionistic but the hypothesis could be formulated that the acceptance of medical intrusion into so many aspects of Soviet life—work, recreation, education—is related to the fact that mothers are expected to worry about the well-being of their children, even into adulthood. And in many cultures, societal values dictate that at all ages it is a good thing to listen to your mother; as a child you obey; as an adult you at least should try to comply with her wishes. The image of the health-provider as a mother figure is indeed congruent with family health care patterns in many societies, not just in the U.S.S.R.

Implications for the future of physician authority

A first review of the field data has suggested some answers to the queries which initiated this research. Across two quite different societies, individual as well as societal characteristics modify the knowledge-power model of the physician's role. Education of the patient does make a difference in acceptance of physician advice, and in some instances interacts with age to undermine authority. Level of bureaucratization of the medical care delivery systems seems, however, to have less meaning for physician power than the way in which medical workers are used by bureaucratic structures as gatekeepers and enforcers of the system. Although the level of bureaucratization of health care varied between the two social systems, in both cases the practitioner's position was strengthened as a result of his or her control over access to non-medical benefits.

The more salient factors affecting medical practitioners' authority and status were, on the other hand, not included in the original knowledge-power model or reflected in the original research questions. These are the historical, cultural, and ideological variables.[6] Traditional imputations of power based on social-class position, the impact of experiences like a devastating war, and institutionalized beliefs in individual health responsibility, appear to have major consequences for the role and authority of the physician. Finally, the sex of the practitioner may have a social-psychological meaning unlike that originally expected, for being a woman may undergird physician authority rather than diminish it, by invoking a mother image.

Doctors have been viewed as the prototype of the occupational category, profession, approaching on all parameters the ideal-typical end of the continua of professional characteristics. What then are the implications of these findings for the future relation of knowledge and authority among professionals, and particularly physicians?

Consider first the key characteristic of the physician's autonomy, the right granted by society and validated by licensure to define and carry out his tasks. The expression and realization of this autonomy shifts from the *societal* level to that of *individual* transactions with clients at the point of actual task performance. While at this stage physician autonomy is operationalized as authority over patients, theoretically it continues to be grounded in the characteristics of the occupation. The findings here tend to nullify that contention. Degree of authority over clients depends in part on *client* characteristics rather than occupational characteristics alone, i.e., on age and education of the patients. Although these variables affect authority through the instrumentality of patient claims to knowledge conflicting with and undermining physician claims to knowledge monopoly, the fact remains that client characteristics have not heretofore been included in the core model of profession,[7] and have been neglected in the concept of the

[6] For a more detailed discussion of these issues with reference to Great Britain, see Haug (in press).

[7] One exception to this generalization is the work of Terence Johnson (1972). In *Professions and Power* he suggests that in the case of corporate clients, authority may flow from client to professional instead of vice versa. Unfortunately, this monograph is little known in the United States, and not too easy to secure.

sick role. Indeed when such characteristics are given weight in studies of compliance with physicians' treatment recommendations, they are viewed as obstacles to obedience rather than source of challenge (McKinlay, 1972).

From another perspective, the critical role of knowledge monopoly is negated by examination of the physician's gatekeeper activities. Professional power is based less on special knowing than on assignment of authority by an organization, and conclusions are reached less on medical than on interactional and bureaucratic grounds. When a doctor is confronted with a worker who has taken a few days off and wants to be paid, the decision to grant the leave has virtually nothing to do with the professional's special expertise. Consideration of his own time pressures at the moment of the request, implications for later requests, the importance of keeping the worker's good will, the possible reactions of the employer, the number of such requests previously granted and their cumulative effect, all enter the decision-making process of the gatekeeper. They equal if not exceed the issue of the actual medical situation of the applicant.

Similarly when a physician becomes a facilitator for housing, phone service, vacations, and the like, he is not as a rule calling up any particular medical expertise. It does not take years of training to recognize that an old lady living alone will need a telephone in the event of an illness emergency. However, the welfare system has been set up to require the physician's validation of a request for this scarce resource, and his power comes from that bureaucratic arrangement rather than from his medical degree.

The variables of history, culture, and ideology are also outside the parameters of the medical model as generally conceptualized. The data on the meaning of traditional class position for compliance with physician authority in Britain reveal that the possession of specialized knowledge is a *post hoc* explanation and justification for a social reality with roots in the past.[8] The findings that medical technology can have differing impacts on physician power depending on cultural setting—in Britain it is said to detract, in the U.S.S.R. to enhance, a doctor's authority—again imply that it is not claims to specialized expertise per se, but societal in-

---

[8] Krause (1971:111),one of the few occupational sociologists to include the historical perspective, makes a similar point concerning the medical profession.

terpretations of the significance of these claims which are governing.

As for the ideological variable, there have been a few indications in the recent literature that this is an important factor in physicians' status. The ideological content of the "new professional" movement and attendant demands for professional accountability is quite explicit, as are the deprofessionalization exhortations addressed to medicine in the sparse information out of mainland China (Haug, 1973). The validity of this factor is reinforced by the present research, particularly in the data from the U.S.S.R., where the ideology of citizen responsibility for health maintenance and for illness treatment is the rationale for public acquiescence to a pervasive system of medical oversight, and explains the formal obligation to accede to physician advice. Although not necessarily incongruent with the theory of profession which distinguishes certain occupations as having special knowledge, humanitarian concerns and derivative autonomy, it adds a new dimension to the theory, redefining the circumstances under which the core characteristics provide a meaningful definition of the concept.

It is possible to summarize these findings and their theoretical implications by stating that data from both Great Britain and the U.S.S.R. confirm the American-based impression that professional authority is eroding, at least in part as a result of client education, and that the medical profession is no exception to this development, although the pace of change varies in different societies. Perhaps more important, it can be said that the model of profession and of medicine based on occupational characteristics is at best incomplete and at worst erroneous. Factors such as client characteristics, societal structure, and ideology may match if not outweigh the occupational parameters.

The hypothesis takes shape that the segments of the division of labor currently entitled "profession" in the West are simply a range of occupations which require greater or lesser degrees of training and expertise, and in which clients, also with greater or lesser knowledge of the tasks that occupation performs, negotiate a course of action designed to accomplish some individually or socially desirable end. Factors affecting this negotiation are the bureaucratic structures in which the transactions occur, the ideological themes which place values on different transactional styles and outcomes, and the historical events and traditions which in various social and cultural settings have patterned practitioner and client beliefs and behaviors. The underlying model is one of expert and consumer, without the moral and evaluative overtones of the professional model. While the data presented here cannot support this hypothesis, they at least suggest the theoretical utility of systematic exploration of its validity.

Marie R. Haug, PH.D.
Department of Sociology
Case Western Reserve University
Cleveland, Ohio 44106

This is a revision of a paper prepared for presentation at the annual meeting of the American Sociological Association, Montreal, Canada. This research was supported in part by the National Science Foundation Grant #GS-41347.

References

Balint, Michael
1957   The Doctor, His Patient and the Illness. New York: International Universities Press, Inc.
Becker, Howard S.
1962   "The nature of a profession." Pp. 27–46 in Education for the Professions, Sixty-first Yearbook of the National Society for the Study of Education, Part II. Chicago: The University of Chicago Press.
Boston Women's Health Book Collective
1973   Our Bodies Our Selves. New York: Simon and Schuster.
Eulau, Heinz
1973   "Skill revolution and consultative commonwealth." American Political Science Review 62 (March):169-191.
Freidson, Eliot
1961   Patients' Views of Medical Practice. New York: Russell Sage Foundation.
1970   Professional Dominance. New York: Atherton Press, Inc.
Geiger, H. Jack
1972   "The new doctor." In Gross, Ronald, and Paul Osterman (eds.), The New Professions. New York: Simon and Schuster.

Goode, William J.
1969   "The theoretical limits of professionalization." Pp. 266–313 in Et-
        zioni, Amitai (ed.), The Semi-Professions and Their Organizations.
        New York: The Free Press.

Haug, Marie R.
1973   "Deprofessionalization—an alternative hypothesis for the future."
        The Sociological Review Monograph No. 20 (December):195–211.

1974   "Computer technology and the obsolescence of the concept of
        profession." Paper presented at the 8th World Congress of
        Sociology, Toronto (Canada) August (Session II of the Research
        Committee on Work).

1975   "The deprofessionalization of everyone." Sociological Focus 8
        (August): 197–214.

in press "Issues in general practitioner authority in the National Health Ser-
        vice." In Stacey, Margaret (ed.), The Sociology of the National
        Health Service. Monograph of the (British) Sociological Review.

Haug, Marie R. and Marvin B. Sussman
1969   "Professional autonomy and the revolt of the client." Social
        Problems 17 (Fall): 153–161.

Johnson, Terence J.
1972   Professions and Power. London: The Macmillan Press Ltd.

Klein, Rudolf
1972   Complaints Against Doctors. London: Charles Knight & Co. Ltd.

Krause, Elliott A.
1971   The Sociology of Occupations. Boston: Little, Brown and Com-
        pany.

Lefkowitz, Annie, and Marlene Ausmus
1970   "Opportunities in subprofessional health occupations." Oc-
        cupational Outlook Quarterly 14 (Winter): 6–18.

Marston, M.
1970   "Compliance with medical regimens: a review of the literature."
        Nursing Research 19 (July-August): 312–323.

McKinlay, John B.
1972   "Some approaches and problems in the study of the use of ser-
        vices—an overview." Journal of Health and Social Behavior 13
        (June): 115–152.

Mechanic, David
1970   "Correlates of frustration among British general practitioners."
        Journal of Health and Social Behavior 11 (June): 87–104.

Moore, Wilbert E.
1970   The Professions: Roles and Rules. New York: Russell Sage Foun-
        dation.

Muller, James E., Faye G. Abdellah, F.T. Billings, Arthur E. Hess, Donald Petit, and Rober O. Egeberg
1972   "The Soviet health system—aspects of relevance for medicine in the United States." New England Journal of Medicine 286 (March 30): 693–702.

Parsons, Talcott
1951   The Social System. New York: The Free Press.

Perrow, Charles
1972   Complex Organizations, A Critical Essay. Glenview, Illinois: Scott Foresman and Company.

Reeder, Leo G.
1972   "The patient-client as consumer: some observations on the changing professional client relationship." Journal of Health and Human Behavior 13 (December): 406–412.

Reiff, Robert
1971   "The danger of the techni-pro: democratizing the human service professions." Social Policy 2 (May-June): 62–64.

Schwartz, W.B.
1970   "Medicine and the computer: the promise and problems of change." New England Journal of Medicine 283 (December 3): 1257–1264.

Sidel, Victor
1968   "Feldshers and feldsherism I and II." New England Journal of Medicine 278 (April 25): 934–939, and (May 2): 987–992.

U.S. Bureau of the Census
1972   Statistical Abstract of the United States. 93rd edition. Washington, D.C.

Wilensky, Harold
1964   "The professionalization of everyone?" American Journal of Sociology 70 (September): 137–158.

Professional Licensure, Organizational Behavior, and the Public Interest

HARRIS S. COHEN

This paper analyzes the close nexus between professional associations and the process of state licensure. Licensure is viewed as an extension of the concern for self-regulation that characterizes professionalism. Notwithstanding the important mission of protecting the health and safety of the public, in many cases, licensure has provided a means of according status and recognition to a body of specialized knowledge, resulting in a "state-protected environment" wherein the profession is virtually autonomous.

Several recent proposals that may have far-reaching impact on the natural insularity of licensing boards are critically discussed. These include public representation, reorganization of boards, institutional licensure, and jointly promulgated regulations. In the context of a growing demand for greater public accountability and responsiveness in the credentialing of health manpower, these proposals may be of pivotal importance if innovative developments in the utilization and distribution of manpower are to be realized.

The past few years have witnessed a growing sensitivity to the problems associated with state licensure of health practitioners. Numerous articles have been written critical of one or another facet in licensure (Hershey, 1971; Forgotson, Roemer, and Newman, 1967; Carlson, 1970; Akers, 1968; Grimm, 1972; Cohen, 1973; Sadler and Sadler, 1971). States, professional associations, and health organizations are seriously addressing the issues of licensing and credentialing. In 1971, the Department of Health, Education, and Welfare submitted to the Congress a comprehensive report on the subject (U.S. Department of Health, Education, and Welfare, 1971). However, despite the broad interest in these issues, they are rarely examined in a context in which the major legislative struggles of "to license or not to license"—to borrow an expression of William Curran's (1970)—as well as the specific jurisdictional boundaries that are defined (or left undefined) in the practice acts might be more meaningfully analyzed. This paper will attempt to develop a conceptual framework of licensure as a political process critical to the organizational autonomy and self-regulation of the health professions.

The Professions and the Licensing Process

A view that is gaining wide acceptance in the sociology of pro-

Milbank Memorial Fund Quarterly, Winter, 1973.

fessions is that professional status results from an interactive process based upon the profession's claims to specialized competence. As Bucher and Stelling (1969: 4) note, the professional "claims that he, uniquely, possesses the knowledge and skills to define problems, set the means for solving them, and judge the success of particular courses of action within his area of competence. To the extent that others accept these claims, the professional is accorded the license and mandate that Hughes has written of as being central to being professional." Freidson (1970: 137), too, describes the autonomy and special privilege accorded professions as predicated upon three claims: "First, the claim is that there is such an unusual degree of skill and knowledge involved in professional work that nonprofessionals are not equipped to evaluate or regulate it. Second, it is claimed that professionals are responsible—that they may be trusted to work conscientiously without supervision. Third, the claim is that the profession, itself, may be trusted to undertake the proper regulatory action on those rare occasions when an individual does not perform his work competently or ethically."

The profession's autonomy is critically linked to the credentialing system, wherein the basic prerequisites and standards of competence are established for professional practice. This system includes—but is by no means limited to: (1) *licensing* by the state, (2) *certification* by the professional association, and (3) the *accreditation* of educational programs. The professions traditionally have sought exclusive control of each component in the credentialing system; and they have succeeded in many instances in forging the three processes of licensure, certification, and accreditation—and other processes as well—into "one comprehensive health-manpower credentialing system" (Grimm, 1972: I1). Thus graduation from a program approved by the profession's accrediting arm is often a prerequisite for taking the certification or licensure examinations.

Autonomy in the credentialing system is tantamount to self-regulation, as reflected in most of the health practice acts in this country which delegate authority to the licensed profession to regulate itself. To quote Freidson (1970: 44), "the state uses the profession as its source of guidance, exercising its power in such a way as to support the profession's standards and create a sociopolitical environment in which the profession is free from serious competition from rival practitioners and firmly in control of auxiliary workers. Within that state-protected environment, the profession has sufficient power of its own to control virtually all facets of its work without serious interference from any lay group."

Professional Autonomy

In analyzing professional autonomy, it is important to emphasize that the individual health professions possess *varying* degrees of autonomy even when their members are credentialed by the licensure process. The literature on professions and professional behavior tends to focus upon the specific, and in some ways unique, role played by organized medicine—as exemplified by the American Medical Association and state medical societies—without calling attention to dramatic differences in the degree of autonomy possessed by other professions. In the final analysis, the measure of a profession's control and self-regulation in the licensure process will depend on its relative political strength vis-à-vis other professional and interested groups in the state. Thus, the literature on professions tends to describe "ideal types," modeled on the status and authority already accorded by the state to *certain* health professions to regulate their own professional practice. Other health professions will tend to pattern their credentialing procedures upon the older and more established professions.

The disparate statutory composition of licensing boards in the health field illustrates this variability. Practice acts in most health disciplines require either that all or a majority of board members be licensed practitioners in the respective licensed category. Other categories—including dental hygienists, nurse midwives, and, in some states, practical nurses—are regulated by boards that do not include a single member of the particular licensed category, but rather are dominated by members of another related profession (Pennell and Stewart, 1968). Thus, while the character of the board is in essence the same in both instances with the majority of membership "having direct professional and economic interests in the areas regulated by the boards" (Grimm, 1972: 118), the relative autonomy of the *licensed* profession is rather varied.

Another aspect of professional autonomy in the licensing process relates to the basic motivation behind the establishment of

234

state licensure. In 1972, legislative bills were introduced in 30 states to consider the merits of licensing one or more of 14 categories of health personnel that were not previously licensed.[1] Some of this legislative activity may have been initiated by essentially external sources, such as in the case of ambulance attendants and emergency medical technicians, with the primary motivation being the protection of the public safety. These bills generally vest the licensing authority in departments of health or other state agencies, and only rarely provide for the establishment of a specialized board of examiners. This pattern, however, is relatively uncommon in the licensure of health personnel. More often than not, the professional associations themselves are the key actors in generating licensing legislation. There are even instances in which state associations were founded for the express purpose of promoting such legislation, although (Akers, 1968: 465) "sometimes in a defensive move to prevent other, already established, professions from regulating them."[2] As Moore (1970: 125) has pointed out, professions have sought governmental licensure (1) as a means of public recognition, (2) as protection from competition by the relatively untrained, and (3) "to establish a preemptive jurisdiction over services that may in fact be in considerable and justified jurisdictional dispute."

As noted above (U.S. Department of Health, Education, and Welfare, 1971: 28), licensure also fulfills the "fundamental role of establishing minimum standards to protect the health and safety of the public." However, there has yet to be developed an objective

---

[1] This information is based upon a study by this writer of the response by professional organizations and states to a recommended moratorium on the further licensure of health occupations. (See U.S. Department of Health, Education, and Welfare, 1971: 73-74.) The following are the categories of personnel considered in 1972 for licensure: ambulance attendants and emergency medical workers, chiropractors, dental technicians, directors of clinical laboratories, EEG technicians, medical technologists and technicians, naturopaths, nurse anesthetists, opticians, physical therapy assistants, psychologists, psychotherapists, radiology technicians, and speech pathologists and audiologists.

[2] See also Stevens (1971: 105). These statutes, at first "permissive," i.e., persons may work in the field without being licensed but may not use the protected title, and later, as the profession becomes more established, "mandatory," i.e., only persons licensed may practice at all, have been dubbed "friendly" licensing laws. See Forgotson and Roemer (1968: 347).

measure of the range of health services that pose substantial threat to the public safety to warrant governmental licensure. Certainly an argument could be made for licensing all health practitioners without exception, insofar as the health of the public is at stake. But this would mean the possible licensing of scores of different occupational categories which, of course, would be untenable on numerous grounds. The issue of public safety, remaining as it is a very imprecise and ambiguous concept, is often secondary to other considerations, such as a profession's desire for autonomy and self-regulation. Thus, while numerous practice acts are formally justified in terms of protecting the public safety, the actual factors accounting for the promotion of such legislation may have had more to do with the above sociopolitical considerations than with the profession's concern for protecting the public from the charlatan or undertrained practitioner.[3]

[3] The language in two recently introduced bills illustrates the use to which the element of public safety is put in justifying legislation:

AN ACT . . . to provide for the licensing and regulation of psychotherapists, to impose a penalty on persons practicing psychotherapy without a license, and generally related to psychotherapists and the practice of psychotherapy.

WHEREAS, Individuals with mental and emotional problems from time to time have sought the help of certain persons conducting either individual psychotherapy or group psychotherapy; and

WHEREAS, Some of the individuals operating as psychotherapists lack the training and experience necessary to recognize existing and developing mental illness, or to recognize when the methods and techiques which they use are having harmful effects on the personality structure or the emotional or mental health of the individual; and

WHEREAS, The State, in the interest of the public health, safety, and welfare, wishes to protect individuals from psychotherapy which endangers their emotional and mental health; and

WHEREAS, it is realized that some persons operating as psychotherapists, although they do not have an academic background in psychology or psychiatry and although they employ heterodox methods, can perform necessary and needed services for the residents of this State, and

WHEREAS, It is not in the interest of the State or its citizens to limit the practice of psychotherapy entirely to persons of certain academic backgrounds, but only to assure that persons with existing or developing mental or emotional disorders be protected from destructive psychotherapeutic

Another facet of professional autonomy in the credentialing process is evident in the close collaboration between the professional association and the governmental agency charged with administering the practice act, particularly when the agency is a specialized board of examiners (Akers, 1968: 470–472). As with the initiation and promotion of the practice acts, the professions themselves generally were the driving force behind legislation to establish specialized boards. David Truman (1951: 418) has noted that when groups have sought regulation, such as in the licensing of occupations, the independent examining board or commission has typically been regarded as the most appropriate form for their purposes, because it assures privileged access for the initiating group. The tendency of regulatory agencies to become the ally or public sponsor of the regulated interest has been noted even when the demand for government regulation originated from outside the profession. As Truman (1951: 418) remarks, "Experience indicates . . . that the regulated groups will have more cohesion than those demanding regulation, that they can therefore keep close track of the work of the commission, and that consequently little will be done by a commission beyond what is acceptable to the regulated groups."[4]

Professional Associations

The associations' access to the examining boards is facilitated in

methods and techniques and be referred to appropriate psychotherapists; now therefore . . .

Maryland House Bill No. 1068 (1972)

AN ACT Providing for a Board of Registration of Radiologic Technologists.

It is declared to be the policy of the Commonwealth of Massachusetts that the health and safety of the people of the state must be protected against the harmful effects of excessive and improper exposure to ionizing radiation. Such protection can, in some major measure, be accomplished by requiring adequate training and experience of persons operating ionizing radiation equipment in each particular case under the specific direction of licensed practitioners as defined herein. It is the purpose of this article to establish standards of education, training and experience and to require the examination and certification of operators of ionizing radiation equipment.

Massachusetts House Bill No. 4099 (1972)

[4] In this respect, the state licensing agency has much in common with other forms of regulatory agencies. See Krislov and Musolf (1964: chapters 3 and 4).

those states and professions where board members are appointed by the governor from a list of nominations submitted by the professional associations, or, as in medicine, where the laws of 23 states provide that the medical society shall have a *direct* voice in the appointment of board members (Derbyshire, 1972: 161). Commenting on the latter method of board appointment, Derbyshire points out that "politics is theoretically removed from the board in that the members of the medical society are in a better position to judge the qualifications of the doctors than is the governor." *Medical politics,* however, is hardly eliminated in the process. Again quoting Derbyshire (1972: 161), "the medical societies are by no means always likely to recommend the most highly qualified people for appointment. All too frequently, they ignore professional and educational attributes, endorsing some faithful political stalwart who has worked his way up in the councils of the medical society."

The organization's ability to nominate or appoint members to the examining boards—who, in most cases, will constitute the majority discipline on the board—is clearly another means of perpetuating the profession's autonomy and self-regulation. Conversely, in cases where this is lacking and the profession is either not represented on the board at all or comprises a minority of the board, the regulated profession will tend to be apprehensive of a process in which decisions related to quality are determined by groups external to the profession. In a recent article, examining the pros and cons of licensing in the field of occupational therapy, one author (Crampton, 1971: 207) cited the composition of the examining boards "which, by law, may turn out not to be comprised in whole or in part of the professionals for whom the law was enacted," as a major problem facing the profession.

The association's interaction and influence with the examining board does not cease at the point of selecting board members; in conjunction with the boards, the associations initiate moves for new legislation, decide what provisions should be added, deleted, or changed to correct inadequacies in existing laws, and work for the passage or defeat of bills that relate to the profession's jurisdictional boundaries and credentialing mechanisms (Akers, 1968: 467; Gilb, 1966: 151–153). Similarly, the associations participate in the formulation of the administrative rules and regulations that govern the conduct and practice both of the boards and of individual practitioners licensed in the state. In fact, some of the major political struggles in the area of manpower licensure continue well after the debate and controversy have been resolved in the legislative branch only to be resumed with equal or greater vigor in the administrative branch in determining the meaning and effect of the enacted legislation.

Recent Proposals for Change

Several recent proposals have been made that would introduce countervailing interests in the governance of licensing boards. This is not to imply that the professions typically function in such a way that the interest of the general public is ignored. Certainly, as indicated by Kaplin (1972: J33), when the profession applies "its special expertise in order to protect the public from professional incompetence, its decision may benefit rather than harm society."

However, there has been deep concern for some time with the effects of specific group biases in limiting the social responsiveness and accountability of professional associations. As Robert MacIver (1966: 53) wrote, in a paper first published in 1922: "The possibility that there may still be an inclusive professional interest—generally but not always an economic one—that at significant points is not harmonized with the community interest is nowhere adequately recognized. The problem of professional ethics, viewed as the task of coordinating responsibilities, of finding, as it were, a common center for the various circles of interest, wider and narrower, is full of difficulty and far from being completely solved. The magnitude and the social significance of this task appear if we analyze on the one hand the character of the professional interest and on the other the relation of that interest to the general welfare."[5] This concern is reflected in some of the current literature which describes professional credentialing as a sociopolitical process dealing not only "with narrow, clear-cut questions of professional competency but also with issues of broad social concern." Consequently, as Grimm (1972: I19; see also U.S. Department of Health, Education, and Welfare, 1971: chapter 1)

[5] For another early, but still timely, critique of professional self-regulation, see Fesler (1942: 46-60).

points out, "the infusion of ideas from the community would help to combat the natural insularity of the boards."

The Public and Licensure

One approach to credentialing that is receiving considerable attention is to expand the composition of licensing boards to include public members with interests outside the respective fields being licensed. A leading proponent of this approach, William Selden (1970: 125; see also Grimm, 1972: 118–120), suggests that the addition of nonmembers of the professions on licensing boards "would provide greater and more consistent assurance that the public welfare is the overriding criterion on which its decisions are made." The Department of Health, Education, and Welfare (1971: 76), in its recent report on licensure, went even further to recommend that several interests be added to the boards which might be representative of: consumers; other health professions; various modalities of health care delivery, such as group practice and public institutions; educators; and others in policy-making positions in health care.

As a direct response to these proposals, numerous bills have been introduced within the past year to amend certain practice acts for the purpose of adding public members to the boards. This certainly has important potential in the direction of infusing greater public accountability in the licensure process. However, the effect of such changes in board composition will ultimately depend on a number of factors, including the status and autonomy of the public members; the extent to which public members are permitted to challenge decisions made by professional members of the boards; the extent to which they accept the responsibility of challenging such decisions; and the availability of an organized constituency or power base from which to exert leverage on other board members when it is felt that they are not acting in the public interest. In light of these considerations, a recent Labor Department report (Shimberg et al., 1972: 379-381) recommended the inclusion on licensing boards of a technically competent representative of a state government agency instead of a nonprofessional public member.

Another critical factor that should be considered with regard to lay representation is the *number* of positions to be designated for public members. Some proponents of public representation on licensing boards are urging (Derbyshire, 1972:161) that a single position be granted to a public member. Indeed, a good number of the legislative bills recently introduced for the purpose of restructuring board composition would expand the present boards by adding *one* or *two* public members to the total board membership. The net effects of such token structural change would probably not be very far-reaching, especially in boards that traditionally have been dominated by the licensed profession. Other commentators (Selden, 1970: 124) are quite emphatic in urging that a *substantial* number of public members be placed on the boards. It would appear that unless board composition were to be *dramatically* altered, the considerable influence of professional associations on the governance and decision making of licensing boards would continue unchecked by other interests. What is suggested, therefore, is a means of introducing greater pluralism in the credentialing system.

Reorganization of Licensing Boards

A related proposal aimed at broadening the perspective of licensing boards and enhancing their potential accountability to the public would centralize the licensing function within a single departmental unit, such as a state health or education department. In the words of a recent monograph (U.S. Department of Labor, 1969: 3), "With administration centralized, occupational groups can continue to be major forces in establishing and enforcing regulatory policies, but through a state agency which can reconcile the interest of the general public with those of the private associations." (See also Shimberg et al., 1972: 372-373.) In this connection, William Selden proposes a single state licensure board for all of the health professions that would be organized with subcommittees for each of the professions. The subcommittees, with majority membership from the licensed profession and including members from related professions and the general public, "would be charged with responsibility for developing policies regarding licensure for their respective professions, subject to the approval of the state board" (Selden, 1970: 126; see also Carlson, 1970: 871–872). As we pointed out elsewhere, however, this form of reorganization might prove ineffective in regulating the professions or even in mandating coordination or joint planning. State licensing boards tend to have considerably stronger links to their respective professional associations than to other public agencies—even when these boards are located within state departments of health or education (U.S. Department of Health, Education, and Welfare, 1971:30).[6]

An alternative model of board restructuring would establish a single licensing board with but *one* representative of each licensed profession. Thus, instead of perpetuating the profession's autonomy and influence by delegating major policy responsibility to subcommittees—which for all practical purposes would probably function as boards—this approach would alter very dramatically the pattern of professional self-regulation that has developed in the health field. We are not suggesting that this approach is politically feasible; it does, however, provide an alternative that at least merits public consideration in weighing the pros and cons of the state-protected environment that presently characterizes licensure in the health professions.

Institutional Licensure

A third proposal, that has been labeled "institutional licensure," and is currently receiving much attention, would introduce a clearly interdisciplinary character to licensing. The implications of a system that delegated the responsibility for competence and quality of practitioners to institutions have been critically examined from several perspectives, including (1) the opportunity for greater legal and administrative flexibility in allocating responsibilities within institutions, and (2) the effects that such a system might have on the present status of the health professions. These issues are largely unresolved at this time and are certainly well-deserving of the discussion that has been generated by both the Department of Health, Education, and Welfare recommendation calling for the further study and demonstration of institutional licensure (U.S. Department of Health, Education, and Welfare, 1971: 77), and the treatment of this concept in the literature (Hershey, 1969a: 71–74; Hershey, 1969b: 951–956; Carlson, 1970: 872–878; Roemer, 1971: 50–51; Tancredi and Woods, 1972: 103).

A point that is sometimes underemphasized is that institutional licensure conceivably could provide the opportunity and impetus for greater interprofessional coordination. Ideally, the

[6] This writer was co-author of the Report on Licensure.

basic credentialing policies in such a system would emanate not from any one discipline, but rather from a representative committee or commission that would reflect the views of several disciplines—including medicine, nursing, hospital administration, allied health, labor unions, and other interests in personnel credentialing. Such an approach might lessen the autonomy of certain or all of the professional associations (depending on how broadly one conceives of institutional licensure)[7] in regulating the professions. But it might also increase the scope of professional policy making, insofar as individual professions would be afforded the opportunity of contributing meaningful inputs in defining the scope of other related professions—an end product that could be extremely valuable to the public, but that is probably unattainable under the present system of licensure. Thus, the "team approach" to licensure may be viewed not only as a means of providing for flexibility within the health care institution, but also as a means of introducing countervailing interests to the existing system wherein professional associations control their respective credentialing systems (Roemer, 1971: 51).

Joint Regulation

Legislation recently enacted in a few states is consistent with the above proposal and its implications for interprofessional coordination and policy making. These laws mandate the responsibility for promulgating scope of practice regulations for emerging fields and expanded roles, such as the case of nurse practitioners, to *both* the medical and nursing boards of examiners.[8] While it is too soon to evaluate the net effects of such cooperative efforts in credentialing, a rather strong argument can be made to justify this approach as being responsive to the cracks that are beginning to appear in the present system of licensure. The joint regulation approach may also be viewed as a prototype of joint boards or some variation on

[7] For a discussion of institutional licensure, see U.S. Department of Health, Education, and Welfare (1971: chapter 10).

[8] See Idaho Code, sec. 54-1413 (1971), "An Act . . . authorizing a professional nurse to perform acts recognized as appropriate according to rules and regulations promulgated by the Idaho State Board of Medicine and the Idaho Board of Nursing"; and Maryland House Bill No. 468 (enacted May 31, 1972), "An Act . . . to exempt individuals to whom duties are delegated by licensed physicians from the necessity of obtaining a license to practice medicine."

the theme of board restructuring, as examined above. There is, however, some indication that when jurisdictional issues are at stake, professional associations may prefer a private approach rather than resorting to statutory or administrative definitions of jurisdiction which "may fence the profession in as well as others out." As Gilb points out, "some professions, such as psychologists in some states, have found it so difficult to arrive at an enforceable definition of their work that they have had to forgo licensing and rely on registration, certification, or the licensing of use of a title, with no clear-cut definition of the work it describes" (Gilb, 1966: 182; Moore, 1970: 124–125).

In sum, these four approaches—public representation, reorganization of boards, institutional licensure, and jointly promulgated regulations—would provide a system of professional checks and balances in the states' regulation of health practitioners. The fundamental issues in credentialing would be addressed from a perspective broader than that of a single interested profession. The pros and cons of these alternatives will undoubtedly continue to be debated both within and among the professions. This is natural; credentialing traditionally has been, and continues to be, of central concern to the professions. As the professional associations and the public become more cognizant of the imposing public responsibilities that have been granted the professions by the state, measures to infuse greater pluralism and public accountability may need to be adopted, by both the public and private sectors, to ensure the public safety as well as the continued contribution and viability of the professions.

Harris S. Cohen, PH.D.
Acting Chief
Political and Legal Analysis Branch
National Center for Health Services Research and Development
Health Services and Mental Health Administration
Rockville, Maryland 20852

References

Akers, Ronald L.
  1968   "The professional association and the legal regulation of practice."
          Law and Society Review 2 (May): 463–482.

Bucher, Rue *and* Joan Stelling
1969 "Characteristics of professional organizations." Journal of Health and Social Behavior 10 (March): 3–15.

Carlson, Rick J.
1970 "Health manpower licensing and emerging institutional responsibility for the quality of care." Law and Contemporary Problems 35 (Autumn): 849–878.

Cohen, Harris S.
1973 "State licensing boards and quality assurance: A new approach to an old problem." Pp. 49–65 in U.S. Department of Health, Education, and Welfare. Quality Assurance of Medical Care. Washington, D.C.: U.S. Government Printing Office.

Crampton, Marion W.
1971 "Licensing of occupational therapists." American Journal of Occupational Therapy 25 (May–June): 206–209.

Curran, William J.
1970 "New paramedical personnel—To license or not to license?" New England Journal of Medicine 282 (May 7): 1085–1086.

Derbyshire, Robert C.
1972 "Better licensure laws for better patient care." Hospital Practice 7 (September): 152–164.

Fesler, James W.
1942 The Independence of State Regulatory Agencies. Chicago: Public Administration Service.

Forgotson, Edward H. *and* Ruth Roemer
1968 "Government licensure and voluntary standards for health personnel and facilities." Medical Care 6 (September–October):345–354.

Forgotson, Edward H., Ruth Roemer, *and* Roger W. Newman
1967 "Legal regulation of health personnel in the United States." Pp. 279–541 in Report of the National Advisory Commission on Health Manpower, II. Washington: U.S. Government Printing Office.

Freidson, Eliot
1970 Profession of Medicine. New York: Dodd, Mead.

Freidson, Eliot *and* Buford Rhea
1965 "Knowledge and judgment in professional evaluations." Administrative Science Quarterly 10 (June): 107–124.

Gilb, Corinne Lathrop
1966 Hidden Hierarchies: The Professions and Government. New York: Harper and Row.

Grimm, Karen L.
  1972   "The relationship of accreditation to voluntary certification and state licensure." SASHEP Staff Working Papers, II., I1–I42. Washington: National Commission on Accrediting.

Hershey, Nathan
  1969a   "An alternative to mandatory licensure of health professionals." Hospital Progress 50 (March): 71–74.

  1969b   "The inhibiting effect upon innovation of the prevailing licensure system." Annals of the New York Academy of Science 166 (December): 951–956.

  1971   "New directions in licensure of health personnel." Economic and Business Bulletin 24 (Fall): 22–35.

Kaplin, William A.
  1972   "The law's view of professional power: Courts and the health professional associations." SASHEP Staff Working Papers, II. J1–J37. Washington: National Commission on Accrediting.

Krislov, Samuel *and* Lloyd D. Musolf (eds.)
  1964   The Politics of Regulation. Boston: Houghton-Mifflin.

MacIver, Robert M.
  1966   "Professional groups and cultural norms." P. 53 in Howard M. Vollmer and Donald L. Mills (ed.), Professionalization. Englewood Cliffs, New Jersey: Prentice-Hall.

Moore, Wilbert E.
  1970   The Professions: Roles and Rules. New York: Russell Sage Foundation.

Pennell, Maryland Y. *and* Paula A. Stewart
  1968   State Licensing of Health Occupations. Washington: U.S. Government Printing Office.

Roemer, Ruth
  1971   "Licensing and regulation of medical and medical-related practitioners in health service teams." Medical Care 9 (January-February): 42–54.

Sadler, Alfred M. *and* Blair L. Sadler
  1971   "Recent developments in the law relating to the physician's assistant." Vanderbilt Law Review 24: 1193–1212.

Selden, William K.
  1970   "Licensing boards are archaic." American Journal of Nursing 70 (January): 124–126.

Shimberg, Benjamin, Barbara F. Esser, *and* Daniel H. Kruger
    1972   Occupational Licensing and Public Policy, Report to U.S. Department of Labor. Princeton: Educational Testing Service.

Stevens, Rosemary
    1971   American Medicine and the Public Interest. New Haven: Yale University Press.

Tancredi, Lawrence R. *and* John Woods
    1972   "The social control of medical practice: Licensure versus output monitoring." Milbank Memorial Fund Quarterly 50 (January): 99–125.

Truman, David R.
    1951   The Governmental Process: Political Interests and Public Opinion. New York: Knopf.

U.S. Department of Health, Education, and Welfare
    1971   Report on Licensure and Related Health Personnel Credentialing. Washington: U.S. Government Printing Office.

U.S. Department of Labor
    1969   Occupational Licensing and the Supply of Nonprofessional Manpower, Manpower Research Monograph No. 11. Washington: U.S. Government Printing Office.

PSROs, The Medical Profession, and the Public Interest

ODIN W. ANDERSON

The federal legislation mandating Professional Standards Review Organizations to monitor the decision making of physicians regarding their patients is a method unique to the United States to control medical care costs according to prevailing professional criteria. Other countries, so far, depend largely on health service structures, reimbursement methods, and arbitrary government budget limitations. Our dislike of highly structured delivery systems has pragmatically moved us in the direction of monitoring diagnostic and therapeutic decision making. PSRO is mandated at a time when there is no systematic methodology with validated criteria for monitoring medical practice. This will likely lead to subtle sabotage of PSRO by the medical profession justified by quality standards which are the professions' prerogative.

It is conceivable that quality standards will rise and, therefore, costs. The drive for monitoring physician decision making is understandable even when there is no methodology. It then behooves medical schools to conduct research on methodologies of monitoring services, a possible favorable side-effect of the legislation. An unfavorable side-effect may likely be that the criteria will be based exclusively on technical medical considerations and ignore the personal and social attributes of patients which should affect the decision making of physicians. Medicine will then become even more technocratic than it is now. All countries are converging at various degrees of intensity in establishing planned limits to expansion, examining possibilities of monitoring physician decision making and capping this off with arbitrary budget ceilings. The state of the art of health services management appears to permit no other recourse.

Introduction

The federal legislation mandating Professional Standards Review Organizations deserves some examination as to its implications for medical practice, the patient, and the sources of financing of health services in this country. I have the temerity to attempt this, inspired by one of the Nine Laws of the Disillusionment of the True Liberal. One of these laws (Levy, 1970) is: "Anticipated events never live up to expectations."[1] Still, we cannot just stand there; we must do

[1] Another law is: "Good intentions randomize behavior," i.e., it is not possible to deal rationally with randomized behavior. It is too unpredictable. Levy's view is that in wicked intentions "there is a strong possibility, in theory, of handling the wicked by outthinking them." The PSRO law is well-intentioned, and the PSRO committees will be "wicked."

something! PSRO is a prime example of this very American, activist philosophy. I start with an international perspective.

In the management of the health services delivery system the United States is unique among countries in that we are moving directly into monitoring the decision making of doctors. I believe this is so because we lack the health services organizational structures and relatively closed-ended financing true of European health insurance or health services systems, particularly that of Great Britain or Scandinavia. Even with more structure than in the United States, costs in all countries have gone up faster than other segments of their economies. It may seem an anomaly that I find no relationship between ownership, sources of funding, the organizational structure of health, and the amount a country spends for health services. The factor establishing the limits is the implicit and explicit public policy on how much a country wants to spend for health services. This amount is in the main a political decision in the murky area of tradeoffs in resource allocation among parties at interest. Until very recently the sky seemed to be the limit, but now health services expenditures are beginning to nudge both governmental and private budgeting limits. Even so, only one country is actually retrenching—Great Britain—and mainly because of the difficulties that country is having with its economy. Great Britain would actually spend more if it could in relation to other priorities. Other countries are not yet retrenching, but agonizing over slowing the pace of increases in expenditures even though their Gross National Products (GNP) may still be expanding. No country has dared to find out what the saturation level of demand would be. It seems reasonable, however, to assume that there is such a saturation level as is true of all goods and services. The country which appears to be closest to the saturation level is the Soviet Union as measured by the lavish number of units of service provided per person as compared with North America and Western European countries. In general, countries in North American and Western Europe reveal about four to six visits per person a year to physicians, whereas the Soviet Union reports 10 visits and is making projections to 16 in the near future (Anderson, 1973; Pu. 'ovoy, 1975), with a commensurate increase in resources. The Soviet norms are set by medical professionals and such norms are inherently generous.

I wish to elaborate on my first statement, i.e., that the United States is unique in moving directly into monitoring the decision making of doctors. The reasons for this, I believe, are that costs were rising rapidly at the same time that some form of national health insurance was being considered seriously, plus our painful expenditures experience with Medicare. These took place in a context of very vague organizational and fiscal boundaries. We do not like visible boundaries and structures with visible limits on budgets, although we are—as are other countries—moving ineluctably in that direction. The pace in each country is a matter of degree.

It seems that we are hoping that a properly functioning PSRO mechanism will establish for us the proper level of expenditures, rather than have the level of expenditures determined arbitrarily from year to year by the processes of government budgeting, competing with the national priorities. It is then ironical that in this country the medical profession faces more direct monitoring of its decision making prerogatives than do its colleagues in government systems elsewhere. This is due in part—if you can believe it—to greater deference shown to doctors in European systems. Nevertheless, health administrators and politicians in Europe are looking enviously at the PSRO developments in the United States and naturally exaggerating their impact here. Their attitudes are somewhat analogous to our penchant for overidealizing the government systems abroad. What universal government systems abroad and in Canada have accomplished is to free the citizens from high-cost episodes of serious illnesses, an accomplishment which appears to be forgotten after other problems emerge, both unintended and unexpected. Now cost containment is the political battle cry elsewhere as it is here. To contain cost, we start with PSRO, the descendant of utilization review mandated by the Medicare Act as a device to shorten length of stay and eventually to limit admissions. The trend may continue to monitor office visits as well—not to mention admonishing patients to see the doctor only when necessary (a presumably precise judgment), and to strike a balance between hedonism and asceticism in their life styles.

The PSRO development is, indeed, remarkable. At first the profession fought it; now predictably it is likely to co-opt it; and I personally see no other alternative unless doctors are handed a manual of instructions to follow. This hardly seems either likely or tenable. If, in their judgment, the doctors are pressed too hard, they will sabotage the monitoring system by many subtle or not so subtle means at their disposal or threaten to strike on the seemingly unassailable reason that good patient care is being jeopardized. Witness house officers in hospitals across the country—preceded by nurses—

who brilliantly intrude into their bargaining processes the issue of proper professional standards for proper patient care. This is a tactic which has not been thought of, for example, by automobile assembly-line workers—who might claim that the quality of workmanship is being jeopardized and in turn the quality of the cars coming off the assembly line.

In attacking the cost imperative through the PSRO mechanism, I agree with Havighurst and Blumstein (1975:25), as they put it in their cogent article, that Congress has not sufficiently faced the *quality imperative*, a powerful weapon in the professional arsenal: "Because the quality imperative dictates that no one should very obviously enjoy better health care than anyone else on the basis of income, the ideal to be striven for is likely to be higher." Further (Havighurst and Blumstein, 1975:41), "A great deal of the discussion surrounding the PSRO concept in the period since its enactment has been rendered almost unintelligible by operation of the quality imperative in a highly charged political and professional environment."

The Situation

After this rambling introduction, where are we? In my more rational moments I deplore broadside legislating for a performance-monitoring mechanism such as PSROs before there is even the semblance of a systematic methodology to monitor performance according to validated criteria. At the same time, in my more pragmatic moments, I agree that we need to work toward some form of performance monitoring, and the issue is then not the principle but the pace and form the performance monitoring will take. I will also observe that, admitting the desirability of some form of performance monitoring, it is unlikely that the profession and the medical schools would voluntarily initiate action and research on performance criteria other than the ones they share informally among themselves in day-to-day practice. At least PSRO is forcing systematic attention to medical performance criteria which may not have come about otherwise. May the medical schools and organizational research agencies respond to the call for research on performance indicators!

In this connection, I recall an interview I had with that brilliant political strategist Wilbur Mills during the maneuvering surrounding the enactment of the Medicare Act in 1965, particularly Part B, physicians' services. I talked with him a year later. The question I posed to him was that in the preamble to the Act there was an explicit statement that the Act should not interfere with the private practice of medicine. Then a few paragraphs later there was spelled out and mandated utilization-review committees in hospitals to monitor length of stay. Is this not interfering with the private practice of medicine? He grinned and said no, the mandating of utilization-review committees was simply to make the doctors talk to each other. Presumably, it was hoped that this legislation would stimulate the formulation of more explicit professional criteria.

This is quite a charge considering the very considerable portion of medical practice which is considered an art rather than a science. It is a reasonable assumption, as Eliot Freidson (1970) puts forth forcefully in his writing, that the medical profession (indeed, any profession) is inclined to exaggerate the extent to which performance is beyond systematic monitoring, given the quality and equality imperative. A reasonable observation is that we do not know at present to what extent medical practice is capable of being monitored according to validated criteria, short of cookbook medicine, which nobody wants. Perhaps, the best that can be done is the strengthening of formal and informal peer review as is presumed to be done in well-organized group practices.

Very little research has been done on the methodology of monitoring physicians' services. A great deal of routine data needs to be collected on physicians' decision-making profiles. In Ontario, for example, the province compiles a tremendous data bank of physician decision-making profiles (Badgley et al., n.d.), but so far has done little with it in terms of comprehending decision-making in medical practices. The monitoring system exposes gross deviations from the average and calls the doctors so exposed into account. Similar methods are in use in the medical care foundations in California. I get the impression that the deviations are so gross that the deviant doctors would be known to their colleagues anyway, without the elaborate record system entailed to isolate these very few.

Medical decision making is, of course, a very difficult problem to analyze, not to mention developing a methodology for application. Medical practice is essentially a one-to-one relationship between a doctor and a patient, and doctors face understandable dilemmas in making decisions on individual patients on the basis of group statistics. The tendency, I would assume, would be to err on the side of safety. Referring again to Havighurst and Blumstein (1975:23): "It seems that sooner or later, government will have to face the dilemma of how to place limits on the commitment of funds to catastrophic disease. Its unwillingness to address this dilemma in the case of renal disease seems directly traceable to the advocates' ability to frame the issue in terms of *identifiable* rather than *statistical* lives." (Italics added.) Yes, indeed, it will take very sophisticated public policy decisions *not* to do something to save the lives of a few in favor of the many when the technology is present. Somehow in personal health services we do not like to deal with statistical lives, although we accept this concept in the carnage on our highways in order to have and drive our automobiles.

On a large-scale basis there appears to have been only two attempts to set up monitoring standards for hospital admissions. Both studies took place in the 1960s. Anticipating the interest in physician decision making as it applied to hospital admissions and discharges, I conducted a survey with Paul Sheatsley (1967) and the National Opinion Research Center (NORC), University of Chicago, of a representative sample of 2,000 surgical, medical, and diagnostic discharges in the state of Massachusetts for a 12-month period. Obstetrical cases were excluded. We queried the patients and their referring and attending doctors about the chain of events and decisions that led to hospital admission and discharge within a few weeks after discharge.

One table stands out in that survey, relating to the doctors' judgments after the fact as to degrees of urgency in admitting their patients to the hospital. We established four categories of urgency-nonurgency as determined by the attending doctors: (1) hospitalization absolutely necessary, the procedures could not have been carried out except in the hospital; (2) quite urgent, would have been difficult to carry out procedures except in the hospital, although maybe possible outside; (3) would have been possible to carry out procedures outside of the hospital, but desired to reduce the margin of error; and (4) finally, made no difference.

The other survey (Fitzpatrick et al., 1962) was conducted on a representative sample of 5,000 discharges in Michigan. The Michigan study selected 18 diagnoses (including maternity cases) which were relatively clear-cut disease entities and for which it was quite easy for committees of physicians to arrive at a consensus for each diagnosis regarding appropriateness of hospital admission and discharge. These 18 diagnoses comprised 46 percent of all general

Surgical Cases

Absolutely necessary	74%	⎫	89% necessary
Quite necessary	15%	⎭	
Safety margin	7%	⎫	11% could be
No difference	4%	⎭	eliminated

Medical Cases

Absolutely necessary	46%	⎫	83% necessary
Quite necessary	37%	⎭	
Safety margin	14%	⎫	17% could be
No difference	3%	⎭	eliminated

Diagnostic Admission

Absolutely necessary	45%	⎫	77% necessary
Quite necessary	32%	⎭	
Safety margin	15%	⎫	23% could be
No difference	8%	⎭	eliminated

hospital admissions. For the purpose here it is sufficient to summarize that "overuse" represented 2.3 percent of the admissions and 6.8 percent of the days. The Michigan study criteria were either/or instead of a range as formulated in the Massachusetts study. It is seen that in relying on professional criteria, there was very little purely wasteful use of hospital services.

I refer to these old—but still new—surveys, because they are the only ones that have been done which give some idea of the "softness" of decision making among doctors for hospital admissions and, given a control mechanism, what proportion of admissions might be eliminated before both doctors and patients would begin to protest in visible numbers. I make the prediction that costs will continue to rise so that stabilized PSRO criteria will not be possible. Rising expectations and the quality imperative will continue to affect expenditures. Criteria need to be revised and tightened periodically unless the body politic is willing to accept what the medical profession as a whole and the public who seek their services regard as appropriate medical care.

Observations and Conclusions

The legislation and discussion regarding PSROs appear to emphasize exclusively the role of doctors in decisions regarding their patients. The tendency is toward purely technical medical decision criteria and the ignoring of extenuating factors regarding the social and family environment of the patients and the patients' psychological state.[2] PSROs will, therefore, make medical practice even more technocratic and their alliance with administrative staffs of hospitals will allow patients even less to say about decision making in the enlarging bureaucracy than now. Can patient points of view be brought into the PSRO-type of decision monitoring? I am not sanguine. We are certainly entering a period of tensions and possible standoffs among patients, doctors, hospital managers, and government funding agencies. Due-process suits from doctors are already appearing (Blum, 1976).

While the United States tries to contain costs by monitoring physician decision making, the country is also laying the groundwork for a structure to contain supply as well in the newly implemented National Health Planning and Resources Development Act of 1974 (Public Law 93-641), following the failure of the comprehensive health planning and regional medical legislation in the late 1960s. In other countries the idea of monitoring physicians is following the creation of organizational structures, because costs are not contained by that means either. Thus, all countries are heading at various degrees of intensity in the direction of establishing planned limits to expansion, examining possibilities of monitoring physician decision making, and capping this with arbitrary budget ceilings.[3] The actors can then sort themselves out in these contexts and arrive at some politically tolerable equilibrium. This seems to be the fate of health services delivery systems.

[2] In a study of 252 admissions to a teaching hospital (Mushlin and Appel, 1976), 79 percent of the patients were judged to be admitted for purely biomedical factors. The remaining 21 percent were admitted for extramedical reasons.

[3] These impressions were gained from my attending three international conferences on the rising costs of health services everywhere. In October 1974, a conference (Ehrlich, 1975) was held in Geneva, Switzerland, sponsored by the International Red Cross through the Henry Durant Institute. This conference was attended mainly by administrators. In June 1975, the John E. Fogarty International Center for Advanced Study in the Health Sciences sponsored the Conference held in Bethesda, Maryland, attended mainly by academicians. In September 1975, the American College of Hospital Administrators sponsored a European seminar on health services in the nine countries belonging to the European Economic Community, in Brussels and Bruges, Belgium. This was attended mainly by hospital administrators. The seminar was arranged by Jan Blanpain, MD, and staff of the Institute for European Health Services Research, Leuven, Belgium.

Odin W. Anderson, PH.D.
Center for Health Administration Studies
University of Chicago
5720 South Woodlawn Avenue
Chicago, Illinois 60637

This article was given in substance at the Annual Convention of the American Public Health Association, Chicago, Illinois, on Wednesday, November 19, 1975.

References

Anderson, Odin W.
1973   Health Services in the USSR. Selected Papers No. 42. Chicago: University of Chicago Graduate School of Business.

Anderson, Odin W., and Paul Sheatsley
1967   Hospital Use—A Survey of Patient and Physician Decisions. Research Series No. 24, Center for Health Administration. Chicago: University of Chicago.

Badgley, Robin F., Catherine Charles, and George M. Torrance
n.d.   The Ontario Health System. Unpublished manuscript.

Blum, John D.
1976   " 'Due process' in hospital peer review." New England Journal of Medicine 294 (January 1) : 29–30.

Ehrlich, David A. (ed.)
1975   The Health Cost Explosion: Which Way Now? Bern, Switzerland: Huber.

Fitzpatrick, Thomas B., Donald C. Riedel, and Beverly C. Payne
1962   "Character and effectiveness of hospital use." Pp. 361–591 in McNerney, Walter J., and Study Staff, Hospital and Medical Economics; A Study of Population, Services Costs, Methods of Payment, and Controls. Vol. I. Chicago: Hospital Research and Educational Trust.

Freidson, Eliot
1970   Professional Dominance: The Social Structure of Medical Care. New York: Atherton Press.

Havighurst, Clark C., and James F. Blumstein
1975   "Coping with quality cost tradeoffs in medical care: the role of PSRO's." Northwestern University Law Review (March-April): 23, 25, 41.

Levy, Marion
  1970   "Levy's nine laws of the disillusionment of the true liberal." Midway 10
          (Winter): unpaged.

Mushlin, Alvin I., and Frances A. Appel
  1976   "Extramedical factors in the decision to hospitalize medical patients."
          American Journal of Public Health 66 (February): 170–172.

Pustovoy, Igo V
  1975   Health Care Planning in the USSR; Its Role in Improving Medical and
          Preventive Services. The 1975 Michael M. Davis Lecture, Center for
          Health Administration Studies. Chicago: University of Chicago Graduate
          School of Business.

Physicians
as Guiders of
Health Services Use

PAUL M. GERTMAN

It is frequently said that the physician is the key decisionmaker in the health-service system. One authority recently commented: "Most observers agree that once the patient has made initial contact with the medical care system, the physician becomes the principal decisionmaker and allocator of medical resources. He, in effect, decides how much and what types of additional medical services the patient should receive" (Shortell, 1972:2). If there is agreement with such statements, then it would seem that the physician's role as a guide to the use of health services would have priority in any discussion of health policy.

Yet the impact of physicians' decisions on the use of medical services and the reasoning behind them has been subject to relatively little scientific investigation or analysis. There is no real body of research literature specifically directed at the question. The following discussions will therefore be aimed at briefly reviewing four selected areas of physicians' actions and reasoning, some implications and trends of each, how their interactions may affect health-services utilization, and some questions for future research. The objective will not be to present a comprehensive analysis—nor is it possible to do so—but rather to provide a few perspectives on how the physician may guide health-services utilization.

In *Consumer Incentives for Health Care*, edited by Selma J. Mushkin. New York: PRODIST, 1974.

Paul M. Gertman

Ambulatory Medical Care: Physician Direction

In a single year, patient contacts with physicians number about one billion. The premise, both explicit and implicit, in many discussions and analyses of ambulatory utilization-pattern dynamics is that patients' initiation of demand is and will continue to be the dominant force in determining patient-physician contacts. Examination, however, of some of the information about ambulatory practice and of trends in medical care should raise some questions about the validity of that premise.

To explore the current and future role of the physician in determining utilization, some data on physician visit rates and their relationship to incidence of illness are presented, and a few studies on referral patterns and patient disposition practices are then reviewed. In 1970, there was a national average of 4.6 physician visits per person (White, 1972). White and his colleagues (1961) estimated from national data sources that in each month seven hundred fifty out of every one thousand adults will recognize and recall an episode of illness or injury; two hundred fifty of the one thousand will consult a physician at least once during the month, and five will be referred to another physician. More recently, Richardson (1971) studied ambulatory use of physicians' services in response to illness episodes of a low-income population in Brooklyn served by a neighborhood health center operated by the Office of Economic Development. In his study, seventy-four percent of the patients with an illness episode contacted a physician. Although the figures at first seem dissimilar, in the low-income group only thirty-four percent recalled an episode of illness, and thus a corrected rate of physicians' visits for the total sample interviewed might be estimated to be approximately twenty-five percent.

The physician's role in directing ambulatory health-services utilization can be examined from two different perspectives—how the patient came to the physician and what disposition the physician made after the initial contact. Preliminary results from the United States samples of the World Health Organization/International

Collaborative Study of Medical Care Use (Kohn, 1973) indicate that approximately 28 percent of all ambulatory patient-physician contacts were scheduled or initiated by the physician. Recent data collected by Mushlin and Barr (1973) at the Columbia Medical Plan—a prepaid group practice affiliated with Johns Hopkins—showed that 47.2 percent of the visits were initiated by practitioners. Investigations of specialist practice referral sources also showed a substantial degree of physician-initiation. In a study of 4,608 "new" patients seen by internists in New York State, Johnson and his colleagues (1965) found that 63.6 percent were self-referred or referred by someone other than a physician, 18.2 percent were referred by general practitioners, 17.1 percent were referred by specialists, and in 1.1 percent of the cases, the source of referral was not determined; the total referral by physicians thus amounted to 35.3 percent.

Creditor and Creditor (1972), in examining the referral sources of 2,090 new patients seen in the private practices of specialists at the Michael Reese Hospital in Chicago, found that 53.7 percent were self and lay referrals (4.3 percent and 49.4 percent, respectively), 27.3 percent were referrals from other specialists or staff of the Michael Reese Hospital, 15.2 percent were from outside medical providers, and 4.4 percent were referrals from other sources.

After the patient has seen the physician for the first time, the latter can either (a) recommend no further care and discharge him; (b) continue to provide care by seeing him again; or (c) recommend care from another provider.

It is then that the physician probably directs almost totally the utilization of further physician services. Richardson's study (1971) indicated that 52 percent of initial patient visits led to a recommendation for a revisit. Initial results from the World Health Organization/International Collaborative Study of Medical Care Use (Kohn, 1973) show that of all persons who had a medical contact in a two-week recall period, 53 percent were scheduled for a revisit or referred to another physician. In Johnson et al.'s (1965) study of internists' "new" patients, almost 85 percent were directed to seek additional physician services; 55.3 percent were given further appointments with the same physician, 18.5 percent were returned to their referring physician for followup care, and 11.1 percent were referred to another specialist. Last and White (1969), studying the content of five primary or general practices located in Vermont, found that over a three-month period each patient illness "condition" resulted in an average of 1.5 physician contacts, which may be interpolated as a 50 percent revisit rate.

The general issue of how economic factors, particularly in the aggregate, affect utilization of physician services is beyond the intent of this paper. With respect, however, to the preceding discussion, one tangential issue might be briefly considered: "Does the physician consciously schedule unnecessary revisits, referrals, or tests to increase his personal financial gain?" Although there are no "hard" data that answer the question, the following speculative thinking might be considered.

First, it is self-evident that all physicians, to some degree, practice medicine to earn money, although most observers would agree that this is not usually the incentive affecting the manner in which they practice and their direction of patient consumption of medical services. Based on the studies mentioned earlier, a large part of a physician's income in ambulatory practice is derived either from revisits that he has directly initiated or from referrals of other medical care providers.

Second, in an ambulatory practice, a physician is essentially selling his time, and thus a significant incentive to schedule unnecessary patient visits might be expected only if there were less than one hundred percent demand for his time. Most information points, however, to a marked excess in today's ambulatory health-care marketplace of demand for physician services over supply. Recent survey data from the American Medical Association (Walsh, 1972) show that average total patient visits per week for all physicians was 132.5, with average office visits numbering 95.5 per week and average hospital visits 38.3; the general practitioner in a nonmetropolitan area averaged 210.8 patient visits per week. Salaries for employed physicians have escalated to the point where some organizations are offering over $75,000 a year to doctors just out of residency training. Discussions with physicians newly established in private practice related to primary care indicates that within six months of setting up shop they are so busy that they are turning away patients. Thus, at the current time, it does not appear that the average physician needs to or does schedule unnecessary visits to increase his income. This limited exposition does not deal, of course, with the issue that the overall demand pattern may have been so "revved-up" by medical practitioners in the past that the individual physician no longer has to act in a consciously self-serving fashion.

Another relatively unexplored area of what may be unnecessary medical-services utilization that might be affected by a physician's interest in personal gain is the ordering of ancillary services in his own office. A recent study by Childs and Hunter (1972) found that physicians providing direct X-ray services to their patients ordered diagnostic radiography for almost twice as many patients as did physicians who referred patients to radiologists for all X-rays. Additionally, the pattern of X-ray work ordered by a physician varied independently of the patient characteristics studied. The authors raised, with appropriate caveats, the following point: "We assume that a physician providing direct X-ray services owned, or had equivalent economic interest in, radiographic or fluoroscopic apparatus and that he operated it in his office. This economic interest would include the capital investment in the apparatus and the income that its use would generate. The physician with X-ray apparatus, therefore, would be motivated to use that apparatus in order to amortize the capital cost as well as to produce income."

There may be other explanations for their findings. A possible one is simply that once the physician has bought a piece of diagnostic equipment, he tends to use it frequently, not primarily to recover the capital investment or increase his income but simply because it is at hand. Bailey (1970) argues that since most ancillary services are available from other "firms" that specialize in them and since he finds that "the individual physician's productivity is not affected by possessing such equipment," the decision to produce the services internally should and can be analyzed separately from the basic decision of whether to order tests at all. That is another area for future investigation of the effect of physician behavior on medical utilization and one that may have some direct implications for attempts to control and regulate physician office fees.

One special aspect of patient disposition is the referral of patients from one physician to another. Williams et al. (1960;1961) in North Carolina found that only 3 percent of the patients seen in general practice were referred to other physicians. Last and White's (1969) study of Vermont general practices showed that the mean referral rate for both specialist and diagnostic examinations was 11.2 for every 1,000 visits or approximately 1.1 percent. The studies suggest that most primary practitioners were attempting to handle the vast majority of their patients' problems without recourse to referral. Evaluations by Peterson et al. (1956) and Clute (1963) of general practitioners in North Carolina and Eastern Canada were both highly critical of the lack of referral. Clute felt that 30 percent of the physicians saw and treated patients who should have been referred to specialists.

Referral rates between specialists appear to be considerably higher than those of general practitioners. In a study of an average week's practice by internists in the Chicago area, Shortell (1972) found that approximately 9 percent of all patient visits led to a referral to another physician. Penchansky and Fox (1970) in a study of prepaid group practice physicians learned that, on the average, 7 percent of the patients seen by urban internists and 9.5 percent of those seen by suburban internists were referred to other physicians. In the study by Johnson et al. (1969), New York internists referred 11.1 percent of their "new" patients to another physician. Given the general similarity of the results, it may be estimated that approximately 10 percent of patient contacts with an internal medicine specialist lead to a referral to another specialist.

The massive increases of future physicians currently in the medical education pipeline and the projected disappearance of general practitioner training make it probable that by the late 1980's American medical practice will consist almost entirely of specialty practice. Thus, it is likely that physician-to-physician referrals will be an increasing factor in determining the overall causal patterns of ambulatory health use.

Several other factors that may tend to increase the relative role of physician guidance in utilization practices are efforts to increase preventive-services utilization, to make health systems more comprehensive, and to increase patient compliance. All involve a more aggressive approach by practitioners to initiate ambulatory-service contacts, both from the outset and in followup care. Therefore, at some future time, a crosscut utilization survey of ambulatory visits may well show that the large majority are initiated by physicians (or other health practitioners) rather than by patients. Finally, one might speculate on the effect that might have on attempts to control patient initiation of services through economic mechanisms, such as deductibles and coinsurance.

Hospital Admissions

In 1971 there were more than thirty million community hospital admissions and expenditures of over twenty-nine billion dollars on hospital care (Cooper and Worthington, 1973). Since 1950 the average expenses per patient per hospital day have risen sixfold. The rise represents not only inflation and changes in hospital care but also a rise from 110.9 to 147.6 admissions per one thousand population per year (Source Book of Health Insurance Data, 1972–73, 1972). The issue of hospital utilization and costs ranks as the priority health-policy problem for public officials.

Physicians are almost totally responsible both legally and functionally for admission of a patient to a hospital, the care he is given, and the length of stay. Research about the physician's role has been largely concerned with the effect of practice organization on admission rates and with the variation in length of hospital stay. Most studies in the former category in recent years have focused on the lower admission rates of prepaid group practices compared with fee-for-service practice (Anderson and Sheatsley, 1959; Densen et al., 1962; 1960; Klarman, 1963; Perrott, 1971; Shapiro and Brindle, 1969). With the exception, however, of a study of federal employees under multiple-option plans (Perrott, 1971), few of the studies to date have large comparable populations and none have adequate measures of "out-of-plan" hospital use. With respect to the individual physician's role, there is no study that has tried to determine whether differences in admission rates are due to variations in patients' disease problems or to variations in physician behavior when faced with similar patient problems. Many studies have also been done on the wide variations in average length of stay for similar disease problems and for variations from physician to physician (McNerney et al., 1962; Hearman, 1964; Jones, 1964; Acheson and Feldstein, 1964; Riedel and Fitzpatrick, 1964).

In a recent study of Indiana Blue Cross-Blue Shield data, Praiss found that " . . . there tends to exist a pattern of providing patient care, as indicated by the length of hospitalization, which is relatively consistent within individual physicians regardless of the hospitals in which he practices, or of patient age group or, to a lesser degree, of the patient condition category" (1971:ii).

The Social Security Administration Medicare Analysis of Days of Care (MADOC) shows that average length of hospital stay in the Northeastern United States is approximately twice as long as that of the West Coast. Regional practice variations are often referred to (although Praiss's data indicate that there are also intraregional physician-related variations) but no explanation is given. Conceptually, it is hard to find a plausible explanation for the differences in physician behavior. United States medical education is highly standardized (compared with other forms of education), and there is significant national migration of physicians. In short, the information to date raises more questions than it answers. A key future research question must be: "What causes the variations in length of stay?"

The only major work exploring physician-decision rationales for hospital admission is Anderson and Sheatsley's study, *Hospital Use: A Survey of Patient and Physician Decisions* (1967). Their findings on a sample of 1,628 general admissions are thus worth reviewing in some detail. Their survey (see Fig. 1) indicated that

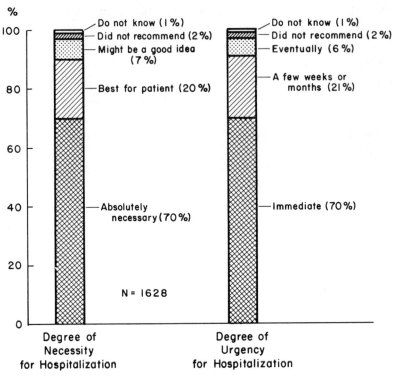

Figure 1. *Attitudes of Recommending Physicians toward Degree of Necessity and Urgency for Hospitalization,
Massachusetts, 12 Months, 1960–1961*

SOURCE: Anderson and Sheatsley (1967).

physicians believed that ninety-seven percent of the admissions
were medically warranted and also that ninety-seven percent of the
cases would either immediately, in the near future, or eventually require admission. Additionally, they felt that only three percent of
medical and four percent of surgical admissions could have been
treated equally well outside the hospital (see Fig. 2). Even with respect to "diagnostic" admissions, physicians reported that only eight
percent could have been treated just as well on the outside. Since
the study was made in 1961, one wonders whether, with the advent

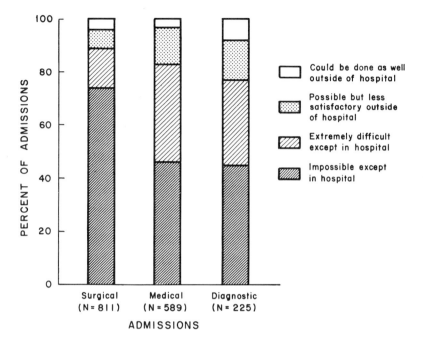

Figure 2. *Classification of Hospital Admissions by Possibility of Outside Treatment, Massachusetts, 12 Months, 1960–1961*

SOURCE: Anderson and Sheatsley (1967).

of Medicare and utilization-review requirements, even these low figures of "unnecessary" admission would be disclosed by physicians today. Another interesting finding was that different sources of payment had no apparent effect on the physician's determination of either the necessity for admission or the length of hospital stay. Clearly, much more probing is needed of the casual dynamics of physician-directed utilization of hospital services. Since the advent of Medicare, however, with its denial of reimbursement for medically "unnecessary" admissions, physicians may be reluctant to disclose information that would increase our understanding of their rationale in hospital-admission decisions.

Medical Decision Practices

The most important factors in understanding the physician's role as a guide to health-services use and the dynamic impact physicians have on overall utilization patterns are the medical-decision concepts upon which diagnosis and treatment are based.

Ledley and Lusted (1959) in their classic paper, "The Reasoning Foundations of Medical Diagnosis," point out that a medical diagnosis is basically a probabilistic determination under conditions of uncertainty because diagnosis "can rarely be made with absolute certainty." Simplistically, in trying to determine between "wellness" and "sickness," a physician can take one of four actions:

(1) dismiss a patient as "well" when the patient is actually *well;*

(2) dismiss a patient as "well" when the patient is actually *sick;*

(3) treat (or continue to investigate) a patient as "sick" when the patient is actually *sick;* or

(4) treat a patient as "sick" when the patient is actually *well.*

Statisticians would label the second decision (i.e., rejecting a hypothesis that is true) as a "type 1" error, and the fourth decision (i.e., accepting a hypothesis that is false) as a "type 2" error.

The single largest element in a physician's judgment affecting medical-services utilization is his desire to avoid committing a type 1 error. Scheff (1963:97–107) made the following comment on that point: "Although there is some sentiment against type 2 errors (unnecessary surgery, for instance) it has nothing like the force and urgency of the sentiment against type 1 errors. A physician who dismisses a patient who subsequently dies of a disease that should have been detected is not only subject to legal action for negligence . . . but also to moral condemnation from his colleagues and from his own conscience. . . . Nothing resembling this amount of moral and legal suasion is brought to bear for committing a type 2 error. Indeed, this error is sometimes seen as sound clinical practice, indicating a healthily conservative approach to medicine." Thus, it is probable that type 2 errors far outnumber type 1 errors in medical practice. A study by Garland (1959), for example, of 14,887 X-ray diagnoses of tuberculosis, found 1,216 false positive readings (type 2 errors) in contrast to only 24 false negative readings (type 1 errors)—a ratio of over 50 to 1.

Even the availability of "hard" data to guide decisionmaking may have little influence on physician behavior. Bell and Loop (1971), for example, published an excellent analysis of clinical criteria for determining whether skull X-rays should be taken in cases of trauma. Use of their "high-yield" criteria would detect ninety-nine percent of all skull fractures and would eliminate the need for doing thirty percent of all X-rays currently performed for suspected skull fractures. Those criteria might save 320,000 persons each year from X-ray exposure and reduce medical-care expenditures by fifteen million dollars a year. When the data from the study were presented, however, to the senior resident staff of a major municipal teaching hospital (who make the decisions on ordering X-rays), every single house-officer stated that he would still continue to order X-rays for all patients who were in the "low yield" category because they could not take the one percent chance of missing a skull fracture!

The implicit and overriding decision norm—"When in doubt, suspect illness and treat (or follow) the patient"—produces a consistent bias for physicians to direct patients to utilize, and overutilize, their own services, hospital services, tests, ancillary services, medication, etc. Although the effect of the bias may be difficult to measure in an individual case, its aggregate impact on health-services utilization is probably enormous.

Ironically perhaps, the more "concerned" or "humanistic" physician may have a greater tendency to commit type 2 errors that lead to higher utilization costs than the "poor" doctor. While the latter may dismiss a patient having vague symptoms with a five-dollar prescription for tranquilizers, the former may schedule multiple tests and followup appointments that cost hundreds of dollars.

An area of great concern related to overtreatment has been the issue of unnecessary surgery. The concern is warranted because, of all general classes of physician procedures, surgery is the one that carries the greatest concomitant risk of death—even when a patient is well. Bunker (1970), Lewis (1969), and others (Anderson and Feldman, 1956; Cope, 1965) have pointed out that there are significant geographic (see Table 1) and socioeconomic variations in rates of surgical procedures. Once again, a solid medical rationale for the wide variation in rates of surgery for procedures like tonsillectomies and herniorrhapies is hard to find. Some critics of the analyses point out that while the U.S. has a greater rate of mastectomies than England and Wales, it also has a higher rate of five-and-ten-year survivals among women who have undergone the procedure.

Another effect of type 2 errors is to unnecessarily put patients in a "sick" role. One study by Bergman and Stamm (1967) illustrates a form of potentially negative results. They screened twenty-five thousand school medical records in Seattle, Washington, for children with heart murmurs. Of one hundred ten positive records, ninety-three chidren were examined; eighteen children had murmurs and organic disease, and seventy-five either had functional murmurs without organic disease or had no murmurs and no organic disease. Thirty of the seventy-five children without disease (or thirty-two percent of the total sample) were found, however, to be psychologically or physically restricted as a consequence of having been labeled as having cardiac disease.

In summary, the implicit decision norm in medical practice—to avoid the error of not detecting and/or treating a patient's illness —strongly influences the direction of health-services utilization. Additionally, it has several serious negative consequences. First, it produces a consistent bias for physicians to overutilize services. Second, to the sorrow of social scientists, it may make aggregate cost-benefit planning and allocation of medical services practically impossible. Finally, it often tends to obscure the potentially harmful effects to an individual of type 2 errors—particularly the serious hazards involved with some diagnostic procedures and therapeutic regimens, and the danger of having a well person entering a "sick" role and becoming eventually disabled or even developing organic disease.

TABLE 1 **Comparative Rates for Selected Operations: the United States and England and Wales**

RATE/1000,000 POPULATION

OPERATION	USA (1965)		England & Wales (1966)	
	Male	Female	Male	Female
Thyroidectomy	9.8	68.5	8.7	42.3
Inguinal herniorrhaphy	508.0	51.1	294.0	29.2
Appendectomy	217.0	180.0	220.7	223.5
Cholecystectomy	94.5	273.0	32.2	89.9
All operations on eye	220.0	223.0	180.6	193.0
Extraction of lens	65.3	82.5	47.2	69.1
Tonsillectomy with or without adenoidectomy	637.0	641.0	322.7	321.9
Adenoidectomy without tonsillectomy	20.7	15.2	49.9	35.6
Hemorrhoidectomy	162.0	137.0	60.5	31.4
Circumcision	96.7		110.0	
Hysterectomy (including subtotal, total & vaginal)		516.0		213.2
All operations on breast	10.9	278.0	5.8	171.7
Partial mastectomy	6.5	196.0	3.0	100.6
Complete (simple) mastectomy		15.0	1.8	27.2
Radical mastectomy		51.0	0.5	25.1
Other operations on breast	4.4	16.0	0.5	18.8

Source: Bunker (1970).

271

Quality of Care

Increasing attention in recent years has been given to the measurement and regulation of the quality of care rendered by physicians. That concern has now been officially expressed in the establishment of Professional Standards Review Organizations (PSRO's) under section 249F of the 1972 Amendments to the Social Security Act (P.L. 92-603). The purpose of the PSRO's, as defined in the law, is " . . . to promote the effective, efficient, and economical delivery of health care services of proper quality . . . through the application of suitable procedures . . . [so] that services for which payment may be made . . . will conform to appropriate professional standards for the provision of health care. . . ." Additionally, it states that each PSRO " . . . shall apply professionally developed norms of care, diagnosis, and treatment based upon typical patterns of practice in its regions (including typical lengths-of-stay for institutional care by age and diagnosis) as principal points of evaluation and review."

The implications are serious both for the physicians—how they will direct utilization of health services—and for the health of patients. Additionally, it has two potentially paradoxical aspects: First, it does not recognize that there can be marked trade-offs between "economy and efficiency" on one hand and "effectiveness and proper quality" on the other. Second, it virtually institutionalizes existing regional variations in care and length of hospital stay, for which (as discussed earlier) there is almost no logical scientific or medical basis.

If the PSRO's function along the line that the federally funded prototype EMCRO's (Experimental Medical Care Review Organizations) have, they may well increase total utilization of health services. The "norms of care" concept has been translated by many of the organizations into the establishment of specific criteria of services that should be rendered for a defined diagnostic condition. Thus, any one physician who does not provide all the services outlined by a "minimal" criteria set will be judged to have rendered poor quality of care. The result will be to establish a floor of utilization for all patients that may be higher than current average utilization. Payne and Lyons (1972) in a study of medical care in Hawaii found that their criteria showed an underprovision (or underutilization) of indicated services of about twenty-five percent.

Another "process" criteria approach, particularly with respect to hospital care, has been to establish "maximal" service criteria, above which no reimbursement would be given. Unfortunately, that approach may produce a tendency for physicians to give or order all services that could be reimbursed; one study (Gertman, 1971) of such a maximal criteria set estimated that it could produce a thirty to fifty percent rise in hospital costs. Additionally, many observers are concerned that such criteria will force upon physicians a rigid uniformity in the provision of services.

Finally, studies by Brook and Stevenson (1970), Brook (1972a), Williamson et al. (1968), and others (Starfield and Scheff, 1971; Codman, 1916) raise serious doubts whether criteria of "good" medical-care process can validly and reliably be related to measures of "good" end results (or outcomes) of care. In a recent review of the research evidence for the Office of the Secretary of Health, Education, and Welfare, Brook made the following conclusion: "The assessment of quality of care based on process data must be dependent on physician judgment in terms of either establishing a list of process criteria statements, reading the medical record, or reading a case abstract. In terms of the studies noted above, this judgment is likely to include many tests and procedures whose benefit in preventing future impairment is questionable. *The end product of a system assessing process is likely to be higher medical care costs without major improvement in the health of the population*" (1972b:25).

Summary

The interacting effects of the factors discussed in this paper are likely to have a considerable and unidirectional impact on the utilization of health services. More care in the future is likely to be initiated at the direction of physicians, rather than by consumers. Initiation of care by physicians will tend to be biased towards overutilization because of a desire to avoid type 1 decision errors. And finally, despite an implicit bias to overutilize, we may have a national regulatory system that will set even higher patterns of health-service utilization. It seems that increasing physician guidance of health-care use in the United States, based on what little we currently know about the behavior of physicians and their rationale for medical utilization decisions, could drive national health-care expenditures to undreamed-of levels (particularly if financing is liberalized under a form of national health insurance).

Therefore, if our society wishes to have control over utilization of health care, it seems imperative to develop a better understanding of the mysterious behavior of that key decisionmaker—the physician—and the rationale he employs in guiding the use of health services.

References

Acheson, E. D. *and* M. S. Feldstein
    1964   "Duration of stay in hospital for normal maternity care." British Journal of Medicine 2: 95–99.
Anderson, O. W. *and* J. J. Feldman
    1956   Family Medical Costs and Voluntary Health Insurance: A Nationwide Survey. New York: McGraw-Hill Book Company.
Anderson, O. W. *and* P. B. Sheatsley
    1959   Comprehensive Medical Insurance: A Study of Costs, Use, and Attitudes Under Two Plans, Research Series No. 9. Chicago: University of Chicago, Center for Health Administration Studies.
    1967   Hospital Use: A Survey of Patient and Physician Decisions, Research Series No. 24. Chicago: University of Chicago, Center for Health Administration Studies.
Bailey, R. M.
    1970   "Economies of scale in medical practice." Pp. 255–273 in

Klarman, H. E. *and* H. H. Jaszl (eds.), Empirical Studies in Health Economics. Baltimore: The Johns Hopkins Press.

Bell, R. S. *and* J. W. Loop
  1971   "The utility and futility of radiographic skull examinations for trauma." New England Journal of Medicine 284: 236–239.

Bergman, A. B. *and* S. F. Stamm
  1967   "The morbidity of cardiac non-disease in school children." New England Journal of Medicine 276: 1008–1013.

Brook, R. H.
  1972a   A Study of Methodological Problems Associated with Assessment of Quality of Care. Baltimore: Johns Hopkins University, Department of Medical Care and Hospitals.
  1972b   "The quality of medical care received by poor people: A proposition paper." Unpublished paper.

Brook, R. H. *and* R. L. Stevenson
  1970   "Effectiveness of patient care in an emergency room." New England Journal of Medicine 283: 904–907.

Bunker, J. P.
  1970   "Surgical manpower: A comparison of operations and surgeons in the United States and in England and Wales." New England Journal of Medicine 282 (January 15): 135–144.

Childs, A. W. *and* E. E. Hunter
  1972   "Non-medical factors influencing use of diagnostic X-rays by physicians." Medical Care 10: 333–334.

Clute, K. F.
  1963   The General Practitioner: A Study of Medical Education and Practice in Ontario and Nova Scotia. Toronto: University of Toronto Press.

Codman, E. A.
  1916   A Study of Hospital Efficiency: The First Five Years. Boston: Thomas Todd Company.

Cooper, B. S. *and* N. L. Worthington
  1973   "National health expenditures, 1929–1972." Social Security Bulletin 36: 3–19.

Cope, O.
  1965   "Unnecessary surgery and technical competence: Irreconcilables in the graduate training of a surgeon." American Journal of Surgery 110: 119–123.

Creditor, M. C. *and* U. K. Creditor
   1972   "The ecology of an urban voluntary hospital: 2. The referral chain." Medical Care 10: 88–92.
Densen, P. M., et al.
   1960   "Prepaid medical care and hospital utilization in a dual choice situation." American Journal of Public Health 50: 1710–1726.
   1962   "Prepaid medical care and hospital utilization: Comparison of a group practice and self-insurance situation." Hospitals 36: 63–68.
Garland, L. H.
   1959   "Studies on the accuracy of diagnostic procedures." American Journal of Roent. 82: 25–38.
Gertman, P. M.
   1971   "Effect of process criteria on hospital costs: A working paper." Washington, D.C.: President's Advisory Council on Management Improvement.
Hearman, M. A.
   1964   "How long in hospital." Lancet 2: 539–541.
Jones, F. A.
   1964   "Length of stay in hospital." Lancet 1: 321–322.
Johnson, A. C., H. H. Kroeger, I. Altman, D. A. Clark, *and* C. G. Sheps
   1965   "The office practice of internists: III. Characteristics of patients." Journal of the American Medical Association 193 (September 13): 916–922.
Klarman, H. E.
   1963   "Effect of prepaid group practice on hospital use." Public Health Reports 17: 955–965.
Kohn, R.
   1973   Personal Communication.
Last, J. M. *and* K. L. White
   1969   "The content of medical care in primary practice." Medical Care 7: 41–48.
Ledley, R. S. *and* L. B. Lusted
   1959   "Reasoning foundations of medical diagnosis." Science 130: 9–21.
Lewis, C. E.
   1969   "Variations in the incidence of surgery." New England Journal of Medicine 281: 880–884.

McNerney, W. J., et al.
1962   Hospitals and Medical Economics. Chicago: Hospital Research and Educational Trust.

Mushlin, A. I. *and* D. Barr
1973   Personal Communication.

Payne, B. G. *and* T. F. Lyons
1972   "Methods of evaluating and improving personal medical care quality: Office case study." Ann Arbor: University of Michigan, February.

Penchansky, R. *and* D. Fox
1970   "Frequency of referral and patient characteristics in group practice." Medical Care 8: 368–385.

Perrott, G. S.
1971   "The federal employees health benefits program: Enrollment and utilization of health services—1961–1968." Washington, D.C.: Government Printing Office.

Peterson, W., et al.
1956   "An analytical study of North Carolina general practice." Journal of Medical Education 31 (Part 2): 121.

Praiss, J.
1971   A Study of the Variations in the Use of Hospital Services Within the Practices of Individual Physicians. Baltimore: Johns Hopkins University, Department of Medical Care and Hospitals.

Richardson, W. C.
1971   Ambulatory Use of Physician Services in Response to Illness Episodes in a Low-Income Neighborhood, Research Series No. 29. Chicago: University of Chicago, Center for Health Administration Studies.

Riedel, D. C. *and* T. B. Fitzpatrick
1964   Patterns of Patient Care. Ann Arbor: University of Michigan.

Scheff, T. J.
1963   "Decision rules, types of errors, and their consequences in medical diagnosis." Behavioral Science 8: 97–107.

Shapiro, S. *and* J. Brindle
1969   "Serving Medicaid eligibles." American Journal of Public Health 59: 635–641.

Shortell, S. M.
    1972   A Model of Physician Referral Behavior: A Test of Exchange Theory in Medical Practice, Research Series No. 31. Chicago: University of Chicago, Center for Health Administration Studies.

Source Book of Health Insurance Data 1972–1973
    1972   New York: Health Insurance Institute.

Starfield, B. *and* D. Scheff
    1971   Assessment of Patient Care: Process and Outcome. Baltimore: Johns Hopkins University, Department of Medical Care and Hospitals.

Walsh, R. J.
    1972   Socioeconomic Issues of Health. Chicago: American Medical Association, Center for Health Services Research and Development.

White, E. L.
    1972   "Current estimates from the Health Interview Survey, United States, 1970." Vital and Health Statistics 10 (72).

White, K. L., T. F. Williams, *and* B. G. Greenberg
    1961   "The ecology of medical care." New England Journal of Medicine 265: 885–892.

Williams, T. F., K. L. White, L. P. Andrews, E. Diamond, B. G. Greenberg, A. A. Hamrick, *and* E. A. Hunter
    1960   "Patient referral to a university clinic: Patterns in a rural state." American Journal of Public Health 50: 1493.

Williams, T. F., K. L. White, W. L. Fleming, *and* B. G. Greenberg
    1961   "The referral process in medical care and the university clinic's role." Journal of Medical Education 36: 899–907.

Williamson, J. W., J. Mitchell, *and* S. Kreider
    1968   Outcomes of Medical Care: A Study of Heart Failure Management in Emergency Rooms. Baltimore: Johns Hopkins University, Department of Medical Care and Hospitals.

Alternative Physician Payment Methods: Incentives, Efficiency, and National Health Insurance

Jon R. Gabel and Michael A. Redisch

Health Care Financing Administration,
U.S. Department of Health, Education, and Welfare;
and U.S. General Accounting Office

O NE REASON that the long and sometimes acrimonious debate concerning National Health Insurance (NHI) continues is that NHI means different things to different persons. While there is general agreement among proponents that NHI should provide financial protection against catastrophic medical expenses, there is a wide divergence of opinion as to broader objectives. Some view NHI's principal purpose as removing financial barriers to care, while others see NHI as the vehicle to reorganize our health care delivery system on a more efficient basis.

For those individuals concerned with reorganizing our health delivery system, few issues have greater importance or generate as much controversy as the method for paying physicians. Each payment method raises philosophical questions regarding the freedom and independence of the individual physician. Moreover, because the physician is the dominant individual in the health care system, physician payment methods will affect not only the quality, quantity, and intensity of services in the $32 billion U.S. physician sector, but also those in the $131 billion non-physician health sector (Gibson and Fischer, 1978).

0026-3745-79-5701-0038-22/$01.00/0 © 1979 Milbank Memorial Fund

This article's intended audience is not the well-published health economist, but the interested health professional who wishes to familiarize himself or herself with some of the implications of alternative methods of paying physicians. We are well aware that physicians are both social and economic beings, and that many non-economic factors are important in determining their behavior patterns and in defining the scope of health policy goals. We have chosen to confine ourselves, however, primarily to analyzing the reactions of physicians to changes in their economic environment.

In the first section, the three major physician payment methods (fee-for-service, capitation, and salary) will be described. The second section will review physician pricing behavior. In the third section, the implications of alternative payment methods will be explored with respect to five dimensions of medical practice: 1) utilization of physician and nonphysician services; 2) treatment setting; 3) location decision; 4) specialty choice; and 5) efficiency of an individual physician's practice. The concluding section will discuss the present and future role of physician reimbursement within the current Washington health policy environment.

Three Methods of Paying Physicians

Fee-for-service is the predominant physician payment method in the United States. We estimate that, with interns and residents included, 71% of the U.S. non-federal, patient-care physicians are paid by this method. The alternative payment systems, salary and capitation, account for an estimated 28% and 1%, respectively. Combination methods, utilized by certain health maintenance organizations (HMOs), encompass a very small proportion of the nation's physicians.

Under the fee-for-service method, the physician charges a fee for each rendered unit of service, such as an office visit, chest X-ray, appendectomy. Approximately 61% of the physician payments in fiscal year 1976 were financed by third-party payors, and 39% came directly from patients (Gibson and Fischer, 1978). With fee-for-service payment, the third-party payors reimburse the physician for each service provided using either one of two methods. Twenty-four state Medicaid agencies, a minority of U.S. private health insurance plans, and most of the other nations of the Western world use *fee schedules* to determine the maximum level of reimbursement for each service (Burney and Gabel, 1979). Medicare, 26 state Medicaid agencies, and a majority of the private health insurance plans use a system unique to America, called *"customary, prevailing and reasonable* (CPR) reimbursement."

Fee schedules designate the maximum level of third-party reimbursement for a specific service, with the physician's actual payment level being the lesser of the billed charge or the fee schedule level. The fee schedule may be established prospectively through negotiations between insurance companies and medical societies, as it is done in most Western European nations, or on the basis of a survey of physician's billed charges (Glaser, 1977). State Medicaid agencies usually establish their schedules by applying a conversion factor to a relative value system. For example, if an initial office visit has a relative value of three units, and the conversion factor is $10, then Medicaid would pay a physician a maximum of $30.00 for an initial office visit.

The CPR method establishes a separate fee schedule for each individual physician and requires that the third-party payor maintain a "profile" on each physician for each unit of service he or she provides. The physician is then reimbursed for each of these units of service or procedures on the basis of the lowest of his *actual* charge, his *customary* charge, or the area's *prevailing* charge. Under Medicare, the customary charge for a procedure is the physician's median billed charge for that particular procedure during the previous calendar year. The area prevailing charge for each procedure is the 75th percentile of the distribution of all customary charges of "similar" physicians within a given "market area" during the previous calendar year weighted by the number of times each physician has billed for that given service or procedure. Definition of the terms "similar" and "market area" are left to the discretion of the Medicare carriers. Under Blue Shield, the equivalent of the Medicare prevailing charge is typically set at the 90th percentile of the distribution of physician charges. Commercial insurers generally set their prevailing rate at the 92nd percentile of the distribution of physician charges (Dyckman, 1978).

Salary and capitation are the two major alternatives to fee-for-service payment of physicians. The salaried approach pays the physician for a specified period of time, regardless of the number of units of service provided or the number of persons served. This arrangement is usually associated with an organized institutional setting such as a hospital, clinic, medical school or health maintenance organization, rather than an individual practitioner's office. Salaries may be on a full- or part-time basis and vary in accordance with the physician's training, professional skills, seniority, scope of responsibility, and with the financial position of the institution.

Under the capitation payment method, the physician's level of remuneration is determined by the number of persons enrolled, rather than the number of services performed as under the fee-for-service system. Capitation is usually associated with physician groups, including those that resemble health maintenance organizations (HMOs) or their hybrid forms, e.g., "HMOs without walls," such as the Madison Blue Shield Health Maintenance Plan. Under a capitation system, physicians, acting individually or as part of a group, agree to provide a specified level of medical benefits to enrollees for a certain period of time for a predetermined amount.[1]

Physician Pricing—Income vs Utility Maximization

Two alternative models explaining physician pricing behavior appear in the health economics literature. Both models are usually applied to a fee-for-service payment method.

The first, the profit-maximizing model, hypothesizes that physicians set their fees so that they may maximize their absolute incomes. The profit maximization model is compatible with either a competitive or a monopolistic market structure.

The second, the utility maximization model, hypothesizes that physicians price their services at a level different from the one necessary to attain the maximum profit level, but in a manner that will allow them to achieve other goals.[2] A popular variant of this model is the target income hypothesis whereby physicians price their

---

[1]The reader should not confuse lump-sum prepayment for HMO membership by a patient with capitation payment to the individual physician. In the U.S., the majority of physicians employed in HMOs are salaried. Throughout the remainder of the article, capitation payment refers to individual physicians, not organizations.

[2]Feldstein has suggested that physicians set prices to create a situation of permanent excess demand so that they can more easily choose "interesting cases" and pluck them from their long queues. See Feldstein, 1970.

services in an attempt to obtain a predetermined income level.[3] Left unspecified is how the desired level is determined, although presumably it is set by comparison with the local income distribution in general and the local physician modal income, in particular.

Physician pricing models have profound policy implications because they yield conflicting predictions concerning the likely change in physicians' fees should the supply of physicians increase—and approximately one of every five physicians in the U.S. is currently in residency or internship. The income maximization model suggests lower fees in most situations where new physicians pour into the system, whereas the utility maximization model can easily coexist with higher fees.

The physician pricing controversy often centers upon the issue of whether and to what extent physicians can generate or induce demand for their services. A number of structural characteristics in the market for physician services appears to make this possible. Foremost among these is that the fee-for-service practitioner is a for-profit entrepreneur who acts as an agent for the patient, providing information that will influence the patient's future purchases of medical care. The physician's conflict of interest arises from the fact that the agent also provides a part of the medical services.

Second, the medical profession—like its legal, accounting, optometric, and mortician counterparts—has historically limited competition through a code of ethics and through direct restrictions on supply. Among the practices physicians have in the past specified as unethical are the publishing of fee information or the tendering of patient care information to a patient for whom the physician is not the designated attending physician. Violation of the code may result in a loss of referrals from peers or expulsion from the local medical society, with possible loss of hospital privileges (Kessel, 1958; Hsaio, 1975).[4]

These factors render the demand for physicians' already heterogeneous services relatively more inelastic by lowering the

---

[3]For a more complete discussion of physician pricing models, see Reinhardt, 1975; Sloan and Feldman, 1978; Redisch, Gabel, and Blaxall, 1979.

[4]Since 1958 when Kessel wrote his article, there have been a number of court rulings that suggest that local medical society membership is no longer a necessary condition for local hospital staff privileges.

cross-price elasticity of demand for the services of other physicians. That is, a physician's patients become less responsive to changes in fees or other practice characteristics of similar physicians in the community. The greater this inelasticity of demand, the greater is the individual physician's discretion over price, quantity, and quality, and the greater is the physician's potential to behave as a price setter. Economists use the term "monopolist" to describe an individual or firm that can set a price for a product, rather than accept a price determined by an outside market.

While there is growing consensus that physicians are price setters, there is still controversy over the degree to which physicians can influence demand for their products. The extent that physicians can generate or induce demand for their services centers upon three interrelated empirical questions:

1. Does an increase in the number of physicians lead to an increase in the utilization of physician services, on a per capita basis?

2. Does an increase in the number of physicians result in higher or lower fees?

3. Does an increase in physicians result in lower or higher physician incomes?

Evidence to date on the first question indicates that greater numbers of physicians per capita are associated with greater utilization of physician services per capita. This is particularly true for elective surgery involving non-functional tissues. Fuchs (1978) estimated that a 1% increase in the density of surgeons will lead to a 0.33% increase in surgery per capita. Another noteworthy study on the ability of physicians to control utilization was that of Wennberg and Gittelsohn (1973), who found that the probability of tonsils removed by a specific age ranged from 8% to 62% across 13 Vermont areas, and the probability of uterus loss by age 75 ranged from 24% to 52%. The 1975 *Study of Surgical Services for the United States* (SOSSUS) examined surgery rates in four metropolitan areas and found the surgery rate per population positively related to surgeon density (American College of Surgeons, 1975). Mathematica Policy Research (1978) estimated that for males ages 5 to 8 in Quebec, a 1% increase in physician density led to both a 0.61% increase in visits per capita and a 1.54% increase in lower priority surgical payments per capita.

Research results on the second question, how an increase in physicians affects fees, are not as definitive. An increasing body of evidence indicates, however, that physician density and fee levels are positively related. Earlier studies suffered from a number of methodological problems, including small samples of procedures and geographic areas, incomplete data on physicians' incomes and hours, and use of cross-sectional as opposed to time-series data bases. Recent work by the authors using a national census of Medicare prevailing charges and a national sample of physicians' actual charges, hours, incomes, and practice costs validate these earlier studies (Redisch, Gabel, and Blaxall, 1979).

Most research on the third question, how an increase in physicians affects physician income, has concluded that increases in physician density results in decreases in real physician income (i.e., adjusting for cost-of-living). The income decrease, however, is not nearly in proportion to the change in physician density. Higher real incomes in lower density areas reflect longer hours and higher levels of patient visits per hour, both of which compensate for lower physician fees (Sloan and Feldman, 1978). Based upon a national sample of 1014 physicians, recent work by the authors tends to support this relationship. Physicians in counties with more than 200 physicians per 100,000 population had incomes nearly 5% greater (unadjusted for cost-of-living) than those in similar specialties from physician-scarce counties. Proper adjusting for living differentials would have reversed the relationship. Physicians in physician-rich areas were able to compensate for the fact that their weekly patient load was nearly 40% lower than their peers from physician-scarce areas. They achieved this near parity in incomes by charging higher fees and by providing and billing for a more intense and complex set of services (Redisch et al., 1979).

Paying the Physician—Implications for Selected Policy Issues

Within each particular payment method, dramatically different incentives are possible according to the specific set of administrative practices employed. For example, fee-for-service in combination with fee schedules could encourage physicians to select surgery as a specialty or primary care, depending upon the relative value system employed. Capitation could encourage or discourage hospitalization of patients depending on the extent to which primary-care physicians bear the financial risk for hospital and specialty care.

The potential effectiveness of any "economic" market strategy for achieving a particular objective, such as remedying geographic maldistribution of physicians or containing rising costs, may be determined by two overriding principles.

The first principle concerns risk-sharing between the individual physician and the remainder of the health sector. Because the physician is the key individual who makes patient-care decisions, guarding access to the system, admitting and releasing the patient from the hospital, ordering diagnostic tests, prescribing drugs, and suggesting and performing surgery, the physician affects not only the $32 billion physician sector, but also the $131 billion non-physician sector. With risk-sharing, the multiplier effect of any physician reimbursement policy is increased, since the cost of the non-physician health sector will be partially borne by the physician. With this approach, hospital services can no longer be regarded as free to the physician, since overbedding, unnecessary hospitalization and excessive availability or use of technology become explicit costs to the physician (Redisch, 1978).

The second principle is that public policy makers may wield greater power to constrain physician expenditures and services under a salary or capitation arrangement than a fee-for-service one. Organized medicine seems well aware of this possibility. With pressure from state medical societies, 46 states have passed legislation outlawing the "corporate practice of medicine." Many states have interpreted this legislation as outlawing the salary arrangement for compensating physicians for patient care activities.

The greater the extent that physicians can induce demand under fee-for-service, the less effective will be the price incentives that policy makers might develop to remedy perceived problems. In Canada, the physician fee index increased only 6.3% per year from 1965–1972, but physicians' net incomes increased by 10.1% per year and per capita expenditures for physicians' services by 12.4% (Lewin and Associates, 1976). West Germany limited fee increases to an average of 2.3% in 1974, but higher utilization of diagnostic procedures resulted in an increase in expenditures of approximately 14% (Reinhardt, 1976). Based upon a sample of 5000 solo-practice physicians in California, the Urban Institute reports that wage-price controls "were successful in controlling the rise in physician fees . . ." but not "the rate of increase in Medicare expenditures for physician services" (Holahan, Hadley, Scanlon et al., 1978). Physicians increased the quantity of services to Medicare patients by approximately 10% per year during the control years. Following the expiration of controls, Medicare reimbursements increased by nearly 11% per procedure, but the volume of services declined slightly (Holahan et al., 1978).

In the next sections, the effect of the three major physician reimbursement methods upon five selected dimensions of medical practice will be discussed: 1) utilization of physician and non-physician services; 2) treatment setting; 3) location decision; 4) specialty choice; and 5) efficiency of an individual physician's practice. For each physician payment method, implicit incentives will be discussed in terms of achieving selected policy objectives.

Utilization of Physician and Non-Physician Services

We noted previously that fee-for-service incentives encourage the physician to provide a larger quantity and more intense mix of services. The financial incentive associated with capitation leads to maximization of patient enrollments while providing the minimal necessary level of services required to the individual enrollee. Under the salary arrangement, the quantity of services provided by an individual physician is unrelated to the level of the physician's remuneration.

This hypothesized behavior is supported by results from a number of studies. The evidence is particularly strong in the area of surgery and hospitalization. In the late 1950s, New York's Group Health Insurance (GHI) and the New York Health Insurance Plan (HIP) both provided a wide range of services to a similar patient population at a marginal out-of-pocket cost of nearly zero. HIP contracted with groups of physicians on a capitation basis while GHI physicians were paid on a fee-for-service basis. The surgery and hospitalization rates for HIP enrollees were almost one-half the rate for GHI enrollees (Anderson and Sheatsley, 1959). Gaus, Cooper, and Hirschman (1976) compared various aspects of HMO performance with that of the non-prepaid, fee-for-service system for the Medicaid population. It was found that Medicaid beneficiaries

enrolled in two medical foundations exhibited no statistically significant differences in hospital use when compared with a matched sample of Medicaid beneficiaries utilizing the fee-for-service system.
These foundations accepted capitation payment for their Medicaid
enrollees, but reimbursed affiliated physicians on a fee-for-service
system. In contrast, Medicaid beneficiaries enrolled in a group of
HMOs with non-fee-for-service physicians were observed to have
356 days of hospital care per 1000 persons per year. This was a
remarkable 62% lower than the 934 days per person per year
measured for the fee-for-service Medicaid control group (Gaus et al.,
1976). On a macro level, the British capitation-salary system
observes a per capita surgery rate about one-half that of the U.S.
fee-for-service oriented system (Bunker, 1970). Similarly, Adelstein
found that the number of X-rays per capita is substantially greater in
the U.S. than in other countries where radiologists (and other
physicians practicing in hospitals) are reimbursed on a salaried basis
(Adelstein, 1973).

Although it may be easier to support empirically the hypothesis
that fee-for-service physician payment leads to higher utilization
levels than salary or capitation, it is more difficult to determine if
there are too many operations, X-rays, and laboratory tests under
fee-for-service, or too few under capitation or salary. As support for
the former notion, we note that many prestigious, high-quality
medical centers—such as the Mayo Clinic—are staffed by salaried
physicians.

Treatment Setting

Glaser (1978b) notes a concern throughout the Western world over
the increasing costs of hospitalization. In the United States, four
aspects of our present fee-for-service physician reimbursement approach can be identified as contributing to the hospitalization rate.

1. More Comprehensive Insurance. Public and private insurance
coverage (but particularly private) tends to be more comprehensive
the more institutionalized the care. Most private insurance companies insure physician services in the hospital, but offer more
limited coverage in ambulatory settings. Within the hospital, physician and other services in the intensive care unit are covered at higher
rates than in non-intensive hospital areas and services provided in

both of these areas are covered more extensively than home health or nursing home care. For example, when a patient is placed in an intensive care unit, he may receive the equivalent of private duty nursing, at near zero out-of-pocket cost to the patient.

Thus, a perverse set of incentives is developed, whereby the lower the cost at the margin to the patient, the higher are the costs to society, and the higher are the marginal revenues to the physician. This encourages the physician to suggest higher utilization of services in expensive treatment settings.

2. Free Hospital Services to Physicians. Hospital inputs, such as equipment, personnel, supplies, are essentially free to the physician. Most third-party payors reimburse hospitals on a cost or full charge basis with no patient cost-sharing after the deductible is met. Of all hospital revenues, 92% is paid by third-party payors, compared to 20% for ambulatory visits (Gibson and Fischer, 1978). Therefore, the mutual economic interests of the patient and physician lie with expensive inpatient care covered by third-party reimbursement.

3. Relative Value Schedules Used by Insurers. Contributing to the strong technological and institutionalized orientation in the U.S. has been the set of values embodied in present relative value schedules (RVS) used by insurers. As noted previously, fee schedules may use RVSs to define the maximum amount of third-party reimbursement for a particular procedure. The CPR systems use relative value schedules to determine payment when an individual physician has performed a specific procedure an inadequate number of times to calculate the customary charge. Traditionally, RVSs used by U.S. insurers have tended to value services provided in institutional settings and technology-related services such as laboratory and radiological services more generously than ambulatory services. For example, the 1964 California Relative Value System, employed by more than one-half of the Medicare carriers, assigns a relative value unit of 1 to a routine office and hospital follow-up visit, 80 relative units to a reduction of a fracture, and 1.2 units for a complete blood count (California Medical Association, 1964). An ordinary office follow-up visit requires 13 minutes of a physician's time, whereas a reduction of fracture requires 120 physician minutes. A complete blood count may require less than 1 minute of a physician's time. Moreover, since the average cost of operating primary care office practices is approximately 60% of the gross revenues (American Medical Association, 1976), and hospital resources are free to the physician, $10 for a follow-up hospital visit provides over twice the net income to the physician as $10 for a follow-up office visit.

4. Fewer Ancillary Personnel in Office Practice. In addition to the rational substitution of "free" hospital resources for explicit and costly office resources, physicians are estimated to employ fewer than the optimal number of ancillary personnel, such as physician assistants, nurses, and technicians for their office practices. Reinhardt explains the failure to hire the profit maximizing number of employees as the physician's aversion to managerial and entrepreneurial risk (Reinhardt, 1975). Since few physicians have any training in managerial skills, this aversion is not surprising.

Degree of Financial Risk for Physicians. Capitation can encourage or discourage physicians to treat patients in an office or hospital setting, depending upon the extent that physicians bear the financial risk for the use of non-office resources. In Britain, primary care physicians are paid on a capitation arrangement, but are not at risk for the hospital sector. If a patient requires extensive services, it is in the physician's economic interest to refer the patient to the hospital where he or she will be cared for by salaried specialists. By doing so, the primary care physician will not have to bear the cost of treating the patient, while simultaneously sacrificing zero income from his predetermined capitated payment. The effect of Britain's capitation of primary care services without institutional risk is to exacerbate the already-existing long waits for hospitalization that are attributable to the limited number of hospital beds per capita. This is countered somewhat by the use in hospitals only of salaried specialists, who do not have a financial interest in seeing patients hospitalized.

Physicians who bear the financial risk for the use of hospital and other institutional resources face a different set of incentives. Since the primary pool of physicians must now pay the hospital and specialists for the care of the hospitalized patient, the primary care physicians' economic interests are to substitute less costly ambulatory care for more costly hospital care and to limit the number of specialty referrals. We feel quality of care could replace cost containment as the dominant policy issue under a "capitation with risk" reimbursement system.

California Medicaid Scandal. The potential abuses of such a system were demonstrated by the recent scandals of the Medicaid program in California. In 1971, the State contracted with prepaid health plans (PHP) on a capitation basis, expecting to lower utilization of resources in general and hospitalization rates in particular. Hospitalization rates did fall to phenomenally low levels. (Some PHPs with enrollments in the thousands had as few as 7 hospitalization days per month!) Subsequent investigations and lawsuits discovered that this was achieved by contracting with proprietary hospitals 30 to 50 miles from the catchment areas, long waits to see primary care physicians (who were usually non-fluent foreign medical graduates), short operating hours, denial of emergency services, and almost total absence of referrals to specialists (Rowland, 1973).

The California PHP scandals may be the other side of the Medicaid mill phenomenon. Both demonstrate the vulnerability of fee-for-service and capitation-type public financing programs to abuse and fraud by medical entrepreneurs, who in these two instances responded to diametrically opposite incentives.

Under the salary method, whether or not physicians will be encouraged to treat patients in ambulatory settings may be dependent upon the criteria that are used to evaluate physicians' pay increases. If compensation is based upon years of service, there will be no incentive to the individual physician to use the most efficient combination of inputs, including the treatment setting.

In contrast to fee-for-service or capitation payment, under the salary method both ambulatory and hospital resources are free to the physician. So, while there is no reward for efficient use of resources, there is also no economic motivation to substitute hospital resources for physician resources. The former, while "free" to the physician, are very costly to society.

Location Decision

A national concern exists over the geographic distribution of physicians in the United States. Physicians tend to concentrate in high-income communities within metropolitan areas resulting in much lower physician-population ratios in the inner city and rural areas than elsewhere in the country. In the 354 counties where the physician-population ratio is lower than 25 physicians per 100,000 population, access to medical care may be limited by the absolute scarcity of physician manpower.

Voluminous research has identified many factors that influence the physician's location decision. Most of this research is in agreement that financial factors are of minor importance in the physician's location choice (Institute of Medicine, 1976). However, these studies usually assess the effect of small changes in financial incentives. The principal lesson from the literature may be that the present system is in equilibrium and that "fine tuning" of the physician reimbursement mechanism will not significantly change the existing physician distribution, unless financial inducements are extremely powerful and the physicians in oversupplied areas are threatened with their very economic survival.

Glaser (1977) has noted that, in Western industrial nations, fees in urban physician-rich areas historically tended to exceed those in rural physician-poor areas. This pattern is found in the United States today. A recent HEW study reports that Medicare prevailing fees in counties with more than 300 physicians per 100,000 population are 33% greater than those prevailings in counties with fewer than 25 physicians per 100,000 population (Burney and Gabel, 1978). Most physician surveys have found that the Medicare fee pattern is representative of the general physician fee pattern.

Under fee-for-service, to encourage physicians to practice in underserved areas, fee schedules (or prevailings) could potentially be set relatively lower in physician-rich areas than in physician-shortage areas. However, if physicians can create their own demand and compensate for lower prices with induced higher quantities of services, this policy will have little effect on total outlays.

Capitation payment has great potential for serving as a self-correcting market mechanism. If payment per patient is set at identical rates throughout the nation, the average physician's income will be directly proportional to the area population-physician ratio. Currently, physicians' incomes for underserved areas such as Benton County, Missouri, where one physician serves 9300 individuals, are slightly higher than in Manhattan, New York, where one physician serves 122 individuals (American Medical Association, 1974). Under the previously described capitation arrangement, Benton physicians' incomes would be approximately 80 times as great as Manhattan's. In contrast to fee-for-service payment, supply-induced demand will result in zero marginal revenue to the physician.

Like capitation, salary payment has the attribute that physician-induced demand will result in zero marginal revenue to the physician. The critical question for a health care system whose physicians are predominantly salaried is the mechanism that allocates the physician slots and salaries. If a central planning agency is responsible for distributing positions, the overall distribution will reflect the competency of the planning agency and the strength of interest groups. If hospitals, clinics, and HMOs retain the autonomy to hire, the physician distribution may approximate the distribution of the financial strength of these employer institutions. If salaries are higher in urban than rural areas, then salary incentives could prove to be as perverse as present fee-for-service ones.

Specialty Choice

Geographic disparities in physician manpower tend to be reinforced by post-war trends in the supply of subspecialty medicine. From 1940 to 1973, there was a decrease in the ratio of general and family practitioners to population from 90.6 per 100,000 to below 30 per 100,000 (Institute of Medicine, 1976). Subspecialists are much more likely than general or family practitioners to locate in urban areas, to be near a large population base and a high technology hospital. The effect has been not only to limit access to primary health care services, but also to increase health care costs through provision of services by higher cost specialists with greater use of technology and hospital services.

With respect to specialty choice, different sets of incentives are possible for each payment method. Under fee-for-service systems, for example, relative value schedules can be designed to reward primary care physicians financially relative to surgeons. As noted previously, present systems favor surgeons and other specialists (radiologists, pathologists) who provide discrete, easily itemizable services.

Glaser observes that throughout the Western industrial world, urban specialists tend to dominate the committees that create relative value systems. Although recently general practitioners have tended to assume a greater role, the committees predictably produce systems favorable to urban specialists (Glaser, 1978a). Previously, it was noted that U.S. relative value systems set physically distinct procedures such as laboratory tests, X-rays, and tonsillectomies higher than non-distinct services such as office visits. Physically distinct tasks are not only more likely to be performed by specialists in their rent-free workshop, the hospital, but are more likely to be covered by insurance. Sloan and Steinwald (1975) estimate that 80% of the surgical services are paid for by third-party payors, whereas only 20% of office visits are so paid. The cumulative effect of these factors is reflected in the specialty income distribution where, according to a 1973 AMA survey, specialists' net incomes averaged 33% higher than incomes of primary care physicians (American Medical Association, 1976).

The income and hour figures for individual specialties emphasize this point. The *Study of Surgical Services for the United States* (American College of Surgeons, 1975) revealed that the average work week for surgeons was 40.2 hours a week, and that surgeons perform an average of 3.5 operations per week. An Arthur Andersen study (1977) of hospital-based physicians' incomes disclosed that in 1975 the average full-time equivalent net compensation for pathologists, radiologists, and anesthesiologists paid a percentage of net or gross department billings, was $138,200, $124,000, and $87,400, respectively. This is in contrast with the average self-reported pediatrician's income of $50,000 and general practitioner's of $44,800 (Sloan, Cromwell, and Mitchell, 1977).

There are no inherent reasons why relative value units should be tilted toward physically distinct tasks. Should policy makers attempt to reverse the existing set of incentives in our RVS systems, however, the result may be a number of distasteful repercussions. The volume of physically distinct procedures, such as laboratory and X-ray tests, and elective surgery, can easily be determined by the physician. If physicians set income targets, the reduced compensation per unit of service may result in significant increases in the volume of diagnostic procedures and elective surgery. With increased volume offsetting decreased price per service, expenditures may remain essentially unchanged, and human suffering from unnecessary surgery and from continued treatment related to diagnostic false positives may increase substantially.

Incentives under a salary system will be strongly influenced by the institutions that retain control over hiring. One possibility is that power to distribute speciality positions and salary levels will rest with a quasi-governmental planning body. Another option is for hospitals, clinics, and HMOs to retain autonomy. The resulting specialty distribution may reflect the financial strength of the employing institutions.

Capitation payment is a payment method for individual physicians and appears to be feasible for primary care services only.[5] Specialty incentives under a capitation system will be contingent on how non-primary care physicians are reimbursed, the extent and nature of primary care physician risk-sharing, and referral patterns in a community. Suppose specialists are reimbursed on a fee-for-service basis, with generous relative values for physically distinct procedures, and no risk-sharing by capitated primary care physicians for specialist services. This system would not encourage primary care as a specialty choice. An alternative system would be salaried specialists, with capitated primary care physicians sharing the financial risk of hospitalization and specialists' services. This arrangement could provide more professional control and entrepreneurial opportunity, and possibly greater net income to the primary care physicians.

Internal Efficiency of Physician's Practice

Few aspects of the market for physician services have been researched more extensively, received more federal support, and generated more inconclusive and contradictory empirical findings than the subject of the internal efficiency of a physician's practice. This research was initiated in the late 1960s and early 1970s, when there was a general consensus that a physician shortage existed and that more physician services were socially desirable. Improving physician efficiency "in the small," e.g., combining inputs in an optimal manner, would be a non-controversial method for introducing change in a sector where direct government intervention was viewed with great hostility. It was thought that improved efficiency would result in a movement toward a new equilibrium with something for everyone: improved access to care at a lower cost for consumers, and higher provider productivity and incomes.

Alternative physician reimbursement methods may have a less direct relationship to physician practice efficiency than to previously

---

[5]One interesting alternative may be to capitate groups of specialists, with individual physicians within the group sharing the net income.

discussed dimensions, such as geographic distribution. One reason for this is the lack of agreement as to the factors that limit costs and enhance productivity of physician practice. We shall concentrate the discussion of alternative payment incentives to three determinants of practice efficiency.

1. How does the payment affect the entrepreneurial function of the physician?
2. Does the payment method provide incentives or disincentives for physicians to join group practices?
3. Does the payment method provide incentives to use paraprofessionals in an efficient manner?

With respect to the first question, the physician is more likely to retain his entrepreneurial role under fee-for-service and capitation arrangements and yield it to a manager under salary. Physicians receive limited formal training in how to manage their practice and conduct their fiscal affairs. Reinhardt (1975) notes they may try to avoid managerial responsibility, even at the expense of reduced practice income. Their aversion to non-physician control is also well-known, however, as many hospital and clinic administrators will attest. So it is difficult to ascertain whether the loss of the entrepreneurial function will raise or lower practice efficiency.

Recent research has failed to demonstrate a strong association of scale economies with group practice. Bailey concluded from his analyses of Northern California internists that returns to scale for time-intensive physician services were constant and returns for capital-intensive services—such as X-ray and lab tests—were increasing (Bailey, 1970). The greater availability of ancillary services in group practices seemed to lead to higher utilization of these services. Today, with the widespread concern over the increasing use of diagnostic services, there is doubt if this efficiency "in the small" (producing ancillary services efficiently and profitably) is translated into efficiency "in the large" (producing the socially desirable number of diagnostic services). Newhouse found that the perverse incentives where physicians shared expenses, but not income, tended to increase unit costs (Newhouse, 1973).

Capitation, when combined with risk for referral and hospital services, implicitly encourages physicians to practice in groups. Salaried physicians by definition are paid by an institution—hospital, medical school, HMO, or clinic. Capitation induces physicians to join groups as a method of spreading risks. Fee-for-service is neutral with regard to practice arrangement.

The answer to the third question is related to the previous two. Salary, directly, and capitation, indirectly, encourage group practice and relinquishment of the entrepreneurial function to non-physician managers who hypothetically are more inclined to hire and substitute paraprofessional labor for physician labor. There is some limited evidence to support this hypothesis. Boaz's study of the skill-mix of 19 family planning clinics revealed that these clinics are paraprofessional-intensive (Boaz, 1972). On the other hand, the National Advisory Committee on Health Manpower, in its study of Kaiser physicians, did not find any "unusual substitution" of paraprofessionals (Reinhardt, 1975).

Conclusions: Physician Payment and National Health Insurance

This paper has assessed the effect of alternative physician payment methods on the physician's specialty and practice location choice, on the utilization of services and treatment setting, and on the efficiency of the physician's practice. The analysis emphasized that incentives embodied within physician payment systems profoundly influence both the physician and non-physician sectors of our health system.

We have attempted to demonstrate the existence of perverse incentives under the fee-for-service system in existence in the U.S. We feel that physicians' demonstrated ability to impact on the demand for their services retards efforts to change specialty and geographic physician distributions and to control the growth in physician and hospital costs. The absence of risk-sharing encourages expensive and intensive institutional care.

National Health Insurance affords policy makers an opportunity not likely to recur for a generation for reorganizing our health delivery systems on a more efficient basis. Yet, a cursory glance at major NHI proposals reveals that the major differences with respect to physician reimbursement are whether to reimburse on a CPR or fee schedule basis. Such proposals are, therefore, more like simple extensions of health care financing to uncovered population groups than major structural reform of the health care system. The one exception is the Kennedy-Corman Bill. Under this proposal, a cap is set on aggregate physician expenditures, but not on those for individual physicians. No NHI proposal restructures the physician reimbursement system so as to make what is efficient and profitable to the physician, efficient and profitable to society. This omission is too costly and consequential to overlook.

References

Adelstein, S. 1973. The Risk-Benefit Ratio in Nuclear Medicine. *Hospital Practice* 8 (January): 141–149.

American College of Surgeons and American Surgical Association. 1975. Manpower Subcommittee. *Study of Surgical Services for the United States. Summary Report (SOSSUS).* Tables III–VIII. Baltimore, Md.: American College of Surgeons.

American Medical Association. 1974. *Physician Distribution and Medical Licensure in the United States, 1974.* Chicago, Ill.: Center for Health Services Research and Development.

––––––. 1976. *Profile of Medical Practice.* Chicago, Ill.: Center for Health Services Research and Development.

Anderson, O., and Sheatsley, P. 1959. *Comprehensive Medical Insurance.* New York: Health Information Foundation.

Arthur Andersen and InterStudy. 1977. *Study of Reimbursement and Practice Arrangements of Provider Based Physicians.* Report in fulfillment of Contract 600-76-0055. Washington, D.C.: U.S. Department of Health, Education, and Welfare.

Bailey, R. 1970. Economies of Scale in Medical Practice. In Klarman, H. E., ed., *Studies in Health Economics.* pp. 255–273. Baltimore, Md.: The Johns Hopkins Press.

Boaz, R. 1972. An Economic Criterion for Determining Skill Mix. *Journal of Human Resources* 7 (2): 66–81.

Bunker, J. 1970. Surgical Manpower: A Comparison of Operations and Surgeons in the U.S., England and Wales. *The New England Journal of Medicine* 282 (3): 135–143.

Burney, I., Schieber, G., Blaxall, M. et al. 1978. Geographic Variations in Physician Fees: Payments to Physicians Under Medicare and Medicaid. *Journal of the American Medical Association* 240 (13): 1368–1371.

––––––, and Gabel, J. 1979. Reimbursement Patterns under Medicare and Medicaid. In *Proceedings of the Conference on Research Results from Physician Reimbursement Studies.* Health Care Financing Administration. Washington, D.C.: U.S. Government Printing Office.

California Medical Association. 1964. *1964 Relative Value Studies.* San Francisco, Calif.: California Medical Association.

Dyckman, Z. 1978. *A Study of Physician Fees: Staff Report of the Council on Wages and Price Stability.* Washington, D.C.: U.S. Government Printing Office.

Feldstein, M. 1970. The Rising Price of Physician Services. *The Review of Economics and Statistics* 52 (2): 121–133.

Fuchs, V. 1978. The Supply of Surgeons and the Demand for Operations. *Journal of Human Resources* 13 (Suppl.): 35–56.

Gaus, C., Cooper, B., and Hirschman, C. 1976. Contrast in HMO and Fee-For-Service Performance. *Social Security Bulletin* 39 (May): 3–14.

Gibson, R., and Fischer, C. 1978. National Health Expenditures, Fiscal Year 1977. *Social Security Bulletin* 41 (7): 3–19.

Glaser, W. 1977. *The Doctor Under National Health Insurance: Foreign Lessons for the United States.* New York: Bureau of Applied Social Research, Columbia University.

————. 1978a. *Health Insurance Bargaining: Foreign Lessons for Americans.* New York: Gardner Press and John Wiley.

————. 1978b. *Paying the Hospital: Foreign Lessons for the United States.* New York: Bureau of Applied Social Research, Columbia University.

Holahan, J., Hadley, J., Scanlon, W. et al. 1978. *Physician Pricing in California: Executive Summary.* Urban Institute. Report in fulfillment of Contract 600-76-0054. Washington, D.C.: U.S. Department of Health, Education, and Welfare.

Hsaio, W. 1975. A Model of Physician Group Pricing Behavior. Unpublished discussion paper. Cambridge, Mass.: Harvard University.

Institute of Medicine. 1976. *Medicare-Medicaid Reimbursement Policies.* Washington, D.C.: National Academy of Sciences.

Kessel, R. 1958. Pricing Discrimination in America. *Journal of Law and Economics* 1 (October): 20–53.

Lewin and Associates, Inc. 1976. *Government Controls on the Health Care System: The Canadian System.* Report in fulfillment of Contract 05-74-177. Washington, D.C.: U.S. Department of Health, Education and Welfare.

Newhouse, J. 1973. The Economies of Group Practice. *Journal of Human Resources* 8 (1): 37–54.

Mathematica Policy Research. 1978. *A Study of the Responses of Canadian Physicians to the Introduction of Universal Medical Care Insurances: The First Five Years in Quebec.* Report in fulfillment of Contract 230-75-0166. Washington, D.C.: U.S. Department of Health, Education and Welfare.

Redisch, M. 1978. Physician Involvement in Hospital Decision Making. In Zubkoff, M., Raskin, E., and Hanft, R., eds., *Hospital Cost Containment: Selected Notes for Future Policy.* pp 217–243. New York: Milbank Memorial Fund.

———, Gabel, J., and Blaxall, M. 1979. Physician Pricing, Costs and Incomes. In Scheffler, R., ed., *Annual Series in Health Economics.* Greenwich, Conn.: J.A.I. Press.

Reinhardt, U. E. 1975. *Physician Productivity and Demand for Health Manpower. An Economic Analysis.* Cambridge, Mass.: Ballinger Publishing Company.

———. 1976. Health Manpower in the United States: Issues for Inquiry in the Next Decade. Unpublished paper presented to the Bicentennial Conference on Health Policy, Philadelphia, Pennsylvania, November, 1976.

Roemer, M. 1962. On Paying the Doctor and the Implications of Different Methods. *Journal of Health and Human Behavior* 3(1): 10.

Rowland, D. 1973. Testimony before Assembly Health Committee of the California State Legislature, Los Angeles, December 13, 1973.

Sloan, F., and Feldman, R. 1978. Competition Among Physicians. In Greenberg, W., ed., *Competition in the Health Sector: Past, Present and Future.* Federal Trade Commission. pp. 57–131. Washington, D.C.: U.S. Government Printing Office.

———, and Steinwald, B. 1975. The Role of Health Insurance in the Physicians Services Market. *Inquiry* 12(4): 275–299.

———, Cromwell, J., and Mitchell, J. 1977. *A Study of Administrative Costs in Physician Offices and Medicaid Participation.* Report by Abt Associates in fulfillment of Contract 600-75-0212, U.S. Department of Health, Education, and Welfare. Washington, D.C.: U.S. Government Printing Office.

Wennberg, J. E., and Gittelsohn, A. 1973. Small Area Variations in Health Care Delivery. *Science* 182 (Dec. 14): 1102–1108.

An earlier version of this paper was presented at the Eastern Economic Association Meetings, Hartford, Connecticut, on April 14, 1977.

The discussion and conclusion expressed in this paper represent solely the views and opinions of the authors, and not those of the Department of Health, Education, and Welfare, or the U.S. General Accounting Office.

Acknowledgments: The authors wish to thank Diane Rowland and Linda Magno for their helpful comments.

Address correspondence to: Jon R. Gabel, Health Care Financing Administration, Department of Health, Education, and Welfare, 330 C Street, S.W., Washington, D.C. 20024.

Decisions to Treat
Critically Ill Patients:
A Comparison of Social
Versus
Medical Considerations

DIANA CRANE

A questionnaire survey shows that physicians in four medical specialties evaluate chronically and terminally ill patients not only in terms of the physiological aspects of illness but also in terms of the extent to which they are capable of interacting with others. A patient's potential capacity to perform his social roles depends upon his "salvageability," i.e., the likelihood that he will be able to resume his roles and the degree of irreversible physical or mental damage which indicates his capacity for resuming them. The priorities in terms of treatment are the following: (1) salvageable patients with physical damage; (2) salvageable patients with mental damage and unsalvageable patients with physical damage; (3) unsalvageable patients with mental damage. Within these categories variables such as patient attitude, family attitude, age, and social class, which define the social environment of the patient, also influence the physician's decision to treat him. Studies of hospital records of cases in two of the specialties were consistent with the survey findings.

The findings suggest that there is a disparity between the traditional ethic concerning the treatment of such patients and the actual behavior of many physicians. As a solution to the inconsistencies between ideal and actual behavior, the development of medical guidelines for the withdrawal of treatment with respect to certain specifically defined conditions is recommended.

In recent years, the subject of death and dying has become increasingly popular in the mass media. It appears that death is no longer, as it was once described (Lester, 1967), a matter of indifference to the average person. Numerous popular articles describe the plight of families facing the dilemmas posed by hospitalization of dying relatives. The number of courses on dying and death offered to college students has multiplied. At the same time, there has been an increase in interest in this subject among physicians and social scientists who have produced a steady stream of articles and books.

What are the reasons for the surge of interest in this topic? One reason is that technology, which has affected virtually every aspect of modern life, has also altered the process of dying. Chronic rather than acute diseases are now the most prevalent causes of death in industrial societies (Lerner, 1970). As a result in part of the nature of chronic diseases and in part of the availability of increasingly sophisticated technology, the physician's control over the exact timing of death has increased. In some cases, if treatment is not withdrawn, the patient can be kept alive almost indefinitely. Unusually difficult interpersonal problems are thus created for the physician, for the patient, and for his family.

As the physician's capacity to treat illness and control the timing of death has increased, the traditional norms that guided medical practice have become more difficult to apply. In the past, when the majority of patients suffered from acute illness, aggressive treatment was almost always appropriate. Gradually it has become apparent that some chronically ill patients do not benefit from such treatment and that they or their families may in fact be adversely affected by such efforts.

Since, to a large extent, it is the physician who makes decisions concerning life and death, it is important to understand the factors which influence his decisions. This article reports the results of an inquiry concerning doctors' attitudes toward the prolongation and termination of life. Under what conditions does the physician do everything possible to save the life of the patient? Under what conditions does he withdraw medical treatment and permit the patient to die? Does the physician, under certain circumstances, actively bring about death—in popular terms, engage in the practice of euthanasia?

Decisions concerning what types of patients should receive aggressive therapy are difficult to make. They have been the subject of considerable controversy in recent years. The literature which explores this problem can be divided into two parts: one which upholds the traditional ethic that decisions should be made entirely on the basis of the physiological aspects of illness and another which suggests that social as well as physiological considerations should play a role in deciding whether or not a patient is treatable. In general, three types of patients are described in this literature: (1) the conscious terminal patient; (2) the irreversibly comatose terminal patient; (3) the brain-damaged or severely debilitated patient whose chances of long-term survival in his present state are good.

The conscious terminal patient who is suffering a slow and painful demise is the most frequently discussed of the three. How actively should such a person be treated and why? The conservative view is that treatment should be continued as long as it is possible to sustain respiration and heartbeat. Social considerations are irrelevant (Karnofsky, 1960). Others have argued that, as these lives become less and less satisfying for the patients and for their families, social aspects of the case should be taken into consideration in decisions to continue treatment (Morison, 1971).

The comatose terminal patient is less frequently discussed in the literature although he is no less of a problem to physicians. Fortunately, the cessation of electrical activity in the brain can be measured unambiguously, and this has become, for many physicians, a criterion for declaring such patients to be dead without waiting for cessation of heartbeat and respirations. This definition has, however, been the subject of considerable controversy.

Probably the most difficult cases are those which are least discussed in the literature on the treatment of the critically ill patient, those of brain-damaged or severely debilitated patients whose chances of survival for a considerable period of time are very good in their present partially functioning state. These patients can be considered to be critically ill, not in the sense that their death is imminent but in the sense that they require considerable medical care and expense in order to maintain their conditions. Into this category fall many senile, severely debilitated geriatric patients as well as mentally defective or severely deformed newborns. Here again, there are differences of opinion concerning whether, for example, severely damaged newborns should be treated. Some physicians argue that such infants should not be treated because it is unlikely that they will be able to participate in the lives of their families in a satisfactory manner (Duff and Campbell, 1973; Shaw, 1972).

There is clearly a dilemma regarding the appropriateness of social as compared to physiological criteria in deciding to treat critically ill patients. Most discussions of this issue are presented in evaluative terms, in other words, in terms of what the physician ought to do rather than in terms of what he actually does. In this article, the criteria which physicians say they use in treating critically ill patients will be examined. Do they evaluate their patients' potential entirely in physiological terms or do social considerations play a role? How much consensus about these matters is there among them? Does analysis of the records of hospital patients confirm or contradict their statements of their attitudes?

The hypothesis being tested here is that physicians evaluate the chronically ill or terminally ill patient not only in terms of the physiological aspects of illness but also in terms of the extent to which he is capable of interacting with others. In other words, the treatable patient is one who, if treated, is capable of resuming his social roles even minimally and temporarily. The untreatable patient is one for whom this possibility must be permanently excluded. For example, the severely brain-damaged patient is completely incapable of performing his social roles while the physically damaged person may be able to resume some of them. For the terminal patient, resumption of social roles is of necessity temporary. For the chronically ill patient, it may be possible for a considerable period of time.

Sociological studies of medicine have been strongly influenced by two models, one which defines the social nature of illness and another which delineates the professional role of the physician. At least in part as a result of Parsons' model of the sick role, there is a sizable literature on the factors affecting the patient's decision to seek medical care (Kasl and Cobb, 1966). On the other hand, there has been very little research on how the doctor perceives the patient and how he decides to treat the patient. What has been lacking is a model which could predict the conditions under which an individual will be likely to receive treatment, given different categories of debilitating conditions, such as acute illness, chronic conditions, and terminal illness.

Both Parsons' sick-role model and his model of the physician's role (Parsons, 1951: Chapter 10; 1958) bypass the ethical issues surrounding the treatment of critically ill patients. The sick-role model emphasizes that it is normative for the patient to seek treatment while the practitioner model emphasizes that the physician should limit his attention to medical rather than social characteristics of the patient. Consequently these models implicitly accept the traditional medical ethic that life should be preserved as long as it is possible to do so.

The patient's potential capacity to perform his social roles can be determined in a number of ways. First, the physician attempts to decide whether or not the patient is "salvageable." Can the patient be restored to health or can a chronic condition be maintained for an indefinite period of time? Alternatively, is the patient's condition one which will sooner or later be the cause of his death? In general, decisions concerning salvageability are based on the known prognoses of various types of diseases. Obviously, from time to time, the prognoses of certain diseases change, but at any particular time there is likely to be a high degree of consensus among physicians concerning the prognoses of most diseases.

A second decision concerns the quality of life which the patient can expect to lead. Is the patient physically damaged or mentally damaged in the sense that he has suffered irreversible physical or intellectual impairment or both?

These factors obviously affect the individual's capacity to perform his social roles. The salvageability of the patient indicates whether it is likely that the individual will resume his social roles; the degree of irreversible damage indicates his capacity for resuming them. If physicians are following the traditional medical norm regarding medical treatment, that is, defining the patient's potential solely in physiological terms, no distinction should be made among cases which differ on these two variables with respect to level of treatment. If the patient's potential is being evaluated in social terms, distinctions will be made depending upon the patient's prognosis and the type of damage which he has sustained. The priorities based on the extent to which the patient is likely to be incapacitated in the performance of his social roles are shown in Fig. 1: (1) salvageable patients with physical damage; (2) salvageable patients with mental damage; (3) unsalvageable patients with physical damage; (4) unsalvageable patients with mental damage.

In addition, certain variables which define the social environment of the patient will be expected to influence the decision to treat within these categories. For example, the attitude of the patient toward his illness, the attitude of his family toward him, the age of the patient, and perhaps his social class might all be expected to influence the physician's decision to treat the patient.

Methods of Research

In order to test these hypotheses, questionnaires were mailed to samples of physicians in internal medicine, pediatrics, neurosurgery, and pediatric heart surgery. After exploratory interviews, questionnaires were developed with the aid of physicians for each specialty using the following format: (a) several case histories; (b)

Prognosis of Patient

Type of damage sustained by patient	Salvageable	Unsalvageable
Physical only	1	3
Mental or Physical and mental	2	4

FIG. 1.   Priorities in the treatment of critically ill patients: Hypotheses

attitude questions; (c) social and professional background questions. The case histories for physicians in pediatrics are concerned with the treatment of infants born with congenital anomalies and severe birth defects. The case histories for physicians in internal medicine examine the treatment of progressive chronic disease. The case histories for neurosurgery and pediatric heart surgery are concerned with the types of cases which occur in the practice of these specialties. The patients described in the case histories vary in terms of brain damage, physical damage, physical pain, patient attitude, family attitude, social class, and age. In order to test the influence of social variables, three versions of the internist questionnaire and two versions of the pediatric questionnaire were developed. The same medical cases were presented in each version, but the social variables were changed.

In neurosurgery, two of the salvageable cases were based on a patient who was described by a neurosurgeon in an interview with the author. The patient had developed a large hematoma (a swelling filled with blood) in his brain. The location of the hematoma in the brain was such that his mental faculties were affected before and after its surgical removal. After recovering from the operation, the patient had an I.Q. of 90, he could no longer practice his profession, and his right arm was paralyzed. If the operation had not been performed, the patient would have died. As a result of the operation, he can be expected to live a normal life span. The informant, a neurosurgeon, said that he sometimes wondered whether or not he had done the man a favor by operating upon him.

Since this condition can affect the physical capacities of the patient rather than the mental faculties, depending upon the location of the hematoma in the brain, a parallel case was constructed in which the patient had suffered visual impairment and some paralysis on the left side of his body but no intellectual or speech impairment.

The neurosurgical unsalvageable cases involved a patient with a solitary metastatic brain tumor. The presence of metastases indicates the transfer of cancer cells from one part of the body to another and is considered to be a sign that the disease is irreversible and terminal. Again, depending upon the location of the tumor in the brain, the patient's physical or mental capacities are affected. Both possibilities were presented to the neurosurgical respondents and they were asked to indicate whether or not they would remove such a tumor in a 40-year-old man. The same pair of cases was repeated with the subject being a 65-year-old man. Another unsalvageable case, that involving a metastatic tumor in the spine which had produced paraplegia in the patient, was also included, since it could be corrected by a fairly simple surgical procedure and therefore was more likely to be performed.

In internal medicine, the salvageable patient with physical damage was suffering from chronic pulmonary fibrosis, a severe respiratory disease. The case is described as follows in one version of the questionnaire:

> A 35 year old man is brought to the hospital by his wife. He has a history of severe chronic pulmonary fibrosis and for three years has been unable to climb stairs or walk more than 10 feet due to shortness of breath. He is found to have pneumococcal pneumonia, but during his first hospital day he becomes cyanotic and semicomatose. If a tracheostomy is performed, he will probably survive without further impairment of lung function. His wife is reluctant to authorize this procedure. Which of the following would you be likely to perform? (Check yes, maybe, or no for each of the following.)
>
> 60. Would you attempt to persuade his wife to authorize tracheostomy?
> 61. Intravenous feeding for dehydration.
> 62. Antibiotics.
> 63. Arterial puncture for blood gas analysis.
> 64. Urine culture for pyuria.
> 65. Urethral catheter for urinary obstruction.
> 66. Appendectomy for incidental suspected appendicitis.
> 67. Small bowel resection for suspected infarcted bowel.

68. If cardiac arrest occurred, would you begin resuscitation?
69. If resuscitation was unsuccessful after 15 minutes, would you continue?

Although the patient is severely debilitated, he is considered salvageable, since patients with this chronic condition can be maintained over considerable periods of time.

The salvageable internal medicine patient with moderate mental damage is described as follows in one version of the questionnaire:

> A 65 year old woman had a severe stroke one year ago. As a result, she cannot walk, eats with difficulty, and has mild difficulty expressing herself. She is admitted to the ward service dehydrated and septic. Her family is unwilling to care for her at home if discharged from the hospital following treatment.

A list of appropriate treatments followed. In two versions of the case, the willingness of the family to care for the patient was presented negatively and positively, respectively.

In a third version of the case, a similar patient with more severe brain damage was presented as "a 65 year old woman with severe cerebral atrophy (who) cannot walk, feed herself, or communicate meaningfully with others."

Two cases of unsalvageable physical damage were presented to the internists. The first case involved a particularly painful form of cancer, cancer of the esophagus (part of the passage through which food is transmitted from the mouth to the stomach). A second unsalvageable case with physical damage presented a man with "melanoma (a type of cancer) of the leg that has metastasized to the spinal cord," causing paraplegia. This case was presented in two versions which varied in terms of the patient's desire to be treated. A third version of this question presented another unsalvageable disease involving physical damage, multiple sclerosis (which causes severe muscular weakness and lack of physical coordination) in order to compare physicians' reactions to a terminal disease which does not have such negative connotations as cancer.

In pediatrics, the salvageable patient with physical damage was an infant who had been born with myelomeningocele, a hernial protrusion of the spinal cord through the vertebral column, usually containing a watery fluid. The infant is described as having "no nerve function in his legs and no bladder or rectal sphincter control." If an operation to close the defect is performed soon after birth, the child's condition can be maintained for many years, although the associated paraplegia and absence of bladder and bowel control remain. If the operation is not performed, the infant may eventually die a slow and painful death.

Two cases of salvageable infants with mental damage were presented to the pediatric respondents. One was an infant with mongolism (Down's syndrome). The other was a case in which, as a result of difficulties during delivery, the infant had been deprived of oxygen. The case is described as follows in one version of the questionnaire:

> As a result of premature separation of the placenta, an infant was without oxygen in the uterus for an indeterminate period. He weighs 1500 grams. Seizures develop within two or three hours of birth and persist in spite of therapy. Marked spasticity and hypertonia develop. An electroencephalogram is highly abnormal. This is the first birth for a professional woman who has had several miscarriages. She wants the child very much. Which of the following would you be likely to perform? (Check yes, maybe, or no for each item.)
>
> 38. Intravenous fluids for maintenance.
> 39. Monitor blood pH and correct as needed.
> 40. Antibiotics for infection.
> 41. If he develops pneumothorax, would you aspirate the chest?
> 42. If he stops breathing for more than two minutes, would you bag-breathe him for two to three hours?
> 43. Would you place him on a respirator if he continues to have apneic spells?
> 44. If he then has a cardiac arrest, would you resuscitate him?

The different versions of these two cases were varied in terms of the social class of the parents and the mother's desire to have the child.

The two unsalvageable pediatric cases were (a) the statistically rare but philosophically interesting case of the anencephalic child, who, because it is born without portions of the brain that control conscious and voluntary processes and coordinate muscular movements, can be considered to be subhuman; (b) the case of a rare and incurable heart defect, hypoplastic left ventricle, which is difficult to diagnose without performing a catheterization, which in turn may be fatal to the patient if he has the condition. The condition, like that of anencephaly, leads rapidly to the demise of the patient.

Finally, the cases which were presented to the pediatric heart surgeons were all cases of salvageable patients with physical or mental damage associated with cardiac defects, since unsalvageable cases are uncommon in their practice. Two cases of children with mongolism were described as having associated heart defects of varying degrees of severity (tetralogy of Fallot is less severe than atrio-ventricular canal). These cases were varied in terms of parental interest in and concern for the child. The same types of cardiac defects were also presented in association with a physical defect, a "severe but treatable urogenital anomaly." In these cases, parental concern and financial resources were varied. Finally, a case of relatively minor cardiac defect, patent ductus arteriosus, combined with rubella syndrome (congenital effects upon the infant of German measles contracted furing pregnancy by the mother) was presented in two parts: with and without associated mental retardation.

Obviously case histories of this sort can only partially simulate the actual medical situation which the physician faces. The details of the cases and the treatments suggested were realistic. However, there is an element of artificiality in the use of such case histories in that the physician generally interacts with a patient over a period of time, during which his assessment of the case gradually changes. On the other hand, regardless of the difficulties involved in using this technique, it is superior to the very general questions on euthanasia which have been used in previous studies (Williams, 1969; Brown et al., 1970).

In the neurosurgery and pediatric heart surgery questionnaires, physicians were asked to indicate whether they would usually, sometimes, or rarely perform such an operation. The internist and pediatric questionnaires provided lists of appropriate treatments for each case. Physicians were asked to indicate which treatments they would use for the patients described in the case histories. They were given three alternatives: yes, maybe, or no. For both the pediatric and internist questionnaires, all items representing hypothetical treatments for the entire set of cases were factor-analyzed as a single group. The factor analysis indicated that each of the cases represented a separate dimension of behavior, although not all items under a single case were included in that dimension. A scale of activism was developed for each question which included only those items which were highly correlated with one another as shown by the factor analysis. The tables which are presented in the following section show the proportions of pediatric physicians who would perform all of the items on a particular scale for the patients described (i.e., a "yes" response) and the proportions of internists who would perform all or all but one of the items on a particular scale. There were fewer items in the pediatric scales than in the internal medicine scales.

Since the specialties of neurosurgery and pediatric heart surgery are small, lists of members of these specialties were sampled. Pediatrics and internal medicine are large specialties, comprising physicians who practice in a wide variety of medical settings. Samples of hospitals were drawn from the American Medical Association's *Directory of Approved Internships and Residencies.* Hospitals were asked to provide lists of their residents in pediatrics and internal medicine and of physicians who had admitting privileges in these specialties. Samples of residents and physicians were drawn from these lists. Since many physicians practice in more than one hospital, respondents in these samples were asked to respond in terms of their practice in the sample hospital which was named in the covering letter.

Questionnaires were mailed to members of all four samples during the winter of 1970-71. Over 70 percent of the physicians returned the questionnaire in all four specialties. The samples are large: pediatrics: 922; internal medicine: 1,410; neurosurgery: 650; pediatric heart surgery: 207.

Results

Prognosis and Type of Damage

It was hypothesized that the following priorities would be observed in the treatment of critically ill patients: (1) salvageable patients with physical damage; (2) salvageable patients with mental damage; (3) unsalvageable patients with physical damage; (4) unsalvageable patients with mental damage. Among the neurosurgeons and the internists, it appears that salvageable patients with physical damage are clearly more likely to be actively treated than any of the other types of patients (refer to Tables 1 and 2). A salvageable patient with physical damage was more likely to be actively treated than a salvageable patient with mental damage. Among unsalvageable patients, a similar distinction was made between those who were physically or mentally damaged.

TABLE 1

Percentage of Neurosurgeons Who Would Usually Operate,
by Patient's Prognosis and Type of Damage
(*N* = 650)

	PATIENT'S PROGNOSIS: SALVAGEABLE		PATIENT'S PROGNOSIS: UNSALVAGEABLE		
	Type of Damage		Type of Damage		
	Physical	*Mental*	*Physical*		*Mental*
			Case 1	*Case 2*	
Percentage Neurosurgeons	89	55	76	50	22
Cause of Damage	Cerebral hematoma		Tumor metastatic from kidney to thoracic epidural space, producing paraplegia	Solitary metastatic brain tumor	

Salv.-Physical vs. Salv.-Mental: Cell 1 vs. Cell 2, z^a = 14.66*

Salv.-Physical vs. Unsalv.-Physical: Cell 1 vs. Cell 3, z = 6.45*
Cell 1 vs. Cell 4, z = 16.33*

Salv.-Mental vs. Unsalv.-Mental: Cell 2 vs. Cell 5, z = 13.37*

Unsalv.-Physical vs. Unsalv.-Mental: Cell 3 vs. Cell 5, z = 22.31*
Cell 4 vs. Cell 5, z = 11.44*

*$p < .01$

[a]In this and subsequent tables, the z statistic measures the difference between correlated means or independent means, depending on which samples or subsamples are being compared (see McNemar, 1962: 80-83).

TABLE 2

Percentage of Internists[a] Who Would Treat Very Actively
By Patient's Prognosis and Type of Damage[b]

PATIENT'S PROGNOSIS: SALVAGEABLE			PATIENT'S PROGNOSIS: UNSALVAGEABLE		
Type of Damage			Type of Damage		
Moderate Physical	*Moderate Mental*	*Severe Mental*	*Moderate Physical*		*Severe Physical*
			Case 1	*Case 2*	
67	30	16	36	28	3
(1,410)	(909)	(501)	(909)	(501)	(1,410)

Salv.-Physical vs. Salv.-Mental:
Cell 1 vs. Cell 2, $z = 28.68$*
Cell 1 vs. Cell 3, $z = 33.13$*
Cell 2 vs. Cell 3, $z = 18.15$*

Salv.-Physical vs. Unsalv.-Physical:
Cell 1 vs. Cell 4, $z = 24.70$*
Cell 1 vs. Cell 5, $z = 20.95$*
Cell 1 vs. Cell 6, $z = 72.30$*

Salv.-Mental vs. Unsalv.-Physical:
Cell 2 vs. Cell 4, $z = 3.57$*
Cell 2 vs. Cell 5, $z = 2.78$*
Cell 3 vs. Cell 6, $z = 3.82$*

Cell 1: Salvageable Prognosis-Mod. Physical: chronic pulmonary fibrosis
Cell 2: Salvageable Prognosis-Mod. Mental: stroke with moderate brain damage
Cell 3: Salvageable Prognosis-Severe Mental: severe cerebral atrophy
Cell 4: Unsalvageable Prognosis-Mod. Physical (Case 1): melanoma of the leg metastized to the spinal cord
Cell 5: Unsalvageable Prognosis-Mod. Physical (Case 2): multiple sclerosis
Cell 6: Unsalvageable Prognosis-Severe Physical: cancer of the esophagus

*$p < .01$
[a]Physicians and residents combined.
[b]There are no cases of unsalvageable prognosis with mental damage in this questionnaire.

However, these physicians were less likely to distinguish between salvageable patients with mental damage and unsalvageable patients with physical damage. For example, a salvageable patient who has suffered severe mental damage (cerebral atrophy) is less likely to be actively treated than a terminal cancer patient with moderate physical damage only (refer to Table 2). This suggests that the mentally damaged, salvageable patient is seen as being less capable of resuming his social roles than the terminally ill, physically damaged patient. Both of these types of cases are more actively treated than the terminally ill, mentally damaged patient. A neurosurgeon commented during an interview:

> If the patient is unsalvageable, you just have to accept it . . . A lot of our patients are severely ill and incapacitated. Frequently death is the better way out.

Among the pediatric cases, a very clear distinction was made between salvageable and unsalvageable patients (refer to Table 3). In this specialty, the physically damaged, salvageable patient was not more likely to be actively treated than the mongoloid, salvageable patient. The explanation may lie in the choice of the physically damaged, salvageable case. The physically damaged, salvageable pediatric patient had a myelomeningocele and was described as having no nerve function in his legs and no bladder or rectal sphincter control. He was thus unlikely to have a more meaningful social existence than the mongoloid infant with whom this patient was compared. However, the expected priorities do appear in the comparison between the infant with a myelomeningocele and an infant whose brain had been damaged at birth as well as in the comparisons between the former and the other two infants in the decision to resuscitate these infants. Twenty-nine percent of these physicians said that they would resuscitate the patient with a myelomeningocele compared to 16 percent who would resuscitate the mongoloid infant and the brain-damaged infant.

Neither the anencephalic nor the infant with incurable heart disease (hypoplastic left ventricle) will live more than a few days on the average unless extraordinary efforts are taken on their behalf. Even so, the infant with physical damage receives more attention than the one with mental damage (refer to Table 3), although this is possibly a result of uncertainties surrounding the diagnosis of the former condition.

TABLE 3

Percentage of Pediatricians[a] Who Would Treat Very Actively by Patient's Prognosis and Type of Damage[b]

PATIENT'S PROGNOSIS: SALVAGEABLE			PATIENT'S PROGNOSIS: UNSALVAGEABLE	
Type of Damage			Type of Damage	
Physical	Mental		Physical	Mental
	Case 1	Case 2		
55 (922)	52 (922)	47 (922)	25 (376)[c]	4 (458)

Salv.-Physical vs. Salv.-Mental: Cell 1 vs. Cell 3, $z = 4.64$*

Unsalv.-Physical vs. Unsalv.-Mental: Cell 4 vs. Cell 5, $z = 47.91$*

Salv.-Physical vs. Unsalv.-Physical: Cell 1 vs. Cell 4, $z = 3.27$*

Salv.-Mental vs. Unsalv.-Mental: Cell 2 vs. Cell 5, $z = 47.85$*
Cell 3 vs. Cell 5, $z = 63.66$*

*$p < .01$

[a] Physicians and residents combined.

[b] Cell 1: Salvageable Prognosis-Physical: myelomeningocele
Cell 2: Salvageable Prognosis-Mental (Case 1): mongoloid with severe respiratory disease
Cell 3: Salvageable Prognosis-Mental (Case 2): seizures with spasticity and hypertonia
Cell 4: Unsalvageable Prognosis-Physical: hypoplastic left ventricle
Cell 5: Unsalvageable Prognosis-Mental: anencephaly

[c] Non-respondents excluded among the residents.

Some of the difficulties involved in making these kinds of decisions were described by a pediatric resident in an interview:

> There are some instances where I would let them all die, for instance, if the child had severe congenital anomalies. But it's hard to draw a line between saving them and not saving them. It's hard to set goals in advance and then follow them. You can't say in the actual situation: "This is one of the kids that I had decided to let die."

The pediatric heart surgeons were presented with case histories of salvageable patients only. They were much less likely to say that they would perform cardiac surgery upon children with an accompanying brain anomaly, mongolism, than upon children with an accompanying severe but treatable physical anomaly (refer to Table 4).

While many physicians appeared to be using social considerations in making their decisions to treat critically ill patients, others upheld the traditional ethic of not making such distinctions. The following statements from interviews indicate the rationales which were used by a neurosurgeon and a pediatric cardiologist respectively for utilizing the traditional approach:

> If one resolves in advance to do *everything* possible for *every* patient, one is spared many of the "difficult decisions" you ask about. Our training is to preserve life and function wherever possible—not only where it is desirable and convenient but where it is possible. We are not trained (and should not be!) to decide who is "better off dead."

> You can't act as God. Someone once said that you treat everybody or nobody . . . I know some cardiac surgeons who won't operate on mentally retarded children. I think it's easier for a physician to operate on everyone.

Attitudes of the Patient and His Family

If a physician is basing his decision concerning treatment in part upon the patient's social situation and not entirely upon his physiological status, the attitude of the patient toward himself and of his family members toward him would be expected to influence the physician's decision. In fact, the effects of these variables are very specific.

Among adult patients, the patient's attitude appeared to influence the physician's decision primarily when the patient was suffering from a terminal illness. For example, in one of the

TABLE 4

Percentage of Pediatric Heart Surgeons Who Would "Usually Operate"
Upon Salvageable Patients by Type of Damage of Patient
and Severity of Patient's Cardiac Anomaly
(*N* = 207)

Severity	Type of Damage		Cause of Damage	Parental Attitude
	Physical	*Mental*		
Mild	93	56	patent ductus arteriosus combined with rubella syndrome and either no developmental retardation (*Physical*) or developmental retardation (*Mental*)	unspecified
Moderate	90	59	tetralogy of Fallot combined with either urogenital anomaly (*Physical*) or mongolism (*Mental*)	favorable toward treatment of patient
Severe	82	50	atrio-ventricular canal combined with either urogenital anomaly (*Physical*) or mongolism (*Mental*)	favorable toward treatment of

Statistical tests are not shown because the sample is not random.

versions of the questionnaire for internists, a terminal cancer patient requests to be treated vigorously. In another version of the questionnaire, he asks that he not be treated actively. Fifty-one percent of the physicians who received the first version of the questionnaire indicated that they would treat this patient very actively. Twenty-two percent of the physicians who received the second version were willing to treat the patient very actively. However, although it was not tested in the survey, it seems likely that the effect of this variable would have been smaller with respect to salvageable patients. A resident in internal medicine expressed this point of view in an interview:

> I had a patient with rheumatoid arthritis who was very uncomfortable and septic. She kept saying, "Let me die," and meant it very much. But I would not let her die because I felt that something could be done to make her more comfortable. But if it was somebody who had metastatic cancer, I would be more sympathetic toward letting him die.

The effect of the patient's favorable as compared to unfavorable attitude toward treatment was much less noticeable in a case where the prognosis was deliberately left ambiguous. While internists indicate that the terminal patient's attitude is an important influence upon their decisions regarding treatment, other studies show that many patients have difficulty communicating their attitudes to their physicians. Those patients who are relatively unsophisticated and inarticulate are not well equipped to engage in the delicate kind of negotiations which are required. Their families are in no better position (Glaser and Strauss, 1965; Kübler-Ross, 1969).

The influence of the family's attitude upon the treatment of the adult patient appears to be much less direct. It has an influence only insofar as it affects the patient's attitude in terminal cases. The family's attitude appeared not to influence physicians' decisions to treat salvageable patients. For example, internists' decisions to treat actively were not influenced by the family's willingness to care for a moderately brain-damaged stroke patient upon her discharge from the hospital. In the case of the physically damaged salvageable patient which was presented to the internists, the family was presented as being opposed to aggressive treatment in all three versions of the questionnaire, but this case was more actively treated by physicians than any of the others. However, the family's attitude may have an indirect influence upon the treatment of unsalvageable patients as is suggested in the following description which an internist gave in an interview of the kind of reasoning that affected some of his decisions:

> If the patient has a chronic incurable illness and has been maintained over a period of years with some kind of meaningful life, there often comes a point when he simply falls apart at the seams. He begins to grumble that his funds are running out and it is difficult for the family. You know there is little that you can do about this. So when the fellow comes to the hospital with an acute illness superimposed upon the chronic illness, you know that if you get him over it, he will have to go to a chronic disease hospital. You tend to let him go. After all, he has probably had five great years.

Surgeons in general are in a very different position from pediatricians and internists in that they cannot go ahead with their procedures without obtaining the legal consent of either the patient or his family. Internists and pediatricians can do a great deal for the patient without obtaining formal consent. Although not tested directly in the neurosurgery questionnaire, there was also some indication in the interviews that the attitude of the patient was important if he was able to participate in the decision to operate. This point of view was expressed strongly by a respondent:

> The most important consideration is that the patient determine what is done on the best available information and that his fate is not decided by the surgeon, family, or society.

If a family does not define a brain-damaged child as socially dead, will the physician's judgment of the case be affected? Table 5 shows that in three medical specialties, pediatrics, pediatric heart surgery, and neurosurgery, the family's concern for a brain-damaged infant or child has a considerable influence upon the physician's decision to treat him. The influence is greatest in the pediatric heart-surgery cases, where the family's rejection of the children was strongest. This was indicated by the fact that the children were described as having been institutionalized. Table 5 suggests that physicians who treat children are aware of the stressful consequences for a family of having a mentally retarded child (Farber, 1968).

However, the effects of parental attitude are once again very specific. For example, these effects are noticeable in cases involving brain-damaged children but much less noticeable in cases which were presented to the pediatric heart surgeons involving

TABLE 5

Influence of Family Attitude Upon the Treatment of
Salvageable Patients with Mental Damage[a]

Medical Specialty	Family Attitude Toward Treatment		Cause of Damage	z Statistic
	Favorable	*Unfavorable*		
Pediatrics[b]	59 (464)	44 (458)	mongoloid with severe respiratory distress (newborn)	10.57*
	58 (458)	33 (464)	seizures with spasticity and hypertonia (newborn)	12.24*
Neurosurgery	47 (650)	32 (650)	hydrocephaly combined with mongolism (newborn)	8.06*
Pediatric heart surgery	59 (207)	18 (207)	tetralogy of Fallot combined with mongolism (child aged 8)	—
	50 (207)	12 (207)	atrio-ventricular canal combined with mongolism (child aged 8)	—

*$p < .01$

[a]Treatment is defined as: percentage who would treat very actively among pediatricians; percentage who would "usually operate" among neurosurgeons and pediatric heart surgeons.

[b]Physicians and residents combined.

physically damaged children with cardiac defects. It seems plausible that the parents' attitude toward a brain-damaged child would be more important than their attitude toward a physically damaged child since a greater effort would be required to establish social relationships with the former.

Age of Adult Patients

Parsons and Lidz (1967) have pointed out that attitudes toward dying in our society differ depending upon whether the process occurs at the end of the life cycle or as a break in the life cycle. The first type of event is considered normal; the second is the object of vigorous intervention. Sudnow (1967) found that in the emergency room of a large county hospital in California the aged were less likely to be resuscitated than young persons.

In the interviews, physicians frequently distinguished between physiological and chronological age, arguing that two patients with same chronological age might have very different physiological potentialities for recovering from illness. They resisted the idea of setting arbitrary age limits for the withdrawal of treatment. The frequency with which physicians indicated that they would treat older patients actively was somewhat lower than for younger patients in two out of three internal medicine cases and in two neurosurgical cases. In these cases, patients in their thirties and forties were compared with patients in their sixties. The largest percentage difference appeared in the internal medicine questionnaire when a 75-year-old patient was compared with a 45-year-old patient.

When the hospital records of a group of patients who had died (some of whom had been unsuccessfully resuscitated) or who had died and had been successfully resuscitated on the clinical service of a university hospital were examined, it appeared that the age variations which had been used in the questionnaries were not wide enough. Physicians apparently distinguish between three age groups: under 40, 40 to 79, and over 79. As Table 6 shows, those under 40 were most likely to have been resuscitated in this hospital. Patients between the ages of 40 and 79 were somewhat less likely to have been resuscitated with no distinction by decade within this group. Those over 79 were much less likely to have been resuscitated. The use of major diagnostic and treatment procedures was also related to age in exactly the same manner.

TABLE 6

Percentage of Patients Resuscitated by Age
in a Sample of Deaths and Resuscitations
on the Clinical Service of a University Hospital

	Age of Patient[a]				
	10-39	*40-59*	*60-79*	*Over 79*	*Total*
Percentage resuscitated	73 (37)	51 (97)	47 (125)	33 (27)	50 (286)

[a] $G = -.29$ (Goodman and Kruskal's gamma).

It is not clear what these three categories of age represent. Do they represent different social values assigned to the various age groups or differential capacities for resuming social roles? Since Western societies place a high value on youth, it could be argued that, with the exception of exceedingly eminent persons, the aged have a low social value.

An emphasis upon chronological age as the criterion for resuscitation would suggest that these age groups have different social values while an emphasis upon physiological criteria would suggest that the important factor is the capacity to perform social roles. If physiological rather than chronological age was affecting their decisions to resuscitate, one would expect that the relationship between age and resuscitation would be lower among patients who died or were resuscitated after their second day in the hospital since it takes time to evaluate the physiological age of an individual. The relationship between age and resuscitation was less strong among patients who were resuscitated after the first two hospital days. Goodman and Kruskal's gamma relating age to resuscitation is $-.43$ for resuscitations performed during the first two hospital days compared to $-.12$ for resuscitations performed after the first two hospital days.

Social Class of Patient

In all human societies, members are ranked according to certain characteristics. Certain classes of individuals are considered more important or valuable than others. Those whom physicians perceive as contributing more to society may be more likely to be the objects of heroic life-saving efforts. In the treatment of a patient with an uncertain diagnosis (myocardial infarction combined with jaundice and history of lung cancer), internists did differentiate to some extent between a patient with a high-status occupation (a banker) and one who was described as an unemployed laborer. However, in the treatment of an unsalvageable patient (cancer of the esophagus) they did not distinguish between a lawyer whose illness was described as "exhausting the family's resources" and a truck driver in the same situation. Both of these cases were treated less actively than that of a lawyer with the same illness whose family had asked the physician "to spare no expense in treating him." This suggests that physicians are responsive to the financial burden of an illness to the family, presumably because of its effects on family relationships. However, when asked to rank the relative influence of social characteristics upon their decisions to treat chronically ill patients, they ranked this factor sixth out of seven.

Further evidence for this interpretation comes from the pediatric and neurosurgical samples. Several physicians suggested in interviews that the family's financial resources would influence decisions involving children with devastating and permanent damage, such as hydrocephaly and myelomeningocele. The child with a myelomeningocele, especially, requires enormous amounts of medical care, since he is very likely to have serious neurological, renal, and bowel problems in addition to paraplegia and mental retardation. Responses to the neurosurgical questionnaire did not suggest that financial factors influenced neurosurgical decisions involving infants with such an anomaly. The case was presented to respondents in two parts, the first one involving "20 year old parents neither of whom have completed high school" and the second part involving parents who were "well educated and financially comfortable." The difference in the proportions usually performing this operation in these two cases was only 2 percent. However, a similar comparison among the pediatricians yielded a percentage difference of 20 percent.

One explanation for the difference between the two specialties may lie in the way the questions were constructed. Since myelomeningocele is often accompanied by mental retardation, the neurosurgical questionnaire included a medical statement which was designed to rule out that possibility for that particular patient. This statement did not appear in the version of the question which was used in the pediatric questionnaire.

Alternatively, the explanation may lie in the relative importance which members of the two specialties place upon the financial burden of an illness to the family. Thirty-eight percent of the pediatricians ranked this factor among the top three on a list of social characteristics of the patient influencing their decisions to treat patients, compared to 21 percent of the neurosurgeons. It seems that the financial burden of an illness to the family is a more important consideration to the pediatrician, and this is reflected in their responses to the two versions of the question concerning the treatment of the myelomeningocele.

However, when social status measured in terms of financial resources was varied together with family attitude on the pediatric questionnaire, the latter appeared to be the more important factor.

The comparison involved two cases which were quite similar: a mongoloid with severe respiratory distress and an infant with seizures combined with spasticity and hypertonia. Brain damage is a very probable result of the latter condition. Table 7 shows that when the family's attitude is favorable, the children are actively treated, regardless of the socioeconomic status of their families. When the family's attitude is negative, socioeconomic status of the family is related to treatment.

Surveys Compared to Hospital Records.

A valid criticism of the type of data which has been presented here is that it does not reflect the actual behavior of physicians. However, the study by Duff and Campbell (1973) cited previously indicates that, in the special-care nursery of a university hospital, decisions to withhold treatment from severely damaged children accounted for 14 percent of the deaths during a two-and-one-half-year period.

In order to validate the findings from the surveys, information concerning the treatment of critically ill adult patients was obtained by examining the hospital charts for all patients who had died (some of whom had been unsuccessfully resuscitated) and all those who had been successfully resuscitated during a calendar year (1969) on the clinical service of a university hospital. On the assumption that each attempted resuscitation in the hospital records sample represented a decision by a member of the house staff, these data were compared with the behavior of those residents in the internal medicine sample who were located in similar types of medical settings. Each case history in the internal-medicine questionnaire included an item on resuscitation. While the number of cases in the hospital records sample which closely resembled the cases described in the questionnaire was small, on the whole, the decision-making patterns in the two samples were similar.

The data suggested that the survey respondents may have exaggerated their likelihood of resuscitating patients, since the proportions of patients resuscitated in the hospital records sample are lower than in the survey. These data suggest that treatment may actually be withdrawn to a greater extent than the survey results indicate.

In a sample of mongoloid children with heart defects who were catheterized in a university hospital during a five-and-a-half-year period, social variables played a more important role than medical

TABLE 7

Influence of Family's Attitude and Socioeconomic Status
Upon Pediatricians' Decisions to Treat Mentally Damaged Newborns[a]
(Percentage of Pediatricians Who Would Treat Very Actively)

Family Attitude	Socioeconomic Status of Patient's Family		Cause of Damage	z Statistic
	High	*Low*		
Favorable	58 (458)	59 (464)	seizures with spasticity and hypertonia (*High*); mongoloid with severe respiratory distress (*Low*)	—
Unfavorable	44 (458)	33 (464)	mongoloid with severe respiratory distress (*High*); seizures with spasticity and hypertonia (*Low*)	2.73*

*p < .01

[a]Socioeconomic status is defined in terms of occupation and financial resources; family attitude is defined in terms of a "precious pregnancy" and maternal rejection of the child.

variables in determining whether or not an operation was performed. Even in this hospital, wher there was a strong normative bias in favor of operating upon these children, these operations occurred less frequently than the questionnaire results would indicate.

Euthanasia and Definitions of Death

Finally, are there situations in which physicians attempt to hasten or to bring about terminal events? Responses to a question in the pediatric questionnaire concerning direct killing of an anencephalic infant were overwhelmingly negative. Among the respondents (both residents and physicians), only 1 percent said that they would be likely to give an "intravenous injection of a lethal dose of potassium chloride or a sedative drug" to an anencephalic infant; 3 percent said that they might do so.

Internists were asked to indicate whether or not they would increase the dosage of narcotics for a patient in the last stages of terminal cancer to the point where it might risk or would probably lead to respiratory arrest. Eighty-one percent of the physicians and 68 percent of the residents were willing to take some risk or high risk of inducing respiratory arrest in the patient by increasing his dosage of narcotics. While the same proportions of both groups were willing to incur some risk of respiratory arrest (38 percent and 39 percent respectively), the physicians were much more willing to incur high risk of respiratory arrest (43 percent) than were the residents (29 percent).

Specific questions to test their perceptions of the act were not included in the questionnaire, but comments in the interviews suggested that some physicians defined this treatment as euthanasia while others argued that this procedure is not a true example of euthanasia since the physician's *intention* is to suppress pain and not to cause death. It is possible, although there is no data to show this conclusively, that the older physician is more likely to make this distinction between intent and action than the younger physician. In other words, for the older physician, the important aspect of the use of narcotics with terminally ill patients is that it suppresses pain. The younger physician perceives both functions equally and is afraid that his action will be interpreted in terms of "hastening" death rather than in terms of pain suppression.

Physicians in all four specialties were asked whether they would consider cessation of brain function, apart from cessation of respiratory and cardiac function, as a terminal event under certain precisely defined conditions. The conditions have been defined by an interdisciplinary committee at Harvard (Ad Hoc Committee of the Harvard Medical School to Examine Brain Death, 1968). In the four specialties, respondents were presented with cases appropriate for their specialties which were described as having the criteria of brain death, as defined by the Harvard Committee. The respondents were given several choices: leaving the respirator running until spontaneous cardiac activity ceased or turning off the respirator either without consultation with other persons or after consulting either colleagues or the patient's family or both. In these four specialties, between 24 and 30 percent of the respondents indicated that they would accept irreversible cessation of brain function as a criterion for death, permitting them to cease maintaining the patient's respiratory functions. In other words for these physicians, irreversible loss of the capacity for social interaction is a more important consideration than the continuation of the physiological indicator of life, heartbeat.

Even among those who accepted the criteria, no more than 18 percent in any of the samples were willing to turn off the respirator without any consultation whatsoever. This suggests that the criteria are as yet not fully accepted, since the agreement of either colleagues or family or preferably both is required by most of these physicians.

The ambivalence which still exists in this area can be seen by comparing the attitudes expressed by pediatricians toward an infant defined as having the criteria of brain death and toward an anencephalic infant whose brain is nonexistent. Both infants lack functioning brains, but pediatricians are much more willing to define as dead the infant whose brain has ceased to function than to withhold treatment from an infant who was born without a brain.

While no more than 2 percent of the pediatricians said that they would resuscitate an anencephalic infant, only 40 percent of the physicians and 31 percent of the residents indicated that they would not use any other forms of treatment. These percentages are substantially lower than the percentages who indicated that they would turn off the respirator when an infant's condition met the criteria for brain death (67 and 80 percent, respectively). It appears that the recent controversy over donation of hearts for transplants has made one type of decision acceptable, while absence of public discussion of another, analogous, type of decision has meant that it remains unacceptable.

Discussion

Evidence from the present study suggests that physicians respond to the chronically ill or terminally ill patient not simply in terms of physiological definitions of illness but also in terms of the extent to which he is capable of interacting with others. The treatable patient is one who can interact or who has the potential to interact in a meaningful way with others in his environment. The physically damaged salvageable patient whose life can be maintained for a considerable period of time is more likely to be actively treated than the severely brain-damaged patient or the patient who is in the last stages of terminal illness. The brain-damaged infant is also not defined as treatable by many physicians, since he lacks the potential to establish social relationships with others.

I have stressed that this study, unlike other treatments of the subject, has been concerned not with what physicians *should* do for the critically ill patient but with their *actual* attitudes and behavior. What are the implications of these findings for those who are concerned with formulating policy in this area and with developing new ethical imperatives for medical practice?

The findings from this study of the treatment which doctors say they would give to critically ill patients suggest that the system whereby this type of behavior is controlled by peers, clients, and other social institutions such as the law is in need of reformulation. The problem arises because there is a disparity between the traditional medical ethic concerning the treatment of these patients and the actual behavior of many physicians. According to the traditional ethic, treatment is meant to be continued as long as life, defined in physiological terms, can be preserved. In fact, as we have seen, treatment is generally withdrawn when the quality of life as defined in social terms has deteriorated or disappeared irrevocably.

In a sense, social control over these kinds of decisions is maintained by stressing the preservation of life, rather than by specifying conditions under which the norm may be relaxed. Informally, social criteria for defining the treatable patient have replaced the traditional ethic, but the new criteria are not universally accepted.

Considerable stress is being placed upon this social control system by the disparity between the formal and informal norms and by the fact that the number of patients for whom application of the formal norms would be undesirable is steadily increasing as a result of improvements in medical technology. At the same time, in other areas, such as abortion and genetic engineering, a similar dilemma of choosing between social and physiological definitions of life is being resolved in favor of the former.

One solution to the problem would be to attempt to alter the formal norms in this area by developing medical guidelines for the withdrawal of treatment with respect to certain specifically defined conditions, since it is clear that physicians prefer to think about these problems in the context of specific cases and not in terms of general rules. In fact, such a set of guidelines has already been formulated to deal with one pressing problem in the treatment of the critically ill patient: the problem of the irreversibly comatose patient whose respiratory functions are being maintained mechanically. As the data presented in this article indicate, this set of guidelines has already been widely although not universally accepted by physicians in four major medical specialties.

Since there appear to be certain cases in each medical specialty which repeatedly cause controversy, some attempt ought to be made to specify the medical and social conditions under which treatment would be desirable. For example, it should be possible to define guidelines for withdrawing all life-saving or death-prolonging treatment from the patient whose capacity for meaningful social interaction has been irreversibly impaired by a stroke. In such cases only the use of treatment which alleviates suffering is appropriate, if the treatable patient is being defined in social as well as physical terms.

Similarly the case of the anencephalic infant would appear to be one where specific guidelines could resolve the inconsistencies which now exist between the treatment of these infants and those whose conditions meet the criteria of irreversible brain death. Treatment can be discontinued in the latter case as specified in existing medical guidelines. Therefore there appears to be no reason to continue it in the former case.

Another example is that of myelomeningocele, a condition which in severe cases produces paraplegia, lack of bladder and urinary control, and brain damage in newborn infants. A recognized medical authority on this type of ailment (Lorber, 1971) has recently stated the criteria for not operating upon certain children with this ailment. Unfortunately such children can live untreated for several months, enduring considerable pain and suffering. Freeman (1972) has recently suggested that this is one instance where withholding treatment should not be considered to be ethically superior to terminating life. In other words, it would be more ethical to kill such a child than to permit it to linger in the hospital for weeks or months untreated, waiting to die. In this type of case, also, specific guidelines for the withdrawal of treatment and even for the termination of life would appear to be highly desirable.

Many difficult medical problems which physicians now face will obviously not be amenable to this approach. However, with improvements in medical knowledge it will no doubt be possible to specify such guidelines for increasing numbers of medical conditions.

What is meant here by medical guidelines is very different from the ethical codes which have been developed in the area of medical experimentation. These codes are stated in such general terms that they provide no useful guidance in dealing with the highly differentiated situations which physicians face. Instead, precise medical guidelines concerning the appropriate levels of treatment for specific conditions or diseases are needed.

The decision to withdraw treatment in accordance with such guidelines should be subject to review by the physician's colleagues. Peer review is already used to monitor ethical aspects of medical behavior in the area of medical experimentation on human beings. Many hospitals also have committees which monitor medical performance with respect to operative procedures and deaths. The individualistic character of medical practice has made any sort of regulation of medical practice extremely difficult. However, now that it has become evident that the rule that life should be preserved in every instance is unworkable, some sort of regulation to resolve the most difficult cases is a necessity.[1]

---

[1] For further information about this study, see Diana Crane. *The Sanctity of Social Life: A Study of Doctors' Decisions to Treat Critically Ill Patients* (New York: Russell Sage Foundation, in press).

Diana Crane
Department of Sociology
113 McNeil-CR
University of Pennsylvania
Philadelphia, Pennsylvania 19174

Address for academic year 1974-75:
Diana Crane
1 rue Huysmans
75006 Paris, France

The research reported in this paper was supported by grants from the Russell Sage Foundation. I thank Dr. Howard Freeman for his advice during the development and conduct of the study.

References

Ad Hoc Committee of the Harvard Medical School to Examine Brain Death
1968   "A definition of irreversible coma." Journal of the American Medical Association 205: 85-88.

Brown, N. K., et al.
1970   "The preservation of life." Journal of the American Medical Association 211: 76-81.

Duff, R. S., and A. G. M. Campbell
1973   "Moral and ethical dilemmas in the special-care nursery." New England Journal of Medicine 289: 890-894.

Farber, B.
1968   Mental Retardation: Its Social Context and Social Consequences. Boston: Houghton Mifflin.

Freeman, J. M.
1972   "Is there a right to die—quickly?" Journal of Pediatrics 80: 904-905.

Glaser, B. G., and A. L. Strauss
1965   Awareness of Dying. Chicago: Aldine.

Kasl, S., and S. Cobb
1966   "Health behavior, illness behavior and sick role behavior." Archives of Environmental Health 12 (April): 246-266.

Karnofsky, D. A.
1960   "Why prolong the life of a patient with advanced cancer?" CA
        Bulletin of Cancer Progress 10: 9-11.

Kübler-Ross, E.
1969   On Death and Dying. New York: Macmillan.

Lerner, M.
1970   "When, why and where people die." In Brim, O.C., Jr., et al. (eds.),
        The Dying Patient. New York: Russell Sage Foundation.

Lester, D.
1967   "Experimental and correlational studies of the fear of death."
        Psychological Bulletin 67: 27-36.

Lorber, J.
1971   "Results of treatment of myelomeningocele." Developmental
        Medicine and Child Neurology 13: 279-303.

McNemar, Q.
1962   Psychological Statistics (Third Edition), New York: Wiley.

Morison, R.
1971   "Death: process or event?" Science 173:694-698.

Parsons, T.
1951   The Social System. New York: The Free Press of Glencoe.

1958   "Definitions of health and illness in the light of American values and
        social structure." In Jaco, E. (ed.). Patients, Physicians, and Illness.
        New York: The Free Press of Glencoe.

Parsons, T., and V. M. Lidz
1967   "Death in American society." In Shneidman, E. (ed.), Essays in Self-
        Destruction. New York: Science House.

Shaw, A.
1972   "Doctor, do we have a choice?" New York Times Magazine (January
        30): 44-54.

Sudnow, D.
1967   Passing On. Englewood Cliffs, N.J.: Prentice-Hall.

Williams, R. H.
1969   "Our role in the generation, modification and termination of life."
        Archives of Internal Medicine 124 (August): 215-237.

III Organizations

Physician Involvement
in Hospital Decision Making

MICHAEL A. REDISCH*

The focus of government health care policy over the past two decades has subtly changed from earlier commitments to provide health care to all who are in need. While assurance of access to care is, of course, still of great concern, the foremost policy issues of today revolve around ways to constrain future increases in health care costs. The major policy battleground is the hospital sector, where the most serious health care cost increases have occurred.

Governmental concern goes beyond the simple figures that show health expenditures rising from 5.2 percent of Gross National Product in 1960 to 8.6 percent of Gross National Product in fiscal 1976 (see Gibson and Mueller, 1977). A similar rise in relative expenditures in the consumer durable sector would traditionally be interpreted as the result of informed choices made in the economic marketplace by consumers of those products. However, medical care in general and hospital care in particular operate in markets so heavily underwritten by public programs and by private insurance that conventional market signals are weak or nonexistent. In 1975, 92 percent of hospital care was paid for by some form of third-party payer, a fact that tends to obscure the cost impact of hospital care on

*Any views expressed in this paper are those of the author and do not necessarily reflect the official position of the U.S. General Accounting Office.

The authors wishes to thank Jon Gabel for a number of comments that were helpful in the preparation of the paper.

In *Hospital Cost Containment: Selected Notes for Future Policy*, edited by Michael Zubkoff, Ira E. Raskin, and Ruth S. Hanft. New York: PRODIST, 1978.

the household budget. Furthermore, the individual seeking care is usually not fully informed of the potential outcomes of that care; instead, he must put his faith and trust in a physician who is allowed to commit the individual to utilize a bundle of scarce health resources. Among them is the physician's own time, and thus a potential conflict of interest is created.

The individual, therefore, typically does not purchase health care through the same mechanism or with the same attitudes as he does other goods and services. The result is governmental concern and intervention as the share of the nation's resources devoted to health care continues to rise.

A number of as yet untested proposals are being offered to combat inflation in the hospital without unduly limiting access to or quality of care. These suggestions include certificate-of-need laws, hospital rate review, various forms of prospective reimbursement, return to the direct wage and price controls of the Economic Stabilization era, or market strategies revolving around the growth of Health Maintenance Organizations.

However, too often in attempts to conceptualize the process by which the hospital sector will react to one or more of these control mechanisms, a central and overriding feature of the U.S. hospital system is omitted. The unique relationship between the hospital and the physician in the production of health care in this country is ignored by many of those attempting to understand or predict the reaction of hospitals to specific government policy. Instead, the hospital is typically viewed as an institution differing from ordinary firms only to the extent that a major portion of hospital care is provided in a not-for-profit setting.

An explanation for the lack of a strong physician figure in most models of hospital behavior can probably be traced to the payment mechanism for health care in the United States. The patient hospitalized here is typically subject to two separate billings; one for "hospital" services and one for "personal physician" services. This dual billing system has led to a conceptually false dichotomy whereby the hospital and physician are often erroneously viewed as independent entities selling services in functionally segmented health markets. Yet from the patient's point of view, "health care" in a hospital setting should be viewed as a single product jointly produced by the combined actions of hospitals and physicians. That patients in fact do take this view is suggested by Yett et al. (1971), who estimate that the demand for hospital care in a state aggregated cross-section is more responsive to changes in a physician surgical fee index than changes in the (more heavily insured) price of a bed day. Davis and Russell (1972) also estimate a demand equation for inpatient care that contains a significantly negative coefficient for the physician fee variable.

This paper will examine the hospital-physician relationship more from a perspective of supply-side response to a set of social and economic incentives than from the perspective of consumer demand for hospital-based health care. It is in the area of modeling supply-side behavior that distortions and erroneous implications can be caused by an improper specification of the role of the physician in determining resource use in the hospital. As Jacobs (1974) has noted, many of the attempts to model hospital behavior either view the hospital as controlled completely by administrators' preferences or lump all decision-making groups into a heterogeneous whole, creating a fictional entity not related to reality. These "organism" models, viewing the "hospital" as the acting body, tend to obscure the way operational decisions are jointly arrived at through the individual actions of patients, trustees, physicians, administrators, and other hospital personnel.

Here we will attempt to delineate more specifically the roles that the physician may play in strategies aimed at controlling cost increases in hospitals. Any effective mechanism for containing the ongoing rapid rises in hospital costs must explicitly take into account the involvement of physicians in hospital decision making. Few administrators like to admit how limited is their control over the operation of their hospitals. They would like to believe that by their efforts alone, order and direction are distilled from anarchy. Yet it is the physician, operating as a separate entity outside the control of the Board of Trustees or the administrator, who directs most of the major resource decisions made in the hospital setting. The physician recommends admission, takes responsibility for ordering diagnostic procedures and therapeutic measures, and determines when the patient is fit to leave the hospital. In addition, it is the physician who typically engages in a lobbying effort with hopes of committing the administrator and trustees to invest in additional bed space, in personnel to help him provide more and better patient care, and in new and expensive technology.

A model of complete physician control, while admittedly an abstraction of reality, is still close enough to be considered a useful tool for analyzing various policy formulations (see Pauly and Redisch, 1973, for a rigorous statement of such a model). The two lines of internal authority in the hospital can lead to inevitable conflict between administrators and physicians. Yet the administrator has little stake in opposing physicians, particularly under a regime of unconstrained cost reimbursement. In fact, the administrator typically finds his own job security most closely tied to his ability to satisfy the demands of the medical staff. Viewed in this light, the administrator's role is simply to provide labor, supplies, and facilities to independent physicians. It is the physician who directs the actual provision of care in the hospital.

Trustees are also organizationally structured to exert external control on physician behavior. In a not-for-profit hospital there are no stockholders or owners of equity capital. The Board of Trustees presumably represents the public interest and bears some form of legal and moral responsibility for all activities, professional and otherwise, that occur within the institution. However, while each member of a typical board is a competent individual in his own field, he is unprepared for participation in the types of issues and decisions involved in the management of the hospital. Ordinarily he has limited knowledge of the medical profession, and his knowledge of the hospital is usually restricted to personal contact as a patient or as a relative of a patient.

A group of laymen without training in medicine thus may find it difficult to fulfill adequately responsibilities related in any way to quality of care, the practice of medicine, or the evaluation of medical staff. Almost all resource-related decisions in the hospital can be classified under one or more of these "medical" rubrics. It is therefore not surprising to see a tendency in most hospitals for the board to abjure direct responsibility and to delegate authority to some internal physician group. This tendency is, of course, actively supported by the American Medical Association, which suggests that "the responsibility of the hospital governing board is to provide the foundation for self-governance by the organized medical staff" (American Medical Association, 1974b:12). Once again de facto physician control over resource-related decisions is not hard to establish.

We will discuss in some detail the physician's role in the hospital cost inflation process and examine the impact of hypothesized physician behavior on the expected relative success of alternative policies for containing hospital costs. First, however, a description of the way inflation has taken place in the hospital will prove helpful.

The hospital cost inflation process will be examined with the patient day (or adjusted patient day, accounting for outpatient department care, American Hospital Association, 1969:466) as the reference unit of output. We feel that a specific illness incident treated as a case is a more meaningful measure of hospital "output" in the social welfare sense than the number of days of varying services devoted to patient care. However, use of the patient day is a more tractable measure and will allow us to explain relationships involving resource use (for example, factor input utilization decisions, a hospital investment function, the operational inflationary mechanism in the hospital environment) as well as or better than the case. This is particularly true since there is yet no precise, generally agreed upon way to measure the economic or medical aspects of "case mix."

The 10 to 20 percent annual increases in per diem hospital costs since 1965 are critically related to changes in the quantities, qualities, and sophistication of the services that are lumped together under the output designation of a patient day. Previous efforts to document the rise in cost per patient day have broken down these cost increases into four basic components: (1) rising wage levels of employees; (2) increased personnel per patient day; (3) rising cost of nonlabor inputs; and (4) increased use of nonlabor inputs per patient day. M. Feldstein (1971a), Davis and Foster (1972), and Waldman (1972) have all independently estimated that rising unit input costs and increased real input use have contributed approximately equal amounts to the rise in per diem costs in the late 1960s and early 1970s.

The American Hospital Association has claimed a recent change in the proportionate share of hospital cost increases related to rising unit input costs (Council on Wage and Price Stability, 1976:13). It estimates that pure factor price increases accounted for over 70 percent of hospital cost increases from January 1974 until June 1975. This reversal, if true, was due to expanded minimum wage laws and collective bargaining, increased malpractice insurance premiums, and higher energy costs. While hospital input prices may temporarily move faster than the general rate of inflation, it is still expected that increases in real inputs have led and will continue to lead, unless checked, to the growing share of hospital care in our national product accounts.

The origin of the rise in the volume of labor and nonlabor inputs utilized per patient day can be traced in part to the ability of the physician over time to reduce his own input or operating costs by transference of functions and costs to the hospital. Examples of this trend include the obstetrician who relies more and more on nursing staff and who rushes in at the last minute for the actual delivery, or the attending physician who utilizes house staff to care for his patients on Wednesdays and Saturdays. Johnson (1969) notes that nurses now perform many tasks that until two decades ago were limited to physicians, for example, the starting of blood transfusions, introduction of intravenous fluids, and injections. Such transference will continue into the future as attending physicians are relieved of suturing and many other responsibilities in surgery, coronary care, emergency room duties, and dialysis.

If this transference were done in an economically and socially efficient manner, then society could capture the potential gain generated by substitution of low-cost hospital inputs for high-cost physician time. While hospital costs would register increases, these would be more than compensated for by decreases in aggregate physician bills to patients. However, this does not appear to have happened. Instead, aided by the separation of bills for the costs of joint hospital-and-physician services, the physician has shown a great willingness to bill as much in his "supervisory" capacity over hospital inputs as when he performs services directly. Physicians are thus able to increase output (and incomes) without dramatic increases in fees. As an extreme example, the Medicare program often

finds itself asked to pay under Part A (the hospital side of Title
XVIII) its proportionate share of the salary of the resident who
performs surgery while simultaneously being asked to cover under
Part B (the physician side) the bill submitted by the supervising
physician.

The physician's growing financial stake in the direction of
resources other than his own labor may be seen by examining data
from 1955 to 1971. Over this period physician incomes rose by
around 7.2 percent per year while physician fees (as measured by
the Consumer Price Index) rose by only 4.4 percent per year.
Physician practice hours per week and practice weeks per year fell
slightly (see Leveson and Rogers, 1976). The maintenance of this
high rate of income growth under these conditions was accomplished by increasing physician productivity through dramatic
increases in the nonphysician resource intensity of medical care.

Even if the physician did not continue to bill in part for services
transferred to the hospital, the trend toward a greater and greater
role for hospital inputs has still led to major inefficiencies in the
production of health care. The physician and his patient are usually
not even cognizant of the costs of basic hospital services. The
hospital will typically tend to prorate the costs of all inputs (except
those used to produce ancillary services) over all users of those
inputs, through the use of room rates or daily service charges, which
cover more than 50 percent of daily patient expense in most
hospitals. Thus the utilization of increasing amounts of basic services
by an individual patient will have a negligible impact on that
patient's bill, since these costs are spread over all patients in the
hospital. As the medical staff increases in size, each physician will
tend to become less and less aware of the effects of his actions on
others, since there are large numbers of patients of other physicians
who share in the costs of these basic services. Unfortunately, the
cumulative effect of this myopic behavior results in the rapid
escalation of basic hospital services and of the hospital's room and
board charge. The basic service increase is reflected in the time
trend of the semiprivate room charge component of the Consumer
Price Index, which almost tripled from 1965 to 1975.

The situation is exacerbated by the extent of insurance for

hospital services. Even when the hospital directly bills the patient for use of specific services, the physician is aware that the major burden of that bill will be borne not by the patient but by some third-party payer. To the extent that hospital care is more heavily insured than ambulatory physician care, the physician is likely to suggest a hospital stay for a patient who could be treated as well (and more efficiently) on an ambulatory basis. The practice of admitting patients into the hospital for an overnight stay to run a series of what are essentially diagnostic tests is the classic example of such behavior. But this specific practice has begun to die out as insurors have taken steps both to cover these tests when performed on an ambulatory patient and to reject payments for inpatient admissions whose sole justification is diagnostic testing.

Thus there appear to be three forces at work that mutually tend to reinforce the physician's incentive to utilize hospital services in an economically inefficient manner. The separation of physician and hospital bills for jointly produced health care, the proration of basic hospital service costs over all patients, and the pervasiveness of insurance for hospital services all make the apparent cost to the physician of additional hospital service very small relative to the true social costs of the inputs used to produce that service. Major incentives are created for the physician to oversubstitute hospital inputs for his own labor and to order the production of only marginally beneficial health and hotel services in the hospital.

At the same time, the physician seems reluctant to utilize health care inputs when he himself must bear the full costs and directorial burden of those inputs. For example, Reinhardt (1972) estimates that physicians could profitably employ in their offices more than twice as many physicians' assistants as they now do. Rather than take the risk and the added responsibility of a larger staff to supervise, physicians have chosen to pass up this potentially profitable option. Yet they seem to show no such compunction when it comes to ordering for their patients increasing amounts of hospital inputs, for which they bear no direct financial or managerial burden.

While the number of inputs used to produce basic hospital room and board services have increased over time, the really dramatic increases in hospital resource intensity seem to be largely related to increases in the availability and utilization levels of a set of diagnos-

Michael A. Redisch

TABLE 1   Growth in Selected Hospital Series[a]

	1968	1969	1970	1971	Percent Change 1968-1971
Operating cost	$55.51	$60.89	$69.60	$78.75	41.8
Operating room visits	.05456	.05071	.05223	.05373	-1.5
Pathology tests	.06327	.11652	.11504	.10914	72.5
Nuclear medicine procs.	.00252	.00705	.00690	.00965	282.9
Pharmacy line items	.35610	.79150	.91918	1.0449	193.4
In- & outpatient lab tests	2.2046	2.2964	2.5393	2.8588	29.7
In- & outpatient radiology procs.	.31753	.31604	.33519	.36378	14.6
Therapeutic radiology procs.	.00685	.01394	.01577	.01894	176.5
Blood bank units	.03759	.05881	.05333	.06333	68.5

[a]All figures are reported in whole units normalized on adjusted patient days. Thus in 1968 operating cost per adjusted patient day in the sample was $55.51 and the average number of pathology tests per adjusted patient day was .06327.

Sources: The data were provided by the Health Services Research Center (the Center) of Northwestern University and the American Hospital Association (AHA). They were obtained by the Center from the Hospital Administrative Services (HAS) Division of the AHA. Data are submitted to HAS on a monthly basis by several thousand voluntarily participating hospitals. These hospitals may then compare their performance in providing services with that of similarly situated institutions.

No payment for services is based on the completed HAS forms, and the data are not audited. HAS puts the raw monthly data onto a computer tape and runs some simple statistical checks that are meant to eliminate "order of magnitude" errors. The Center obtained a tape of this monthly data file for close to four hundred hospitals. The tape was than "annualized" on a calendar year basis for the years 1967 to 1971. Hospitals reporting less than nine months of data were eliminated from the sample, and it was assumed that hospitals reporting between nine and eleven months of data would have reported "average" figures (based on months they did report) for the missing months. In addition, statistical checks were performed to eliminate obviously erroneous outliers. There still appear to be some order-of-magnitude errors in the data, and certain hospitals and unreliable variables will have to be removed in later empirical work.

All identifying hospital characteristics (geographic area, teaching status, affiliations, services offered other than those reported on the HAS forms, etc.) were removed by either HAS or the Center. The data were then made available to the author.

It was quickly decided that the data for 1967 were too fragmented and erratic to be of much use. (HAS was just starting up and many hospitals were unfamiliar with the forms.) Also, those hospitals that did not appear in all years (1968 to 1971) were eliminated from the sample. The original sample consisted of 348 hospitals in 1968, 370 in 1969, 379 in 1970, and 375 in 1971. After removing those hospitals that did not appear in one or more years, we were left with a sample of 285 hospitals. These were fairly evenly spaced out over all hospital bed-size groups. The average bed size in the final sample varied slightly from year to year about an aggregate mean of 249 beds.

tic and therapeutic medical services provided in a hospital setting under the direction and control of physicians. The increases can be seen quite clearly in Table 1. Over a period of time (1968 through 1971) in which the number of operating room visits per adjusted patient day actually declined slightly in these sample hospitals, we can see explosive growth in the utilization levels per adjusted patient day of seven medical services (pathology tests, nuclear medicine

procedures, pharmacy line items, inpatient and outpatient laboratory tests, inpatient and outpatient radiology procedures, therapeu-
radiology procedures, and blood bank units). There is no break in
the general pattern when hospitals are grouped into separate bed-
size classes. In a separate paper by the author (Redisch, 1974),
hedonic cost indices are estimated that suggest that the growth of
these seven medical services accounts for more than one-third of the
increase in cost per adjusted patient day in the sample hospitals.
Since approximately one-half of the per diem cost rise is related to
rises in unit costs of basic inputs, these estimates imply that two-
thirds of the increase in real inputs per adjusted patient day in the
sample hospitals were related to increases in the per diem use of
these seven medical services.

Much of this increase can be traced to the growth of highly
specialized treatment centers within hospitals. Coronary care units,
intensive care units for adults and for newborns, burn units, and so
on, contribute to a highly structured form of patient care. (The ratio
of private, not-for-profit hospitals reporting intensive care units
jumped from 11 percent in 1960 to more than 70 percent today.)
There may be a tendency to establish routines in patient monitoring
in these units. Patterns of diagnostic ancillary service use can
develop that may bear little relation to the needs of the individual
patient (see Griner and Liptzen, 1971).

Growth in ancillary service use has also been encouraged by new
hospital technology, such as multiple channel autoanalyzers, that
lowers unit costs of individual tests when operating at a high
volume. However, these scale economies may soon be dissipated
through a "Xerox effect" (in many business offices, the surge in
volume after the introduction of duplicating machines may more
than make up for the drop in unit costs). Physicians who once
ordered a small number of lab tests to confirm their original clinical
diagnosis now order a full range of ten or twenty tests to "see what
comes up." This somewhat spurious demand for laboratory tests can
then be used to justify the purchase of still more automated lab
equipment.

Moreover, rapid growth in ancillary service use is stimulated by
a major new force in the practice of medicine. The rising number of

Michael A. Redisch

dissatisfied patients who choose to sue their physicians and hospitals for malpractice, the decreasing reluctance of physicians to testify against one another in the contest of such suits, and the growing propensity of the courts to award large sums of money to patients who are successful in pursuing these suits have all contributed to an increasing tendency for physicians and hospitals to practice "defensive medicine."

This ancillary service growth, contributing such a large share to the rise in per diem hospital costs, is under the direct control of the physician. Furthermore, it is not at all clear that this intensive use of a fairly common set of hospital services has positively contributed to the overall level of the "quality" of hospital care. Berki, for example (1972:31), notes that it is not known whether the more intensive use of laboratory procedures corresponds in fact to increases in the quality of care or to medically unjustified overuse of convenient, income-generating services. Ofttimes what may emerge from haphazard diagnostic testing is one or two false positives that lead to further testing or to inappropriate treatment. For example, Schimmel (1964) notes that 20 percent of the patients in Yale's Intensive Care Unit suffered complications from diagnostic tests, drugs, and various therapeutic measures.

Until now we have talked about hospital cost inflation primarily in terms of increases in costs per adjusted patient day. Yet government policy should be directed not just at these "unit" or daily costs, but at the aggregate level of hospital expenditures, as reflected in per capita hospital costs. Per capita costs are determined by the product of per diem costs and the number of patient days per capita. And the latter is determined by the per capita hospital admission rate and by the average length of stay for hospital care. Thus far we have examined the influence of the physician on per diem costs. We must now consider his degree of control over the admission decision and the discharge (or length of stay) decision.

Work by Wennberg et al. (1975), concerning several Maine communities at a single point in time, suggests that the admission decision is the most important explanation of variations in per capita hospital costs and expenditures. They find that average length of stay or cost per admission is less important than per capita admissions in explaining those variations. Physicians' uncertainty about the need for service or the value of alternative therapies is the likely cause of large observed differences in age- and sex-adjusted per capita hospital admission rates across what would be considered fairly homogeneous communities. Wennberg and his associates conclude that "the resource implications of differences in management within hospitals are less important than decisions to manage patients at the ambulatory or the institutional level of care" (Wennberg et al., 1975:305).

While growth in per diem costs plays a larger role than growth in per capita admissions in explaining increases in per capita hospital costs over time, it *is* true that the admission decision is a central one in initiating the hospital cost inflation process. The decision seems dominated by a group of socioeconomic incentives aimed at both the patient and the physician, and by the varying perceptions of individual physicians as to what constitutes medical need.

Perceptions of medical need do vary among physicians. In England, medical care is not rationed by the price mechanism and physicians face identical economic incentives across all of their patients. In a study of over three thousand normal deliveries in the Oxford Record Linkage Study area in 1962, M. Feldstein (1968) found that the most important single factor influencing any woman's expected hospital stay during delivery was the standard practice of the obstetrician in charge of the case. This was found to be more important in determining length of stay than the age of the woman, the number of previous children, her social class, or other characteristics.

Physicians have a great deal of discretion in deciding whether the "medical needs" of the patient include admission to a hospital. Their determination of this need may be influenced by a number of social and economic forces not directly related to the medical condition of the patient. For example, Rafferty (1971) has observed that in two Indiana hospitals increases in the general incidence of illness in the community, resulting in increases in the rate of bed occupancy, made physicians reluctant to hospitalize patients for less severe illnesses or for minor elective procedures. Similarly, Davis and Russell (1972) found that rises in occupancy rates lead to treatment of marginal patients in the outpatient department. When beds are relatively scarce, they are saved by physicians for the seriously ill.

The resource decisions that physicians implicitly make in response to perceived social needs do not have to be minor ones. Titmuss (1950) notes that in 1939 almost half the patients in English hospitals (some 140,000 individuals) were discharged in anticipation of war casualties, at a time when there were 200,000 people on hospital waiting lists. Major changes in the way health care is delivered can be accomplished if they are considered part of desirable public policy with a degree of universal public acceptance.

While it is clear that "medical need" is the major determinant of health care utilization, we have shown that various social forces and differences in the medical perceptions of individual physicians also influence the decision to utilize hospital services. In addition, economic incentives to the patient and to the physician produce nontrivial changes in the level and mix of care. Bishop (1973:29) notes that the simplification of an extended care facility (ECF) transfer form and, more important, an agreement by a third-party payer to cover physician services in the ECF led to net savings by the insuror and the ending of a hospital expansion plan.

New York City provides another example of how physicians' personal economic incentives can affect their behavior in a way that is particularly relevant for future health care policy decisions. In the late 1950s, Group Health Insurance (GHI) and the Health Insurance Plan of Greater New York (HIP) both provided a wide range of health services at a marginal out-of-pocket cost of approximately zero to similar sets of subscribers in New York City. GHI paid participating physicians a fee for each service performed, while HIP contracted with groups of physicians who agreed to provide care to HIP enrollees in return for payment on an annual capitation basis. The rates for nonsurgical, nonobstetrical physician visits were similar for each plan, but GHI enrollees had an average of 7.18 hospitalized surgical procedures per hundred persons per year, while the rate for HIP enrollees was only 4.18 (Monsma, 1970:151). It may be that "too many" appendectomies, hysterectomies, and tonsillectomies were performed by GHI surgeons, or it may be that "too few" were performed by HIP surgeons. The only statement that emerges with any clarity is that the financial incentive to the physician somehow seems to have heavy impact on definitions of "medical need" when elective surgery is considered.

The impact of personal economic incentives to the physician can be further viewed in the study by Gaus et al. (1976), which compared various aspects of HMO performance with those of the nonprepaid, fee-for-service system for the Medicaid population. It was found that Medicaid beneficiaries enrolled in two medical foundations exhibited no statistically significant differences in hospital use when compared with a matched sample of Medicaid beneficiaries utilizing the fee-for-service system. The foundations accepted capitation payment for their Medicaid enrollees but reimbursed affiliated physicians on a fee-for-service basis. In contrast, Medicaid beneficiaries enrolled in a group of HMOs with non-fee-for-service physicians were observed to have 356 days of hospital care per 1,000 persons per year. This was a remarkable 62 percent lower than the 934 days per 1,000 persons per year measured for the fee-for-service Medicaid control group.

The authors conclude that the fact that foundations show no major differences in hospital use, despite the financial incentives at the organization level to do so, indicates that the financial incentive of capitation payment to the HMO organization may by itself not have significant impact on the hospitalization practices of affiliated physicians. The major cost impact of HMOs appears to lie not simply in having an organization (the HMO) take the risk for total care of the beneficiary. Instead, it lies in having the physician limit his incentives to hospitalize patients by removing him from the fee-for-service setting, by separating to some extent resource control from the medical staff, and by reconstituting medical practice within the context of a salaried, multispecialty group.

These conclusions are partially confirmed at a wider level by Bunker (1970), who observes a much lower rate of surgical procedures per 1,000 persons in England than in the United States. Similarly, Adelstein (1973) shows that the per capita number of x-ray exams is much higher in this country than in other countries.

Michael A. Redisch

Surgery and radiology in England are performed by salaried specialists working full time as hospital staff members, while surgery and radiology in the United States are typically performed by independent physicians faced with the perverse incentives of a fee-for-service reimbursement system.

This documentation of the pervasive influence of physicians in determining resource allocations within the hospital implies that control measures to hold down the rate of inflation of hospital costs, if aimed solely at the hospital, will be disappointing. Certificates of need, rate review, or alternative forms of prospective reimbursement all *do* provide the administrator with an added rationale for confronting and standing up to the physician staff. Yet the benefits to the administrator of siding with the staff are usually so high that true confrontations are exceedingly unusual.

Most hospital administrators see themselves in competition with other hospitals for physicians, not for patients, since it is only through a physician that an individual may be admitted to a hospital. As long as there are other hospitals that will admit him to practice, a physician is not totally dependent on a particular hospital for his livelihood. But a hospital that cannot retain a satisfied medical staff will soon find its occupancy rate falling, its per diem costs rising, and its ability to function as a health care institution seriously impaired. Furthermore, if cost guidelines are given to a hospital on a per diem basis, many administrators may find themselves in the seemingly paradoxical situation of allowing certain marginal equipment and personnel decisions or capital projects to attract or keep physician staff so that the occupancy rate will be high enough to move the hospital within the per diem cost constraints.

It is not surprising that administrators will put off as long as possible the inclusion of medical staff into any negative budgetary decisions that must be made. Most physicians practicing in a group of Western Pennsylvania hospitals that were being reimbursed on a prospective basis by the local Blue Cross organization were not even aware of this fact (see Applied Management Sciences, 1975). Cost containment was considered an administrative issue, not a medical one.

If hospital budgetary controls are made so tight that they cannot be met by simply eliminating any administrative slack in the hospital, then affiliated physicians will have to become more directly involved in the hospital's budgetary process. However, even when the administrator is forced to confront his medical staff on cost issues, he is at a disadvantage. Physicians can argue persuasively and with a unique degree of authority about medical need and quality of care. It is difficult for the lay administrator to pick and choose among these arguments and make resource decisions that hurt one physician group but not another. Even when these negative decisions are chosen, they are most likely to be based on the degree of power of the various physician specialty groups within the hospital, rather than on criteria based on some nebulous concept of social efficiency norms. There has been a paucity of sophisticated evaluation relating medical care inputs to health outcomes, even for expensive pieces of equipment. Without such evaluation, hospital administrators have little with which to judge competently or counter physician arguments concerning quality of care.

A more effective control mechanism might make an impact on the physician directly, rather than through the administrator. Yet the costs of policing physicians through direct regulation on a case-by-case basis can be excessive. Medical cases are highly differentiated goods. No two patients are ever exactly the same, even if they exhibit the same general set of symptoms. If the decision to hospitalize were based solely on medical reasoning, the physician would be hospitalizing a disease rather than a person with a disease.

The current method of applying case-by-case regulation is through a form of professional peer review structured around local Professional Standards Review Organizations. Yet peer review in this form may prove more effective as a quality control measure than as a cost control device. Historically, peer review in the health care sector seems to have been oriented toward preventing abuse of patients and not toward preventing abuse of resources. Skeptics have claimed that this orientation will continue, and that hospital costs will rise as PSRO-mandated "resource ceilings" quickly become "quality floors."

A more effective form of case-by-case peer review may be simply to have third-party payers provide full funding on a prospective basis for a second opinion by an "impartial" board-certified surgeon whenever a physician feels that nonemergency surgery is indicated. One study in this area, with a one- to four-year follow-up of cases, showed that "in the voluntary programs, one out of four screened patients, and in the mandatory programs, one out of seven and a half screened patients, appear to be permanently 'deferred' from surgery" (McCarthy and Kamons, 1976:7).

However, peer review in any form should not be expected to play a dominant role in strategies aimed at containing health care costs. The history of peer review in fields other than health has been marginal at best, because of an unwillingness or lack of power to impose meaningful controls. The inability of peer review to function effectively as a cost control device in fee-for-service health care settings gains credence from empirical studies of fee-for-service group practices in California. Physicians in these practices share costs but either bill patients directly or share in the net receipts according to a weighting scheme based on volume of the individual physician's patients. Costs have been observed to be as high as or higher than those in similarly situated solo practices (Newhouse, 1973).

The potential economies of sharing paramedical personnel and office equipment have been dissipated by physician behavior. With a large number (N) of physicians in practice together, each physician knows that by prescribing extensive use of the groups' resources he bears the burden of only $1/N$th of the costs but gains a proportionately greater share of the revenues. Even though physicians have a direct economic stake in the actions of their colleagues, peer group pressures in this ambulatory setting have not been effective cost control devices as physician staff size becomes unwieldy.

And the future may be less bright. Noll (1972) has shown that the regulatory process in areas other than health care has quickly degenerated into a system of peer control. This occurs when the only groups competent to evaluate the regulated firms are themselves current or former members of the industry.

Direct government intervention through the regulatory or rate-review process also does not appear to be the panacea that will bring hospital cost inflation in line with price rises in the rest of the economy. Work by Salkever and Bice (1976) and by Hellinger (1976) in evaluating the early impact of certificate-of-need legislation, and the study by Gaus and Hellinger (1976) of prospective reimbursement systems show that even in those few cases where these regulatory devices evoke a statistically discernible effect in the desired direction, the magnitude of this effect, while large in dollar terms, is quite small relative to cost increases in the hospital sector.

The "co-option" of the regulatory process in health care seems to have already begun in some areas. For example, the Center for the Analysis of Public Issues (1974) makes charges relating to health care regulation in New Jersey. On a more inferential level, Cromwell et al. (1975:121) note that only one out of forty-one certificate-of-need applications was denied to hospitals in the Greater Boston area in 1973.

There is thus a real danger that health care regulation will be proposed and supported by members of the industry as a mechanism for supplanting whatever competitive elements remain with a legal, enforceable cartel. This view would allow for state hospital associations to petition their legislatures to put them under the protective umbrella of a state-mandated prospective reimbursement system that is meant to *guarantee* an "adequate" cash flow to each hospital. This view would also encompass the use of comprehensive health planning by local hospital groups as a vehicle for keeping Health Maintenance Organizations from encroaching on their territory.

Even if direct hospital regulation turns out to be a moderate success, its role will have to be strengthened by some basic structural changes in the way physicians are educated and reimbursed. Today the typical physician, acting in the interests of himself and his immediate patients, puts little weight on the larger issues of economic efficiency and social benefit. This attitude has been reinforced by the strong technological imperative instilled in physicians during their medical training programs (and is tacitly encouraged by the present cost-based system for financing hospital care).

The professional training of physicians has traditionally not emphasized the concept of the physician as a manager of health care resources confronted with complex issues of cost and efficiency. Instead, the physician emerges from his training period with a perception of the hospital as a rent-free workshop, a place where he feels justified in pressing administrators and trustees to add those medical care inputs that allow for full, modern treatment of patients while simultaneously enhancing the physician's income and prestige.

Individual physician and patient issues, not social issues, dominate the training process and are carried over into the medical practice. For example, physicians who specialize in treating patients with a given disease will not agree to the exclusion of facilities at hospital A, where they hold staff appointments, unless they are granted staff privileges at hospital B, where the planning agency would like to concentrate all facilities for diagnosis and treatment. The physician not only has a financial interest involved; there is also the matter of the preservation and employment of professional skills.

At times this type of behavior is costly not only to society but to the individual patient as well. The only one to gain is the physician. Rosenthal (1966:109) quotes, as a not so extreme example, the President's Commission on Heart, Cancer, and Stroke to show that in the early 1960s 30 percent of the 777 hospitals equipped to do closed-heart surgery had no such cases in the year under study, and 87 percent of the 548 hospitals that did have cases performed fewer than one operation per week. Furthermore, 77 percent of the hospitals equipped to do open-heart surgery averaged less than one operation per week, and 41 percent averaged less than one a month. Little of this sporadic surgery was of an emergency nature, and the mortality rate of both procedures when done infrequently was far higher than in institutions with a full work load.

This phenomenon is, of course, closely linked to the explosive growth in the opportunities for application of new and high-cost technology in health care. Recent innovations in medical care have been characterized by an emphasis upon complex diagnostic and therapeutic techniques usually requiring hospitalization and the physician-controlled application of complicated, expensive equipment. Examples include cancer radiation therapy and chemotherapy, renal dialysis, organ transplants, open-heart surgery, brain and body scanners, and intensive care units for burn, trauma, and heart patients. The overall cumulative effect of health care technology in this country, in combination with hospital-oriented, cost-based health insurance, has been to shift the focus of the health system from office-based, primary care medical practice toward hospital-based, specialist care medical practice.

Furthermore, this shift in focus is made more acute by the interaction of technological applications in health care and the current orientation of medical training programs. The new high-cost hospital technology necessitates specialization and fosters a narrow professionalism among new physicians. That is, for reasons relating to income, prestige, and the way that modern medicine is practiced, new physicians are drawn toward the practice of specialized medicine within an urban, institutionalized setting. This trend in turn creates ever greater demands from physicians to induce hospitals to adopt still more technology. Thus the cycle is completed and starts anew. And thus delivery of health care has shifted from general practitioners toward high-priced specialists operating in expensive settings. From 1963 to 1973 the overall number of physicians in the United States increased by 32.5 percent. There was a 53.5 percent increase in medical specialists, a 29.8 percent increase in surgical specialists, a 50.3 percent increase in all other specialists, and a 26.5 percent *decline* in the number of general practitioners (American Medical Association, 1967 and 1974b).

The massive movement toward specialization has helped fuel the hospital cost inflation process through the specialist-technology relationship described earlier. M. Feldstein (1971b:871), using a pooled cross-sectional time series for individual states for the period 1958–1967, estimates that the addition of one or more specialists in a state in that time interval would cause hospital costs to increase by $39,000 per year. Conversely, general practitioners were shown to be a substitute for hospital care. Feldstein estimates that the introduction of an additional GP into a state would cause hospital costs to decrease by $39,000 per year. Thus the true costs of producing ever-increasing numbers of specialists must include these induced hospital costs as well as any added educational costs (in part underwritten by public funds) and higher physician fees associated with specialization. These additional costs should be taken into account in any decisions impacting on the extent of public funding for the production (that is, education) of hospital-oriented physicians.

The greatest potential in utilizing the physician to contain hospital costs, however, may lie in the movement, whenever possible, away from fee-for-service as the method of reimbursing physicians and away from a system in which individual physicians control hospital inputs without bearing any responsibility for them. Such a movement, if feasible at all, would probably have to take place in piecemeal, incremental fashion. Capitation or salaried service may marginally increase in popularity, but it seems clear that, even with a major restructuring of the health care system through national health financing legislation, these two methods of reimbursing physicians will for some time appear only as options to physicians who desire alternatives to fee-for-service. Any new system, to be politically feasible, must meet with at least grudging acceptance by physicians. While most physicians see the hospital as an adjunct to their practice and an extension of their office, a vocal minority visualizes the hospital as a threat to the private practice of medicine. The AMA and individual physicians have fought long and hard to maintain de facto control of resource decisions in hospitals to keep this fear from becoming a reality. The AMA (1974b:20) suggests that "a physician should not bargain or enter into a contract whereby any hospital, corporation, or lay body may offer for sale or sell for a fee the physician's professional services." The only exceptions to this stated AMA principle are salaried "educational" staff appointments. The AMA's position has been that hospitals are "exploiting" salaried physicians by making shadow profits on their activities to support other departments (American Medical Association, 1959).

However, physician groups can no longer severely punish individual physicians who are induced to defect from traditional fee-for-service reimbursement. The courts have ruled that hospitals may not deny staff privileges to a physician simply because he is a member of a group practice or is not a member of the local county medical society.

The amount of money society can afford to spend to induce defections may prove to be quite large. From July 1975 to June 1976 hospital costs increased by $7.2 billion (Gibson and Mueller, 1977). This represents 27 percent of the total cost of physician services in that period, or around $23,000 per U.S. physician, and a much higher figure when divided only by fee-for-service physicians.

We have suggested that a large part of these annual hospital cost increases is related to the growing intensity of care caused partly by the method by which physicians are reimbursed and partly by the way they are free from responsibility for hospital inputs. Movement away from the perverse incentives of fee-for-service, in combination with the separation to some extent of resource control from the medical staff, could produce the dramatic drops in per capita hospital utilization similar to the ones associated with HMOs. It is these anticipated savings that society could decide to use to encourage defections from fee-for-service practice.

Adoption of a European-style health care system, with hospitals primarily the domain of salaried specialists, and with general practitioners operating independently in office-based settings, might be a step in this direction. Many physicians are already practicing in hospitals on a straight salary, such as interns and residents (who comprise more than 20 percent of active physicians in many states), full-time salaried chiefs of staff, and other physicians serving educational functions. Still other physicians could be induced to practice on a salaried basis if the salary were high enough. (While many physicians are ideologically opposed to anything but fee-for-service reimbursement, others are concerned not about ideology but about levels of income and hours of work today and in the future.)

However, adoption of a European-style system for the United States would present many problems. The level of physician salaries and of payment responsibilities would have to be determined. State laws against the corporate practice of medicine would have to be redesigned (they are currently being rewritten in many states to allow for the functioning of HMOs). A way would have to be found to gradually allow new staff privileges only to salaried specialists. And more important, while this system removes many of the perverse incentives individual physicians face with respect to the utilization of hospital resources, it does nothing by itself to provide incentives to the hospital to contain costs.

A more practical approach that should be viewed as a movement in this general direction would be to push for salaried status for three specific hospital-based physicians. Anesthesiologists, pathologists, and radiologists often control small fiefdoms within the hospital. They practice under reimbursement methods that are financially very favorable to them (fee-for-service or some percentage of their departments' gross or net revenues). It is suggested that these reimbursement methods contribute simultaneously to their high average income level and to rising levels of hospital costs resulting from the inordinate growth of their departments' services.

There are, of course, other alternatives to full-scale fee-for-service in addition to the European model. New concepts deserve encouragement, such as variants of the reimbursement plan being developed by the Blue Shield organization in Wisconsin. Individuals or groups of primary care physicians can elect capitation for a number of their patients. That is, they agree to provide a basic set of primary care services "on demand" in return for a fixed monthly fee. (The monthly fee and the set of primary care services can vary from physician to physician.) A pool is set up to pay for referrals to specialists and for hospitalization costs of patients. If the pool is not depleted by year end, the remainder is distributed back to the participating physicians.

Other new methods might be tried that attempt to make the physician responsible for the level of hospital costs. Monetary disbursements could be made to all physicians in an area where hospital costs are below projections, and also for residents or other full-time staff in a specific hospital. While this might create some incentives for the physician peer review process to focus in on some financial criteria, there would be many complications inherent in determining both a projected level of costs and a disbursement method. When variants of this reimbursement method have been tried (as in medical foundations), the evidence appears to show that fee-for-service incentives to the individual physician are stronger than peer group pressure (see Gaus et al., 1975).

The major physician-related impetus to cost containment in hospitals may come from the growth and encouragement of nonfoundation-type HMOs. It has already been suggested that these HMOs keep hospital costs in check not by the organization as an entity going at risk to provide medical care, but from the actions of staff physicians who are removed from fee-for-service reimbursement, who practice in multispecialty groups, and who do not operate with complete autonomy in regard to resource control. Encouragement of HMOs could take many forms. For example, a major insurance plan with deductibles for hospital and physician care and a 20 percent copayment provision for physician services (such as Medicare) could offer to drop all deductibles and co-insurance payments for beneficiaries who joined HMOs that agreed to provide care at a cost to the program of 80 percent of the average beneficiary cost in the area.

In the end it must be remembered that the search for a single panacea to contain hospital and other health care costs is likely to be a futile one. There are major forces at work in the health care arena. They are related to the interaction of physician incentives, patient passivity (induced in part by high levels of insurance), new technology, and cost-related hospital reimbursement. These forces are not unique to the American health care system. Costs of hospital care and other forms of health care can be observed to be rising rapidly in many societies operating under a wide range of regulatory activity and financing arrangements. The lesson to be learned is that there does not appear to be a single, simple solution to the health care cost crisis. Instead, the problem is one that will have to be solved (or at least partially alleviated) through a number of small, discrete steps. Utilizing the physician as a lever to help contain hospital costs is one of those steps.

References

Adelstein, S.
> 1973   "The risk-benefit ratio in nuclear medicine." Hospital Practice 8 (January).

American Hospital Association
> 1969   Hospitals, Journal of the American Hospital Association (August, Guide Issue).

American Medical Association
> 1959   "AMA/Acts on hospital-physician relations." Hospitals, Journal of the American Hospital Association (December): 17–19.

> 1967   Distribution of Physicians in the U.S., 1963. Chicago: AMA Managerial Services Division.

Michael A. Redisch

1974a   Distribution of Physicians in the U.S., 1973. Chicago: AMA Center for Health Services Research and Development.

1974b   Physician-Hospital Relations. Chicago, Ill.

Applied Management Sciences

1975   Analysis of Prospective Reimbursement Systems: Western Pennsylvania. Prepared for the Office of Research and Statistics, Social Security Administration, U.S. DHEW, under Contract No. HEW-OS-74-226.

Berki, S.E.

1972   Hospital Economics. Lexington, Mass.: Lexington Books, D.C. Heath & Co.

Bishop, C.

1973   Public Regulation of Hospitals: Summary of a Conference. Health Care Policy Discussion Paper No. 4, Harvard Center for Community Health and Medical Care (March).

Bunker, J.

1970   "Surgical manpower: A comparison of operations and surgeons in the United States and in England and Wales." The New England Journal of Medicine 282 (January): 135–143.

Center for the Analysis of Public Issues

1974   Bureaucratic Malpractice. Princeton, N.J.

Council on Wage and Price Stability

1976   The Problem of Rising Health Care Costs. Staff Report, Washington, D.C. (April).

Cromwell, J., P.B. Ginsburg, D. Hamilton, and M. Sumner

1975   Incentives and Decisions Underlying Hospitals' Adoption and Utilization of Major Capital Equipment. Prepared by Abt Associates, Inc., for National Center for Health Services Research and Development. Contract No. (HSM) 110-73-513 (September).

Davis, K., and R. Foster

1972   Community Hospitals: Inflation in the Pre-Medicare Period. Social Security Administration, Research Report No. 41. Washington, D.C.: Government Printing Office.

Davis, K., and L.B. Russell

1972   "The substitution of hospital outpatient care for inpatient care." Review of Economics and Statistics 54 (May): 109–120.

Feldstein, M.S.

1968   Economic Analysis for Health Service Efficiency. Amsterdam: North-Holland Publishing Company.

1971a   The Rising Cost of Hospital Care. Washington, D.C.: Information Resources Press.

1971b   "Hospital cost inflation: A study of nonprofit price dynamics."
         American Economic Review 61 (December): 853–872.

Gaus, C.R., B.S. Cooper, and C.G. Hirschman
1975   "Contrasts in HMO and fee-for-service performance." Social
         Security Bulletin 39 (May): 3–14.

Gaus, C.R., and F.J. Hellinger
1976   Results of Hospital Prospective Reimbursement in the United
         States. Paper presented to the International Conference on
         Policies for the Containment of Health Care Costs and Expendi-
         tures. Fogarty International Center (June).

Gibson, R.M., and M.S. Mueller
1977   "National health expenditures, fiscal year 1976." Social Security
         Bulletin 40 (April): 3–22.

Griner, P., and B. Liptzen
1971   "Use of the laboratory in a teaching hospital: Implications for
         patient care, education, and hospital costs." Annals of Internal
         Medicine 75 (August).

Hellinger, F.J.
1976   "The effect of certificate-of-need legislation on hospital invest-
         ment." Inquiry 13 (June): 187–193.

Jacobs, P.
1974   "A survey of economic models of hospitals." Inquiry 11 (June):
         83–97.

Johnson, E.
1969   "Physician productivity and the hospital: A hospital administra-
         tor's view." Inquiry 6 (September): 59–69.

Leveson, I., and E. Rogers
1976   "Hospital cost inflation and physician payment." American
         Journal of Economics and Sociology 35 (April): 161–174.

McCarthy, E., and A. Kamons
1976   Voluntary and Mandatory Presurgical Screening Programs: An
         Analysis of Their Implications. Presented at American Federa-
         tion for Clinical Research, Atlantic City (May 2).

Monsma, G.
1970   "Marginal revenue and the demand for physicians' services." In
         H.E. Klarman, ed., Empirical Studies in Health Economics.
         Baltimore: John Hopkins Press.

Newhouse, J.P.
1973   "The economics of group practice." Journal of Human Re-
         sources (Winter): 37–56.

Michael A. Redisch

Noll, R.C.
1971   Reforming Regulation. Washington, D.C.: The Brookings Institution.
Pauly, M., and M.A. Redisch
1973   "The not-for-profit hospital as a physicians' cooperative." American Economic Review 63 (March): 87–99.
Rafferty, J.
1971   "Patterns of hospital use: An analysis of short-run variations." Journal of Political Economy 79 (January–February): 154–165.
Redisch, M.A.
1974   Hospital Inflationary Mechanisms. Presented at Western Economic Association Meetings, Las Vegas, Nev. (June).
Reinhardt, U.
1972   "A production function for physician services." Review of Economics and Statistics 54 (February): 55–66.
Rosenthal, G.
1966   "The public pays the bill." Atlantic 218 (July): 107–110.
Salkever, D.S., and T.W. Bice
1976   The Impact of Certificate-of-Need Controls on Hospital Investment, Costs, and Utilization. Final report to the National Center for Health Services Research, DHEW, Contract No. HRA-106-74-57 (August).
Schimmel, E.
1964   "The hazards of hospitalization." Annals of Internal Medicine 60 (January): 100–116.
Titmuss, R.
1950   Problems of Social Policy. London: HMS Office and Longmans, Green.
Waldman, S.
1972   The Effect of Changing Technology on Hospital Costs. Research and Statistics Note No. 4, DHEW Publication No. (SSA) 72-11701 (February 28).
Wennberg, J., A. Gitteljohn, and N. Shapiro
1975   "Health care delivery in Maine III: Evaluating the level of hospital performance." Journal of the Maine Medical Association 66 (November).
Yett, D., L. Drabek, M. Intriligator, and L. Kimball
1971   A Macroeconomic Model for Regional Health Planning. Presented at the 46th Annual Conference of the Western Economic Association (August).

Physician Participation
in Health Service Management:
Expectations in United States
and Experiences in England

ROCKWELL SCHULZ

DAVID S. GRIMES

T. E. CHESTER

Increasing governmental regulation such as called for in PSRO and health planning legislation, pressures to contain rising costs, physician strikes, and other manifestations of change suggest that traditional hospital organization and management patterns ought to be re-examined. Moreover, as the United States moves toward a governmentally financed and regulated system, experiences in Great Britain and other nationalized systems become more pertinent to us. The 1974 major reorganization of the British National Health Service provides for considerable physician participation in management. A similar participative approach to the management of the hospitals in the United States is worthy of consideration as a way to meet increasing challenges of a governmentally financed and controlled health care system.

In arguing for physician involvement in hospital management the 1968 report of the Secretary's Advisory Committee on Hospital Effectiveness (United States Department of Health, Education, and Welfare, 1968:20) related the following fable to emphasize their point:

> An intelligent visitor from Mars was interrogating a hospital administrator on the purposes, functions and management of a hospital. The Martian was told that the doctors in the hospital order the procedures for patients and thus determine how the resources are used, what work members of staff do and also decide which patients to admit and when to dismiss them.
>
> "And where do these important persons stand in your operation?" the man from Mars asked.
>
> "Actually, they stand outside the organization," the hospital administrator explained. "They are paid by our customers and they must observe certain rules, but by tradition the hospital must not interfere or seek to influence their decisions."
>
> "You must be joking!" the visitor exclaimed. "As anyone can plainly see such an arrangement would be impossible to manage."
>
> The administrator acknowledged that it was not easy.

The intelligent visitor was heard to mutter as he departed, "Impossible...or very very expensive."

The Commission on Health Manpower and others have argued for physician participation in hospital management decisions as important to containing the rise in hospital costs (National Advisory Commission on Health Manpower, 1967: 63-64). Since these reports, however, utilization review requirements have put increased responsibility for hospital costs on physicians. Nevertheless, in 1974 a bill was introduced into Congress (HR 13461) that called for doctors to share in any savings on hospital costs as an incentive to help control them. Reasons other than cost containment have been suggested for physician participation, such as it would help improve relationships within the hospital.

The American Medical Association has promoted the participation of physicians in hospital management by asking for the membership of physicians on the Hospital Governing Board, this request being endorsed by the American Hospital Association in 1973 after years of deliberation.

Reasons for Physician Participation

Management decisions must be distinguished from clinical decisions in which there is essential autonomy for the physician, either individually or collectively through the specialty organization. The physician who participates in management might discuss, deliberate, and help decide major issues such as:

1. The definition of hospital goals and plans, evaluating the success in achieving such goals through review of financial and other management reports.
2. Allocation of resources, whether these be financial, facilities, or manpower.
3. Obtaining resources through fixing the level of charges and determining the facilities to be provided.
4. Certain personnel decisions such as a selection of key administrative staff.

Although the control of rising costs has been said to be a major reason for involving physicians in administration, there are other reasons which do not directly involve expenditure. For example, physicians seem to be concerned about the growing power of hospital governing boards and administrators and want a greater voice in administrative decisions. In her warning about this, Betty

Jane Anderson (1973:4), of the office of the General Council of the American Medical Association, placed particular emphasis on the dangers of lay administration:

> In some institutions, the situation has become so grave as to create a line of authority that goes from the attending staff to a salaried medical hierarchy which in turn is responsible to a hospital administrator often styled as president of the hospital and frequently not only chief hospital executive, but the dominant voice on the hospital governing board. In the institutions where the hospital administrator occupies the role of hospital president and chairman of the hospital governing board, the only line of communication between the governing board and the medical staff is through him. This is lay domination at its zenith a trend that should be aborted as early as possible.

While instances in which the hospital administrator also serves as chairman of the board would be most unusual, concerns about administrative dominance are real.

It has also been suggested by physicians in hospitals that there is a conflict in goal priorities with the physician concerned about the provision of service to the individual and the administration concerned with maintenance of the organization as a whole (Goss, 1963:180). Consequently the physician may be accused about lack of concern with the welfare of the hospital and likewise the administrator and board accused of lack of concern about the welfare of the patient. Participative management is recognized as fostering goal conformity and promoting understanding of the problems faced by others in the organization.

It is expected by national policy makers that an important major result of the involvement of physicians in management will be to help control hospital costs. Some of the ways in which this might be brought about can be summarized as follows:

(a) The physician might be more concerned than the administrator or trustee about the cost to the patient with whose financial situation he may be more familiar.

(b) By understanding the overall problems, the physician might be more supportive of management efforts to reduce costs.

(c) He might become more aware of the financial results of unnecessary utilization of beds and ancillary services.

(d) Participation in decisions regarding allocation of funds and other resources might bring about a more realistic evaluation of requests for more staff, equipment, and new services, and a greater willingness to veto extravagant requests. Lay boards and administrators frequently find it difficult to refute a claim from a physician, nurse or other professional who states that a new service, higher staffing levels, or more equipment will improve quality or that "patients may die" if they do not get what they want.

Reasons Against Physician Participation

Although it is hoped that the main results of physician participation in management will be beneficial, it is possible to see how it could lead to difficulties.

1. It could diminish the influence of administrators, governing board members, and individual physicians by placing unusual power in the hands of a few physicians.
2. The involvement of a practicing physician in management might bring about goal conflict, thus weakening his professional standards when dealing with an individual patient.
3. It could result in more overall goal conformity but thereby minimize constructive conflict which might promote change.
4. It might bring about cost increases even more rapidly than at present. Arguments to support this point of view can be summarized as follows:
    (a) By participating in management activities a physician will have less time to spend on patient care.
    (b) Physicians are frequently believed to be poor managers as their training and orientation is an antithesis to a management role.
    (c) A physician participating in budget matters might use his influence to extract even more costly services and facilities, as it is frequently claimed that the physician is oriented toward a maximum service for his patient irrespective of cost.

A search of the literature found many opinions about physician participation, but no empirical evidence that would shed light on these questions. In 1971, Schulz (1972) surveyed administrators in Illinois and Wisconsin regarding medical staff membership on governing boards and medical staff participation in decisions related to reviewing hospital income and expense statements, budget preparation, selection of key personnel, remuneration of hospital-based specialists, and facility plans. While he found increasing numbers of hospitals had physician membership on governing boards, such membership appeared to be concerned more with representing medical staff interests rather than active participation in decision activities. In the few cases where there appeared to be extensive participation, there was no statistical evidence of major differences in utilization of hospital services or hospital cost indicators.

The British Experiment

While there appears to have been little experience with physician participation in the United States, for reasons described later, Great Britain has recently (i.e., from April 1, 1974) reorganized its health service with physician participation in management as one of the major objectives. (While objectives of reorganization were similar for England, Wales, Scotland, and Northern Ireland, each has distinctive characteristics. Characteristics described refer to England, unless otherwise noted.) The plans and some limited experience in Great Britain may be of interest to those in the United States wrestling with similar issues. Moreover, with the enactment of the National Health Planning and Resources Development Act (P.L. 93-641) in 1974 an organizational structure and planning process seems to emerge in the United States which bears some resemblance to the reorganized British National Health Service. We describe below the reorganized National Health Service (NHS) and will also expose some of the substantial differences between it and the United States medical delivery system. For a description of other facets of the reorganization see Battistella and Chester (1973).

The organization of the NHS had to take account of the existence of three major groups of physicians, that is, the hospital-based specialists, the community-based general practitioners, and the public health doctor whose role has been enlarged to a specialist in community medicine. Throughout England and Wales there are approximately 20,000 general practitioners, 10,000 hospital specialists, 1,500 specialists in community medicine, and in addition to these three groups 15,000 junior hospital doctors in training grades (i.e., interns and residents).

It is the British preference to build on the existing institutions as much as possible. Although this has been criticized as merely putting new wine into old bottles and preserving for longer than necessary deadwood that can be swept away (for example, the preservation of a separate organization for general practitioners), there is the major advantage that the changes have often been accepted by the participants if they could continue to formally play their old roles. Many levels of management are incorporated in the reorganization. At every level there is the participation of the three major groups of physicians and to a lesser extent particpation by house staff. The system takes into account that the medical input will be greatest at the operational level, while economic, political, and social implications will predominate at the national level. For that reason the role (i.e., the power and responsibilities) of the representatives of medicine must be different at the various levels.

Physicians of all groups are to be involved in both an executive-management line and advisory machinery. The executive groups must be small, usually comprising six to nine individuals, whereas the advisory committees may be large and representative, consisting of groups of approximately 20 individuals. At an operational level the physician members of the executive groups are elected by their colleagues, whereas at the national level this would involve an elaborate or cumbersome electoral machinery; the medical officers at such levels are therefore appointed by the democratically elected national government.

The Machinery of Participation

The division of the country into regions for health administration (first introduced in 1938) has been continued. In England there are 14 regional health authorities, which are responsible to the Department of Health and Social Security (DHSS). The regions are divided into 90 areas which are further subdivided into a total of 205 districts. The district is the operational unit, serving a population of about 250,000 people and providing all health service facilities, including a general hospital under the control of a district management team. See Fig. 1 for the organization chart of the English National Health Service.

The District Organization

The District Organization is shown at the top of Fig. 1. A detailed description can be found in Management Arrangements for the Reorganized National Health Service (Department of Health and Social Security, 1972).

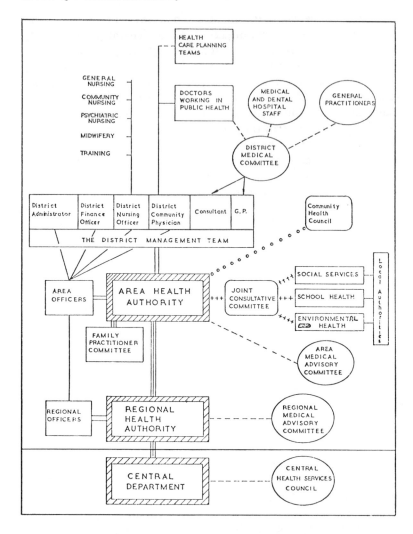

Adapted from *Health Trends,* 1974, Vol. 6.
*Reproduced by permission of the Controller
of Her Britannic Majesty's Stationery Office*

FIG. 1. Organization Chart of Some of the Structure of the Reorganized National Health Service in England

The Organization of General Practice A district may be served by 100 general practitioners, and although some remain in solo practice, more and more are working from health centers in group practices supported by nursing and social work professionals and basic laboratory and X-ray services.

The traditional representative organization of the general practitioners has been the Local Medical Committee (LMC). This is a group of about 20 elected representatives. In this committee practitioners will discuss their views and attempt to reach decisions about how they would like to practice. There is no direct control over general practitioners, as they are legally independent contractors to the National Health Service.

The Hospital Organization   Every district will normally be served by a District General Hospital, which may have 600 beds staffed by about 150 physicians, a third of these being permanent specialists (called consultants in Britain) who have full clinical control of the beds allocated to them and their corresponding outpatient departments. The other two-thirds are in training grades generally comparable to interns and residents in the United States.

Although the latter group is numerically larger, the effective share in medical management is much less. The house staff are transients, mainly concerned with training, and they may not have a hospital specialist career as an ultimate aim. Whereas the basic medical organization for general practitioners is the geographical district, the Local Medical Committee being elected by all doctors within it, the basic unit of organization within a hospital is the "Division" which has emerged fairly generally over the past 10 years (Department of Health and Social Security, 1974a). The division is not an elected body but comprises all specialists working in closely related fields (i.e., all surgeons, all internists, all pediatricians, etc.). One should expect to find in a large district general hospital from five to 10 such divisions. A teaching hospital may have additional divisions of education and research which tend to cut across more traditionally defined clinical areas. Each division elects its own chairman. It discusses matters concerning the work and interests of its members (it must be noted that in most British hospitals specialists are strictly separated from their colleagues in other disciplines). They have their own wards, are supported by their own nurses, and their own house staff. Divisions are responsible for defining developments in terms of expenditure, capital building, and manpower but do not have the authority for implementation of such policies. Recommendations and requests from the divisions are passed to the next level of medical participation, the so-called Medical Executive Committee (MEC) which comprises the chairmen of all divisions. The chairman and vice-chairman of this Medical Executive Committee are not elected by members of the committee itself but by all the consultant staff of the hospital. This is an attempt to fulfill a major recommendation that the administrative work load of physicians be spread as much as possible. It is considered that the chairman of the MEC would be unable to cope with the additional work load of a divisional chairman. The MEC chairman is elected for a period of five years, whereas the divisional chairmen are usually elected for a period of two years. Chairmanship of the medical executive committee necessitates a considerable amount of time devoted to administration. It is thought that there is an increasing tendency for physicians based in service departments such as pathology or radiology to play a more active role in administration than their colleagues in the "bedside" specialities, where the work load is less predictable and the allocation of time for administration correspondingly more difficult. The chairman of the MEC is supported in his task by the provision of special office accommodation, full-time secretarial help, and a reallocation of his work among colleagues without loss of income. It is customary for senior representatives from nursing, finance, and administrative departments to attend the meetings of the MEC as observers, thereby supplying information vital to decision making. The main functions of the MEC can be summarized as follows:

(a) It decides priorities on claims for additional medical staffing.
(b) It coordinates recommendations and requests for equipment and facilities from the divisions.
(c) It authorizes the allocation of study leave for medical staff.
(d) It may act on occasions as a disciplinary body.
(e) Perhaps most important of all, it provides peer control over claims for drugs and equipment. It is the task of the MEC to allocate priorities for these two items within a budget which is given by the management. It has become the practice for the MEC to draw up a list of drugs which can be prescribed without restriction. Drugs not on that list can still be prescribed but only with prior approval of the MEC on the basis of a recent application. In other words, presumably clinical freedom is preserved while there is a check on ill-considered prescribing.
The overall function of the MEC is the determination of priorities of manpower, equipment, and drugs in a

situation of limited resources. Practical experience has shown that when such decisions are made only by lay administrators they readily succumb to the threat of dire consequences by demanding clinicians.

In the United States, of course medical staff organizations are primarily concerned with quality control. It must be pointed out that in England this is not so; there is almost no quality or utilization review at the current time.

The District Medical Committee The next level of medical participation is the District Medical Committee (DMC) which is meant to be an instrument where the views of general practitioners and hospital specialists can be synthesized into a medical view. It also provides a voice for the third major medical group, i.e., the community physicians. It must be stressed that the constitution of this and the other medical committees to be mentioned later have been worked out by the medical organizations themselves and have subsequently been approved and incorporated into the official guide issued by the DHSS (Department of Health and Social Security, 1974b).

The DMC will normally have fifteen members, the size balancing the need for effective functioning with satisfactory representation of the main branches of the medical profession.

It will be composed in equal parts as follows:

(a) Normally five general practitioners selected by the LMC, also to include general practitioners in training.
(b) Normally five hospital-based physicians selected by the MEC, also including house staff.
(c) A similar number of community physicians and physicians concerned with medical education.

The DMC elects its chairman and the vice-chairman of whom one has to be a hospital specialist and the other a general practitioner.

The District Management Team The next stage in the decision-making process is to integrate the view of the DMC, in itself a synthesis of the not always reconcilable, strongly held views of the main parts of the medical profession, into a decision-making group which will take account of the administrative and financial problems involved—together with the views of the other major health care professions. This is the task of the District Management Team (DMT).

The DMT consists of six members and is composed as follows:

•The chairman and the vice-chairman of the DMC, i.e., one specialist, one general practitioner, are automatically members of the DMT for the time they are holding their functions in DMC. This enables them to bring to the DMT the views of their medical colleagues and explain the reasons for them. They can make clear to the other members of the DMT what physicians would like to do and what they are not prepared to accept. This, so it is assumed, may prevent a management decision unacceptable to physicians which may even lead to a confrontation and a breakdown of health care. They remain active clinicians who continue otherwise in their normal role of patient care. Indeed, their credibility with their colleagues rests on this fact. They are part-time managers giving up, normally, only a few hours a week so that they cannot be considered by their practicing colleagues of "having gone over to bureaucracy." They are being compensated for this managerial activity by an honorarium currently about $2,000.

•The District Community Physician is appointed by the Area Health Authority and is not an elected representative of his colleagues. This is a key role to help achieve objectives of the reorganization for identifying needs and integrating health resources to meet needs. It has been constructed in the reorganized service from two main sources:

(a) The former Medical Officer of Health, which all local authorities in Britain have had by statute since the nineteenth century and who was broadly responsible for all public health matters, including vaccinations and control of epidemics.

(b) The Senior Administrative Medical Officer, who since 1948 has been in charge of all hospital planning and medical staffing.

As a new concept which still needs further elaboration in practice, the District Community Physician (DCP) is intended to be a new medical planner and adviser trained in all branches of public health including epidemiology, information systems, etc., and also in such behavioral disciplines as organization theory and social administration. It is anticipated that he will function effectively as a medically trained intermediary between his colleagues in clinical practice and health service managers. It is noteworthy that his role has been recognized from the point of view of the new arrangement as the equivalent status to that of a hospital specialist. He is being represented at all levels of the reorganized service and may often be a specialist in a particular field of community medicine such as child health, environmental health, capital planning, or medical information and research.

- The District Nursing Officer with responsibility for both hospital nursing and nursing services in the community.
- The District Finance Officer who co-ordinates the preparation of budgets, monitors effective use of resources, and provides financial advice to both the DMT and the DMC.
- The District Administrator, who may have previously served in a role roughly comparable to that of a hospital administrator in the United States and who is responsible for the full administrative and clerical staff in the district in all facilities and services, includint the running of the district general hospital, health centers, etc.

The basic principles of the decision-making process of the DMT could be summarized under two headings:

- There is no imposition of a permanent chairmanship. All members are considered to be co-equal partners. They are fully entitled to elect their own chairman if they so wish, and they may even prefer to elect a new chairman for each session according to the expertise which the particular problem may demand.
- Decision making is based on the principle of "consensus management." This means that all six professional members including the two clinicians must find any proposal acceptable before a decision is reached. If any one of the six objects, no decision is taken. In this case the organization provides that the matter may be referred up to the next level of management, i.e., the Area Health Authority, normally composed of about 15 "trustees" (in the American sense), appointed by the region, who can reach a decision by simple majority vote. The main task of the DMT is to coordinate the medical information coming from the DMC with the proposals coming from the Health Care Planning Teams (which are multi-disciplinary and relate directly to community needs) and from other sources so as to work out a district plan determining priority within

a multi-professional framework.

Health Care Planning Team (HCPT) Medical participation in health service planning is now also provided for quite separately from the professional machinery in so-called Health Care Planning Teams (HCPT). It is proposed to set up such teams in every district oriented toward major client groups—for example, for planning the services for the elderly, for children, the mentally ill, and the mentally defective. The composition of these teams is meant to be very flexible but unquestioningly specialists in these particular disciplines are given a prominent place and will clearly play a predominant role with their colleagues in general practice, nursing, social work, etc. It is envisaged that the District Community Physician will play a major role in the coordination of the Health Care Planning Team.

The Area Organization

While the District Management Team is in charge of the Operational Unit, it is on the other hand part of the NHS, and its decisions have to fit into the broad national pattern. This is the main purpose of the hierarchical structure which is being built up for the whole of the Service. In the new organization decisions are first scrutinized by the Area Health Authority (AHA) which attempts to make sure that the district decisions fit into a cohesive area pattern and that priorities are appropriately determined and facilities adequately distributed.

Again there is an input by the medical profession in various ways:

1. The final authority in the area (the AHA itself) consists of about 15 *voluntary members*, as has already been stated, and normally includes a consultant and a general practitioner who, while in no way democratically representing the profession, will nevertheless make the medical viewpoint available.
2. The *professional advisors* of the AHA are the area team of officers: this is composed of four chief officers including the Area Medical Officer (who is a specialist in community medicine) and who is supported by at least three other specialists in community medicine with specific responsibility for child health, communicable diseases, and social services.
3. The Area Medical Advisory Committee is composed of 20 to 30 members representing all branches of the medical profession in

that area. About a third are general practitioners, including general practitioners in training, selected by the Local Medical Committee. There is an equal number of hospital-based doctors including at least one member of the house staff. Other members will be one or more community physicians selected by their colleagues in the area and up to three representatives of medical educational interests, such as postgraduate training, training for general practice, and the undergraduate medical school.

This committee is not concerned directly in management. It is an important means by which the local physicians may be consulted on crucial planning issues and can make their voices heard.

The Regional Organization

The decisions of the AHA again have to be ratified with their corresponding Regional Health Authority (RHA). Each of the 14 RHAs receives medical input for its decision making in a way similar to the area:

1. Through the membership on the Authority of 1 or 2 physicians
2. Through the Regional Medical Officer and his staff of specialists in community medicine
3. Through the Regional Medical Advisory Committee, which consists of representatives of the medical profession determined partly on geographical considerations and partly on the specialities within the region. Its members will be either the chairman or vice-chairman of each of the Area Medical Advisory Committees, together with representatives of hospital house staff (selected by the hospital house staff themselves within the region), community physicians (selected by their colleagues within the region), and representatives of undergraduate and postgraduate education. Regional specialist subcommittees (e.g., in laboratory services, psychiatry, and general practice) will be formed by the profession themselves and the chairman of each subcommittee will sit on the Regional Medical Advisory Committee. The Regional Health Authority and its officers will thereby gain medical advice on crucial issues of planning and the distribution of specialities and manpower in particular.

The National Organization

National policy for the NHS is ultimately, since Britain is a democracy, in the hands of an elected official responsible to Parliament—the Secretary of State for Health and Social Security. Very rarely in England has this official been a physician. On the other hand the medical profession is strongly represented in influencing the decisions which the Secretary of State finally reaches:

1. *The Chief Medical Officer.* Since the middle of the nineteenth century, when the health of the nation became of vital public concern, a physician was charged with the task of advising the Minister responsible. The Chief Medical Officer today is in control of a very substantial department of qualified doctors who themselves are specialists in all topics concerned with the health of the nation. These Medical Officers of course have close contact with the clinical branches of the profession and administrative officers of the DHSS. Rarely is a decision formulated without detailed professional consultation.

2. *The Central Health Services Council (CHSC).* Direct consultation between the DHSS and the medical profession takes place within the CHSC which has been in existence since 1948. The CHSC is composed of elected representatives such as the presidents of the Royal Colleges, the chairmen of the British Medical and Dental Associations, and eight other medical practitioners, together with dental, nursing, pharmaceutical, and social work professionals, other persons with experience in health service management, and those representing the point of view of the public. The CHSC appoints several standing or ad hoc Medical Advisory Committees, which will discuss a wide range of topics such as cancer research, organ transplantation, alcoholism, screening in medicine, etc. The profession through the CHSC advises the DHSS in its production of national policy guidelines.

The Machinery in Practice

1. The machinery described is very new. Clearly it will take some time before the participants will grasp the full implications and thus before a smooth-running process develops. Moreover this running had been delayed in the first year owing to the financial difficulties which have affected the operation of NHS and brought in its wake a confrontation of the hospital specialists with the government.

2. The National Health Service is a large and complex organization, and any machinery for effective participation by the physicians is bound to be complex. The physician working at the bedside still feels that he is a long

way from what he perceives to be the point of ultimate administrative decision. There seem to be too many levels between him and those who have the actual power. As a result, the decision making is rather slow.

3. There is also the difficulty of *keeping in touch with one's elected representative*. Feedback is relatively easy from the specialist to his hospital-based colleagues through a well-developed divisional system. However, the house staff member on the DMC frequently finds it difficult to communicate with his colleagues. Thus, there is still a widespread feeling in the medical profession of remoteness from decisions which vitally affect it. Personal involvement is as yet an elusive goal.

4. It is obviously difficult for specialists or general practitioners to find the *time* to participate in administration while continuing active clinical duties, although it is imperative that they achieve this in order to retain their credibility.

5. A number of voices have criticized the whole idea of team management and would have preferred a system of individual management by a chief executive. It is indeed suggested that team management may "wither away" in practice as strong personalities emerge in the team who will arrogate to themselves leadership and unrestricted decision making. It will be interesting to watch whether these forecasts prove correct or whether the multi-professional approach may not turn out to be the method of the future (Howard, 1973).

6. So far we do not know if general goal conformity can be reached with the widely differing interests and aims of community physicians, general practitioners, and hospital medical staff. At the present time the hospitals have a major and disproportionate share of both staff and financial resources, whereas preventive medical services are extremely undersubscribed.

7. There is finally the fundamental question of *consensus* management itself which is leading to a number of as yet unresolved issues.

    (a) Whereas a delegate involved in political negotiations has to take a line predetermined by his colleagues, a representative in a consensus group must be given freedom to exercise his own judgment while nevertheless protecting the interests of those he represents. This is a situation to which the medical profession has not yet adjusted itself.

(b) Practicing clinicians have now been given a managerial voice equal to that of professional administrators. They may feel themselves outnumbered by the four officers of the DMT, viewing the community physician and the nursing officer as part of the administrative establishment. However, the administrator and finance officer could also feel themselves to be in a minority of four to two, viewing the community physician and the nursing officer as a clinical group with the consultant and general practitioner. As participants become more familiar with the workings of consensus management, the concept of numerical inferiority should become less and less relevant.

(c) When the consensus principle was originally proposed, many people concerned with the administration of the health system felt sincerely that this would be disastrous. After all, what it would mean in practice—so they expected—would be that every professional in turn would exercise his veto so that, instead of efficient decision making, there would be eternal wrangles and at best log-rolling.

Although two years is too short a time for reaching definite conclusions, it can be stated that these woeful forecasts have not come to pass. It might have happened that controversial decisions were deferred from further consultations by the District Management Team, but formal vetoes recording irreconcilable disagreement have been very rare indeed. The reasons for this outcome have been the fact that the DMT, in spite of their heterogeneous professional backgrounds, welded themselves fairly quickly into organic entities. The regular meetings, very often underpinned by common meals, led to greater friendliness and understanding, so that very soon no individual member was anxious to incur the odium of pronouncing a veto which would mean that the decision was taken out of the management team and referred above to the Area Health Authority. Social forces and group behavior seemingly are stronger than organizational constraints.

Implications for the United States

To an American observer it appears that physician participation in management decisions is a good move in England under a nationalized system with very limited resources. Is it to be recommended for the United States? In the recent past it was probably not a feasible alternative. Medical staff members were, by and large, independent individuals and a lay administrator was less a threat to such independence than a physician who took or helped to take responsibility and accountability. Moreover, many physicians in the United States already feel too overburdened with quality- and utilization-review activities to spend more time in management committees.

Most administrators and boards in the United States have been quite receptive to requests for new services and facilities. Because it was possible to raise rates and because new services usually generated more income and prestige for the hospital and lowered unit costs of the departments, administrators and trustees did not need to raise questions as to whether or not the new service or facility really improved quality. Administrators, too, have not wanted participation or interference from others, for a major source of administrative power is control of management information.

The environment for hospital and health management is, however, changing rapidly in the United States. For example, the National Health Planning and Resources Development Act (P.L. 93-641) unifies planning, resource allocation, and regulatory efforts in the United States and increases federal control over local activities. Figure 2 presents the organization and responsibilities called for under this act. This hierarchically related network provides some striking resemblances to the framework of the English National Health Service.

Other trends also portend organizational changes in American hospitals. The independence of the individual physician is diminishing through utilization- and quality-review requirements. Physicians are also becoming more cohesively organized, as evidenced by recent collective bargaining activities and even strikes.

Hospital administrators and trustees too must make harder decisions on allocation of limited resources. Increasingly, decisions will need to be made as to where staffing might be reduced and even which services will be curtailed. Administrators and trustees are

SECRETARY, U.S. DEPARTMENT
HEALTH, EDUCATION AND WELFARE

- Issues guidelines for national health planning policy
- Establishes health areas recommended by governors
- Designates health systems agencies in each area
- Issues regulations governing implementation of the act
- Reviews health plans produced by substate and state agencies
- Administers grant programs to agencies
- Approves most federal assistance plans and project grants

STATE HEALTH COORDINATING
COUNCIL (SHCC)
(a consumer majority council of citizens 60% designated by HSA, 40% designated by the governor)

- Conducts health planning activities for the state
- Implements or supervises implementation of plans
- Prepares preliminary state health plan
- Serves as agency for (S.1122) review
- Administers a state certificate-of-need program
- Reviews and makes findings concerning all new institutional health services in the state
- Reviews periodically all health services offered in the state
- Coordinates all health data activities in the state
- Assists SHCC in its work
- Administers federally assisted facilities construction activities
- Administers optional rate review and approval programs

STATE HEALTH PLANNING AND
DEVELOPMENT AGENCY (SPDA)
(a state agency designated by the governor to carry out activities mandated by the act)

- Reviews and coordinates health planning activities of substate agencies
- Prepares and approves state health plan
- Reviews and comments on annual budget of substate agencies
- Reviews and comments on annual applications of substate agencies
- Advises SPDA on its work
- Reviews and approves all state plans and applications for funds under federal health legislation

HEALTH SYSTEMS AGENCY (HSA)
(A public or private nonprofit agency with a consumer-majority board or advisory body which carries out functions mandated by the act in a defined geographic area. Areas are based on criteria defining minimum population and available health services to meet the needs of the areas residents.)

- Assembles and analyzes data on health status and health programs in its area
- Prepares and publishes a Health Systems Plan (HSP) and an Annual Implementation Plan (AIP) for its area
- Develops specific activities and projects which support plans
- Implements plans through technical assistance and through developmental grants to community agencies
- Coordinates activities with other planning bodies and PSROs
- Reviews and approves each use of federal health funds in its area
- Recommends action on each health service offered in area to state
- Reviews and comments to state agency on all capital expenditures and new service projects in area institutions
- Recommends health facilities projects to state for funding

COMMUNITY INSTITUTIONS AND ORGANIZATIONS

- Submits all new service and capital expenditure projects for review
- Participates in periodic review of existing services
- Submits all applications for federal support for review
- Conducts special projects under developmental grant authorities

Source: Schulz and Johnson (1976: 265).
© *McGraw Hill Inc.*
Used with permission of McGraw Hill Book Co.

FIG. 2.   Planning, Organization, and Responsibilities under P.L. 93-641, National
Health Planning and Resources Development Act.

likely to want physician participation in such decisions.

With increasing influence of Health Systems Agencies, the hospital governing board's role as the link to the hospital's environment becomes less important. In that case hospitals may in the future find internal boards composed in a large measure of physicians and key administrative and professional personnel to be more effective than community representatives (Schulz and Johnson, 1976: 47-65).

Assuming that controls over hospitals and needs for greater control within hospitals will increase, the advantages of the traditional organizational arrangement in U.S. hospitals of almost separate medical staff and hospital trustee, administrator, and employee organizations are diminishing. If such a divided organizational pattern remains, it may result in more formal collective bargaining and confrontation between the two organizations. If medical staffs and hospitals are to be integrated it seems quite plausible for a management team approach to be utilized. The other alternative is for an even more hierarchical approach with a full-time lay administrator or medical director as the chief executive officer, which Great Britain for one found unacceptable.

Experiences with participative management teams in Great Britain should be evaluated as to their effects on costs, quality, attitudes, and feasibility for adaptation to U.S. hospitals. Hospitals in the United States should experiment with such alternative approaches. Certainly traditional hospital organization patterns will need to be re-evaluated in light of health delivery system changes we are experiencing.

While we are in no way suggesting transplantation of the British organizational arrangement to the United States, we do suggest that a management team approach does have application in changing United States health delivery system. Further support for the team approach in the future is suggested by Ansoff (1973), who predicts that demands on managers of complex systems will exceed the capacity and comprehension of any single individual and will call for the concept of the corporate office which replaces the chief executive officer with a team of coequals. While Ansoff is talking about industrial management, his model seems to be particularly relevant to the hospital, which is already one of the most complex organizations in our society.

Rockwell Schulz, PH.D.
Programs in Health Administration
University of Wisconsin-Madison
1225 Observatory Drive
Madison, WI 53706

David S. Grimes, M.B., CH. B., M.R.C.P.
Department of Gastroenterology
Withington University Hospital
Manchester, England

T. E. Chester, C.B.E., D. JUR.
Department of Social Administration
University of Manchester
Dover Street
Manchester, England

References

Anderson, B.J.
1973   Hospital Governing Board Relations. Presented at the North Central Medical Conference Program, Bloomington, Minnesota, October 20. Reprinted in the Milwaukee Medical Society Times.

Ansoff, I.
1973   "The next twenty years in management education." Library Quarterly 43: 293–328.

Battistella, R., and T.E. Chester
1973   "Reorganization of the National Health Service." New England Journal of Medicine 289: 610–615.

Department of Health and Social Security
1972   "The clinicians' role in the management process." Pp. 68–71 in Management Arrangements for the Reorganized National Health Service. London: Her Majesty's Stationery Office.

1974a   Third Report of the Joint Working Party on the Organization of Medical Work in Hospitals in England and Wales. London: Her Majesty's Stationery Office.

1974b   Local Advisory Committees. National Health Service Circular HRC (74)9.

Goss, M.E.W.

1963   "Patterns of bureaucracy among staff physicians." In Freidson, Eliot (ed.), The Hospital in Modern Society. New York: Free Press.

Howard, H.T.

1973   "Doctors in management." Health and Social Services Journal (December 1 and 8).

National Advisory Commission on Health Manpower

1967   Volume 1. Washington, D.C.: Government Printing Office.

Schulz, R.I.

1972   "How effective is physician participation in hospital management." The Hospital Medical Staff (December): 4–10.

Schulz, R.I., and A.J. Johnson

1976   Management of Hospitals. New York: McGraw-Hill Book Company.

United States Department of Health, Education, and Welfare

1968   Report of the Secretary's Advisory Committee on Hospital Effectiveness. DHEW Publication No. 0-295-545. Washington, D.C.: Government Printing Office.

Milbank Memorial Fund Quarterly/*Health and Society, Vol. 57, No. 2, 1979*

Organizational Determinants of Services, Quality and Cost of Care in Hospitals

W. RICHARD SCOTT, ANN BARRY FLOOD, AND WAYNE EWY

Department of Sociology, Stanford University; Organizations and Mental Health Training Program, Stanford University; and Warner-Lambert/Parke-Davis Pharmaceutical Division

FTER MORE THAN A DECADE of research on the structural features of organizations (Blau and Schoenherr, 1971; Pugh, Hickson, Hinings et al., 1968 and 1969), researchers are turning their attention from the determinants to the consequences of organizational structure. In particular, attention has recently been focused on the effects of structure on organizational effectiveness and efficiency (Child, 1974 and 1975; Goodman and Pennings, 1977; Price, 1972; Steers, 1977). Good examples of the latter variables are provided by quality (effectiveness) and cost (efficiency) of health care in hospitals. These variables are also of great interest to policy makers because of the recent rapid increases in hospital costs and uneven quality of hospital care in this country.

A large number of studies have examined factors associated with quality or cost of care in hospitals, but only a small number have examined both simultaneously, and an even smaller number have attempted to relate them to structural features of hospitals (Cohen, 1970; Morse, Gordon and Moch, 1974; Neuhauser, 1971; Rushing, 1974; and Shortell, Becker and Neuhauser, 1976). Results from these and related studies have not been clear or persuasive. Important limitations of previous work include: 1) a lack of effective techniques for taking into account differences among patients that

0026-3745-79-5702-0234-31/$01.00/0 ©1979 Milbank Memorial Fund affect both the cost and the quality of care observed; and 2) a lack of attention to the development of output measures that distinguish the outcome of care received from the quantity or costs of services delivered or from the potential to provide care implied by the elaborateness of facilities and the qualifications of health care personnel.[1] We designed our research approach to deal with both of these difficult issues. To handle the first issue, we adjusted the measures of services and outcomes for hospital patients to take into account variations due to the health status of the patients being treated. To handle the second issue, we developed independent measures of quality of care, quantity of services, costs of care, and structural measures of the potential of the organization to provide care, and examined their interrelationships. Based on this research, we examined in a related paper (Flood, Scott, Ewy et al., 1978) the relations among measures of the average quantity of services delivered and the average quality of outcomes achieved by patients in a hospital. In this paper we focus on a set of structural characteristics of hospitals as predictors of variations in the average intensity and duration of services provided to patients, the average amount of expenditure for patient care, and the average quality of outcomes experienced by patients in the hospital.

Methods

Data Sources

Data used in this study were drawn from 17 acute care hospitals. The hospitals had all previously participated in the prospective study of our research team concerning the organizational factors affecting quality of outcome following surgery (Stanford Center for Health Care Research, 1974). Although some of the data on organizational characteristics was used in our previous study, the patient data in our current study are based on a much broader spectrum of patients, including both surgical and medical patients, and employ information obtained entirely from abstracts of patient records. The study

---

[1]Strengths and limitations of the various classes of measures employed to assess care quality are discussed in Donabedian (1966) and Scott (1977).

hospitals were selected from a roster of 1377 hospitals participating as of 1972 in the Professional Activities Study (PAS) of the Commission on Professional and Hospital Activities (CPHA), a hospital abstracting system collecting and summarizing selected information on all patient discharges from its member hospitals. Thirty-two hospitals were selected randomly from a stratified sample of all short-term voluntary hospitals participating in PAS; of these 32, 16 agreed to participate in the research and a 17th, administratively linked to one of the 16, volunteered to participate at its own expense. Stratification variables included size, teaching status, and expenses. The 17 hospitals are not completely representative of all short-term acute care hospitals in this country. In particular, they do not include proprietary or federal short-term hospitals. Compared to hospitals of a similar type, their average size is greater than the national average (304 vs 164 beds).[2] Six of the study hospitals (35%) were affiliated with a medical school or had an approved and active house staff program, compared to 28% of comparable U.S. hospitals. Costs of care within the study hospitals were similar to the national average: $113 average cost per patient day for our study hospitals compared to $115 for U.S. hospitals. The goal of obtaining substantial variance within the sample along these important dimensions was achieved: for the sample, size varied from 99 to 638 beds, and average costs from $77 to $154 per patient day. Ten states and all major geographic regions within the continental United States were represented.

All patient data were based on information contained in the PAS abstract record, which was available for each of the approximately 670,000 patients discharged from the study hospitals during the period, May 1970 through December 1973. The final set of study patients numbered approximately 603,000; virtually all of the excluded cases were newborns. Data from the patient abstract provided the basis for our measures of services received and outcome, including the number and types of diagnostic and therapeutic services received during the hospitalization, the length of hospital stay and the measure of patient outcome, i.e., death in hospital. In addition, we used information from the patients' abstracts (by means of a procedure to be described below) to adjust the service and outcome

---

[2]Study hospital and national figures are based on 1973 data.

measures for differences in patient mix and in hospitalization experience.

Data on the organizational characteristics of the hospital and medical staff came primarily from our previous study on the quality of surgical care (Stanford Center for Health Care Research, 1974). For that study, interviews had been conducted during the spring of 1974 with key hospital and medical staff personnel who acted as expert informants, describing the structure and operation of their units. Questionnaires had also been administered to the staffs of the operating room, recovery room, and surgical wards, and to selected physicians providing primary care and selected ancillary services. Data on surgeons' training and experience had been collected from either hospital records or American Medical Association (AMA) records. In addition to these data from our earlier study, information was assembled on selected hospital characteristics from the American Hospital Association (AHA) annual survey for each of the 4 years studied.

Measures of Major Variables

The principal measures in this study may be grouped into four categories: 1) outcome of hospitalization; 2) amount and type of in-hospital services; 3) actual hospital costs; and 4) hospital structure.

Measure of the Outcome of Hospitalization. The indicator of quality of care is the rate of *in-hospital mortality* adjusted for patient characteristics—a measure emphasizing the quality of outcome of care for patients.

Measures of In-Hospital Services: Rates of Service Intensity and Duration. We developed indicators to estimate the number or amount of services of varying types received by a patient during a hospital stay. Although it is not feasible to assess all of the many types of services provided by hospitals, we measured seven types of important diagnostic and therapeutic services provided to inpatients. We also assessed the duration of the services, as measured by length of stay. For purposes of this analysis, we limited our attention to a composite measure of these seven services rather than to each service measured independently. An *Index of Service Intensity* reflects the amount and variety of diagnostic and therapeutic services provided to patients, as well as the relative cost of each of these different types of services.[3] An *Index of Service Duration* is based on length of stay. This measure weighs length of stay by the proportion of total hospital charges associated with routine nursing and hotel services provided to all patients regardless of any specific services consumed.[4] The two indexes, their component measures and weights, are summarized in Table 1.

The measures of outcome and of service intensity and duration were first computed at the patient level by detailed analysis of individual records for the 603,000 patients, to permit standardization for individual patient differences. General features of the approach are described in Appendix A; specifics are provided in Forrest, Brown, Scott, et al. (1977). Briefly, using a combination of classification by diagnosis (with 332 diagnostic groupings) and linear regression, and using indicators that characterized each patient's condition and treatment record, including diagnoses, operations, admission test findings, and socio-demographic characteristics, we computed the expected levels of service intensity, duration, and outcome for each patient, conditional on the patient's specific

---

[3]Categories of therapeutic and diagnostic services measured are reported in Table 1. Costliness of services was reflected in a weight assigned to each individual category before combining them into the composite measure. These weights were based on the average proportion of total charges for a hospitalization episode associated with each category of service. The weights were obtained from data on hospital charges supplied by a non-study hospital. Thus, they are not intended to reflect the actual variations in charges among study hospitals, but were uniformly applied to all hospitals. The intent was only to reflect differences in *relative* costliness among the various categories of services provided by hospitals.

Since we were able to assess not only whether a given category of service was used by a given patient but often the amount or numbers of such services consumed as well, the actual weights applied to each service used by a patient took into account these frequencies. Thus, the final weighting for each service consisted of the proportion of total charges for each category of services, as reported in Table 1, divided by the average amount of each type of service consumed by study patients during their hospitalization. For example, since the average number of operations for study patients was 0.545, the final weight assigned was $14.27/0.545 = 26.183$, which was applied to each operative procedure received by a given patient.

[4]For some analyses not reported here, these two composite measures were combined into an overall measure of services. For this reason, a weighting of length of stay was introduced. This weighting does not alter any of the results presented in this paper, but is included to allow a comparison of the relative costliness of specific services and routine care.

TABLE 1
Components of the Service Intensity and Duration Indexes and Their Weights

Items From the PAS Abstract for Patients	Class of Services Being Estimated	Proportion of Patient Charges for Class* (%)	Weighting Factor of PAS Item for Each Patient†
Components of Index of Service Intensity:			
Diagnostic services:			
No. of radiographic procedures performed	Radiological services	7.08	32.627 per procedure
No. of blood tests	Laboratory	8.48	12.676 per test
Therapeutic services:			
No. of operative procedures	Surgery	14.27	26.183 per procedure
Administration of any blood or blood parts	Laboratory	2.83	52.407 if any blood given
Physical therapy	Therapy	2.66	52.157 if physical therapy given
No. of classes of drugs	Medical supplies	8.52	7.992 per class of drugs
Use of intensive care unit	Special care units	4.21	56.892 if special unit used
	Subtotal	48.05	
Component of Index of Service Duration:			
No. of days in hospital	Hotel services	51.95	6.185 per day
	Routine nursing care		
	Total	100.00	

*Based on the proportion of average patient's bill attributable to a given service class using 1973 figures from a non-study hospital.
†To obtain the weighting factor, the proportion of charges for the class is divided by the mean number of corresponding services on the PAS abstract actually used by patients in the study (see footnote 3).

characteristics and physical condition at admission. For each of the three types of measures based on patients—service intensity, duration, and outcome—the expected levels reflected the pattern of utilization or outcome obtained on the average in the set of study hospitals by patients with the same type of disease and physical condition. We then calculated difference scores for each patient, which reflected the difference, whether positive or negative, between the expected level of service intensity, duration, and outcome for a patient of that type and the actual level of service intensity, duration and outcome observed for that patient. To obtain a measure for a hospital, these difference scores were then averaged for the set of all patients treated in the hospital during the study period. Thus, our measures of service intensity, duration, and outcome for each hospital are summary measures of observed departures in the experience of individual patients from expected scores based on the typical experience of similar patients treated in all of the hospitals in our sample.

Measure of Cost Based on Actual Hospital Charges.   Unlike the measures of services and outcomes, the measure of cost was not based on data obtained on individual patients and then aggregated to the hospital level, nor was it adjusted for differences in patient mix among hospitals. Data on actual expenditures on, or charges to, patients were not available. Instead, the cost measure was based on data obtained from the AHA's annual survey of 1973 and consisted of the total annual expenditures of each hospital divided by the number of patients treated during that year, which provides the *average expenditures per patient episode.* We attempted to correct this measure for regional differences in cost by dividing each hospital's score by the Medicare reimbursement index for the county in which the study hospital was located. Clearly, however, because our measure of cost does not take into account differences in patient mix, its usefulness is compromised, and it will not receive much attention in our subsequent analyses.

Measures of Hospital Structure.   Measures of the structural characteristics of hospitals were grouped into two categories, capacity and control, as follows:

1. *Capacity* refers to those aspects of the hospital that represent its potential to supply services. Six types of measures were used. One obviously important measure was that of hospital size or scale. Since

hospitals are organizations heavily dependent on personal services, we used as our indicator of size the *total number of personnel employed.* (This indicator was correlated 0.93 with average daily patient census.) Second, to measure the elaborateness of the therapeutic and diagnostic facilities available, we assessed the *number of different types of facilities* and the *proportion of beds devoted to intensive care* in the hospital. The third set of measures examined the intensity of the staffing, indicated by the *ratio of all staff to the average daily census* and by the *ratio of direct care nurses to average daily census.* Fourth, the teaching status of the hospital was measured by the *ratio of residents to regular medical staff.* Fifth, the qualifications of the staff were determined by several types of measures indicating training, certification, and experience. These included the *ratio of registered nurses (RNs) to other types of nurses* e.g., licensed vocational nurses (LVNs); the *average number of years in nursing* for staff nurses; the *proportion of the surgical staff that was board-certified;* and the *average number of years in practice since residency* for surgeons. A final measure assessed the unused capacity or slack resources of the institution as measured by the *occupancy rate,* the ratio of occupied beds to total bed capacity. It should be noted that occupancy rate measured capacity used.

All of the above measures of the hospital's capacity to supply services were based on data supplied by the hospital administrator for each study hospital, with the following exceptions: information on facilities and intensive care beds was obtained from the AHA annual survey, and information on the average years of nursing experience was compiled from a questionnaire distributed to all ward staff nurses in the study hospitals (average return rate, 75%).

2. *Control* encompassed several features of the organization including the distribution of power or influence over decisions and mechanisms for the control and coordination of work activities. We assessed the distribution of influence among two major sets of actors within the hospital—administrators and staff physicians, coordination at several organizational levels, and controls exercised by the surgical staff over its own members. Brief descriptions of the variables used to assess these control features follow; more detailed information on the measures employed is provided in Appendix B.

Three measures of influence were developed on responses by key hospital informants to a set of hypothetical decision questions. One measure focused on the *hospital administrator's influence on decisions in the administrative area;* a second focused on the *chief of surgery's influence on decisions within his jurisdiction;* and a third examined the extent of *encroachment by physicians on administrative decisions.*

Coordination and control activities were assessed using measures of administrative intensity, clerical support, formalization, and frequency of communication with quality assurance personnel. Specifically, for the hospital as a whole, we assessed the *ratio of supervisory-to-direct care personnel.* At the nursing ward level, we measured the *average number of ward clerks and secretaries* present and, based on questionnaire responses from staff nurses, the *explicitness of general nursing policies.* To assess coordination by special professional units, we determined the *frequency of case discussions between physicians and pathologists* as reported by pathologists.

Finally, to assess the control exercised by the physician staff over its own members, we measured the extent of formalized *control exercised by the surgical staff over new members* as well as the *control exercised over tenured members.* These measures of formalized control were based on the rigorousness of the initial and continuing review of credentials, length of probation, and/or gradations of privileges. A third measure assessed the *proportion of contract (salaried) physicians* on the physician staff, an indicator favored by Roemer and Friedman (1971) as the best single measure of physician staff control.[5]

Predictions

In general, we expect organizational capacity to be positively associated with greater average service intensity and hence with higher average costs per patient episode. It should be noted that, since service intensity was adjusted to take into account differences in patient mix, the argument is not the conventional one that patients with more severe illnesses are more likely to be treated in larger and more elaborate facilities where they receive more services. Rather, we argue that patients served in more elaborate and more

---

[5]The data sources, the techniques employed to standardize service intensity, duration, and outcome measures, and all of the individual measures are described in detail in Forrest, Brown, Scott et al. (1977).

professionalized facilities are more likely to receive more services than expected, taking into account their specific condition. Such services are expected to be provided both because they are "more available" and because they contribute to other valued organizational and staff goals, such as teaching and research. There is no clear rationale for linking organizational capacity in general to duration of services, so no predictions are made concerning length of stay.

Hypotheses relating organizational capacity to quality of care are also somewhat problematic. Since the indicators of care quality vary considerably from one study to another, and since measures of structure, process, and outcome tend to be poorly correlated with one another (Brook, 1973), we restrict attention to outcome indicators of quality. There is some evidence to suggest that quality of outcomes is higher in larger hospitals (Kohl, 1955; Lipworth, Lee, and Morris, 1963; and the Commission on Professional and Hospital Activities, 1969). The relation between the average level of staff qualifications and surgical outcomes was investigated in an earlier prospective study of 9500 patients by the Stanford Center. In her analysis of these data, Flood (1976) reported that better surgical outcomes were associated with hospitals whose surgical staff had completed a greater average number of residencies (e.g., more varied postgraduate training) but, unexpectedly, poorer outcomes were associated with staffs having longer average residencies. Also unexpected was the finding that greater average specialization on the part of surgeons—measured by the types of operations actually performed—produced poorer outcomes, while the proportion of board-certified surgeons on the staff was not associated with quality of outcomes. The same study showed that better outcomes were associated with hospitals whose nursing staff had longer nursing experience, on the average.[6] Whether one should expect the average length of nurse and physician experience to be positively associated with better quality outcomes is unclear: a staff with a higher average level of experience signifies, on the one hand, more practice and exposure to varied medical problems but, on the other hand, increasing age and

---

[6] It should be emphasized that these results were observed at the aggregate level of analysis—i.e., using the average level of training and experience as the independent variables. Different results may be expected and have been observed when the level of analysis is shifted to the individual physician (Flood, 1976; and Flood, Scott, Ewy et al., 1977).

remoteness from training and, perhaps, from contemporary methods of care.

Turning to predictions involving control and coordination systems, we might expect to see greater controls exercised by administrators and physicians associated with reduced services to patients. Such an expectation is probably somewhat utopian since it is not at all clear that, given high influence, hospital administrators or the medical staff have much incentive to curb the services provided to patients and thus to contain the costs of medical care (Fuchs, 1974). Also, we should not expect both service intensity and service duration to be affected in the same manner by administrative and professional controls. Thus, our predictions with respect to hospital coordination and control systems and services are unsure, and we hope to learn from an examination of the empirical relations observed. By contrast, previous research suggests that better quality of medical care is positively related to administrative influence over decisions within its own domain (Flood and Scott, 1978), to coordination of work at the overall hospital and ward levels (Georgopoulos and Mann, 1962; Longest, 1974; and Neuhauser, 1971) and to the ability of the physician staff to regulate its members (Flood and Scott, 1978; Roemer and Friedman, 1971; and Shortell, Becker, and Neuhauser, 1976).

Strengths and Limitations

Before presenting the results, we should note the important strengths and limitations of the present data base and approach. Considerable confidence can be placed in our estimates of differences in services and quality of care among hospitals since they are based on a very large number of observations per hospital. Also, detailed measures of patient characteristics are used to standardize service and quality measures for differences among hospitals in patient mix. Further, unusually varied and detailed measures of the organizational characteristics of the hospitals and their medical staffs are available. These strengths are somewhat offset by several serious limitations. First, our indicator of quality of care—death in hospital—while highly reliable, is severely limited in reflecting only mortality experience. Had the data sources permitted, it would have been greatly preferable to include other outcome measures such as morbidity or return to function,[7] as well as to include information on patient condition after discharge. Second, although detailed measures of hospital and physician staff characteristics are available, there is some discrepancy in the time at which they are measured in relation to the patient data. As noted, patient information covers the period 1970 through 1973, while on-site collection of organizational data occurred in the spring of 1974. One must allow for the possibility that basic structural changes occurred within one or more hospitals during the period under study. A further limitation: since the original data were collected for a study of surgical care, most of the measures of physician staff are based on the characteristics of surgeons and the organization of the surgical staff. Surgeons constitute, of course, only a subset of the full medical staff. Third, although the measures of services and outcomes are based on the experience of a large number of patients, we have only a small number of hospitals on which to test predictions relating hospital characteristics to these dependent variables. Clearly, in presenting these results, our mode must be exploratory, and the results must be regarded as suggestive rather than definitive.

Results

Interrelation Among Service Intensity, Quality, and Cost

Before presenting the data relating to our predictions regarding organizational factors affecting services, cost, and quality of care, we note briefly the interrelations among these aggregated dependent variables. In all cases, except costs, results are based on the standardized measures. There exists a slight negative association between service intensity and service duration (-0.27):[8] hospitals delivering more services to patients than expected tend to exhibit shorter average stays than expected. Longer average service duration

---

[7]An attempt to include in-hospital complications as another indicator of care quality had to be abandoned due to the poor quality of data in this area.

[8]All correlations are Pearson product moment. The significance level adopted for these analyses is $p \leq 0.10$. For an *n* of 17 and a two-tailed test, an $r \geq 0.412$ is significant at this level.

was slightly associated with higher average costs per patient episode (0.37), while the average level of service intensity showed no association with average costs per patient episode (0.07). Most important, a higher than expected level of services within a hospital was significantly associated with a lower than expected mortality rate (−0.43), while longer than expected service duration was significantly associated with a higher than expected mortality rate (0.64).

Analyses of these relations reported in detail in a companion paper (Flood et al., 1978) reveal that both indexes of services and the outcome measure were strongly influenced by regional location of the hospital. When relations among these measures are examined for hospitals within regions, however, the negative association between service intensity and mortality persisted while the positive association between service duration and mortality tended to disappear. In short, it appears that the association between duration of services and poorer outcomes, which was observed for all study hospitals, is probably due to regional variations in medical practice rather than to hospital differences.

Effects of Organizational Capacity on Service Duration, Intensity, Quality and Cost of Care: Zero-Order Associations

Table 2 presents the zero-order correlations among the several measures of organizational capacity and the measures of service intensity and duration, quality, and cost of care. We note that larger hospitals having proportionately more residents and more elaborate facilities tended to provide more services than expected—both intensity and duration—and to be characterized by higher expenses per patient episode. On the other hand, these same measures of capacity were not associated with better than expected outcomes. The only exception to this general pattern was that hospitals having a higher proportion of their beds devoted to intensive care tended to exhibit shorter than expected lengths of stay and better than expected outcomes.[9] Higher labor intensity also was associated with better out-

---

[9]Since the indicator of quality of care used is the hospital's mortality rate adjusted for differences in patient mix, a negative correlation is indicative of better outcomes, hence, higher quality of care.

TABLE 2

Effect of Hospital Capacity on Service Duration and
Intensity, Quality and Cost of Care: Zero-Order Correlations*

Hospital Capacity:	Services		Quality: In-Hospital Mortality	Costs: Expenditures per Patient Episode
	Duration	Intensity		
Size:				
Total no. of staff	0.38†	0.41†	0.00	0.62†
Facilities:				
No. of different facilities	0.16	0.39†	0.02	0.65†
Percent of beds in ICU	−0.36†	0.54†	−0.32	0.29
Labor intensity:				
Ratio of total staff to ADC	−0.29	0.19	−0.44†	−0.05
Ratio of direct care nurses to ADC	−0.17	−0.22	−0.25	−0.48†
Teaching:				
Percent of residents	0.47†	0.18	0.09	0.71†
Qualifications:				
Ratio of RNs to LVNs	−0.31	0.29	0.05	−0.03
Average yrs of experience in nursing	−0.29	−0.31	0.30	−0.26
Percent surgeons with board certification	0.05	−0.08	−0.29	0.37†
Average yrs since residency	0.57†	−0.58†	0.60†	0.19
Extent capacity used:				
Occupancy rate	0.23	0.39†	0.22	0.30

*All measures of services and quality rates have been standardized to take into account patient mix of hospitals. Note that, since quality is measured by death rate, a negative correlation reflects a lower standardized death rate and thus better quality of care. *Abbreviations:* ICU = intensive care unit; RN = registered nurse; LVN = licensed vocational nurse; ADC = average daily census.
†Significant at ≤0.1 for one-tailed test; sample size of 17.

comes, but, at the same time, it was negatively associated with expenses.

The measures of qualifications were, in general, not related to services as predicted, or to quality of care. In general, training levels for both nurses (proportion RNs) and physicians (proportion board-certified surgeons) revealed little association with services and out-comes; costs tended to be higher in hospitals served by more board-certified surgeons. Nursing experience revealed no significant associations with services and outcomes, but length of practice for surgeons was strongly associated with longer service duration, lower service intensity, and poorer than expected outcomes. Finally, we had expected that lower occupancy rates—greater unused capacity—would be associated with higher levels of services and costs, but the data tended to be in the opposite direction: higher occupancy rates were associated with higher service intensity.

Effects of Organizational Control on Service Duration, Intensity, Quality and Cost of Care: Zero-Order Associations

The zero-order correlations among the indicators of influence, coordination, and control within the hospital and physician staff on the measures of services, quality and cost of care are presented in Table 3. Beginning with the measures of influence of administrators and the surgical chief and his staff, we note that higher influence of both groups tended to be associated with longer service duration and

TABLE 3
Effect of Hospital Control Factors on Service Duration and
Intensity, Quality, and Costs of Care: Zero-Order Correlations*

Hospital Control Factors	Services		Quality: In-Hospital Mortality	Costs: Expenditures per Patient Episode
	Duration	Intensity		
Influence:				
Administrative influence in own area	0.66†	−0.27	0.54†	0.37†
Surgical chief's influence in own area	0.33	−0.02	0.28	0.69†
Encroachment by medical staff	0.39†	0.26	0.16	0.31
Coordination within hospital:				
Ratio of supervisors to direct care personnel	−0.19	0.51†	−0.38†	−0.38†
Coordination within wards:				
No. of clerks on wards	−0.29	0.57†	−0.58†	0.06
Explicitness of nursing policies	−0.41†	0.41†	−0.19	−0.13
Coordination by professional units:				
Frequency of case discussions with pathologists	−0.64†	0.36†	−0.33	−0.26
Physician staff controls:				
Control over tenured staff	0.32	−0.61†	0.42†	−0.25
Proportion of contract physicians	0.41†	−0.27	0.38†	0.33
Control over new staff	−0.19	0.10	−0.28	−0.09

*All measures of services and quality rates have been standardized to take into account patient mix of hospitals. Note that, since quality is measured by death rate, a negative correlation reflects a lower standardized death rate and thus better quality of care.
†Significant at ≤0.1 for one-tailed test; sample size is 17.

with greater expenses per patient episode. This pattern was observed both for influence measures within each role group's domain of decision-making as well as for the measure indicating physicians' encroachment on administrative decisions. Administrative influence was also associated with poorer quality outcomes.

The several indexes of coordination also revealed a rather consistent general pattern. Higher levels of coordination within the hospital generally and in the patient care wards tended to be associated with shorter length of stay and lower expenses per patient episode but with a higher level of service intensity and better care outcomes. By contrast, two of the three measures of physician staff control indicated that a higher level of staff control over its own members tended to be associated with longer service duration, lower service intensity, and, unexpectedly, with poorer quality outcomes.

Combination Effects of Selected Measures of Hospital Capacity and Control on Service Intensity, Duration, Quality and Costs of Care: Multiple Regressions

Multiple regression analysis was employed to examine the combined effects of selected variables assessing both organizational capacity and control. Variables were selected in terms of their theoretical interest, the magnitude of their association with the dependent variable, and to provide breadth of coverage of the various types of factors considered. The results of one set of regressions are presented in Table 4. These results are representative of other regressions examined employing various combinations of factors and alternative indicators. Variables in Table 4 are listed in the order obtained in a step-wise regression. In addition to the zero-order association, this table reports the individual regression coefficients (B) for each variable, which are equivalent to their regression slopes partialling out the impact of the other variables in the equation, the standard error for B, and the standardized regression coefficients, or betas (β). Results of F tests are reported, which assess the significance of each partial coefficient as well as the significance of the combination of coefficients included within each prediction equation.

Table 4 *A*. reports results using the index of average-adjusted service duration as the dependent variable. Four variables stand out as very strong predictors of average length of stay: administrators' influence, average years of practice for surgeons, and proportion of

TABLE 4
Effect of Selected Measures of Hospital Capacity and Control on Service Duration and Intensity, Quality and Cost of Care: Multiple Regressions*

Selected Measure	r	β	B	Std. Error B	F
A. Service Duration					
Administrative influence in own area	0.66	0.38	0.96	0.18	27.40†
Average yrs since residency	0.57	0.80	0.35	0.04	78.77†
Total no. of staff	0.38	0.29	0.0006	0.0004	2.79
Control over new staff	−0.19	−0.60	−0.52	0.07	48.69†
Percent of beds in ICU	−0.36	0.59	52.45	9.59	29.90†
Explicitness of nursing policies	−0.40	−0.23	−0.59	0.20	8.15†
Percent of residents	0.47	0.35	4.87	2.61	3.49
Multiple R = 0.99		R^2 = 0.98		Overall F at final step 38.25†	
B. Service Intensity					
Average yrs since residency	−0.58	−0.03	−0.038	0.35	0.01
Total no. of staff	0.41	1.03	0.006	0.003	3.31
Percent of residents	0.18	−0.52	−19.24	22.73	0.72
Ratio of supervisors to direct care personnel	0.51	0.32	20.20	16.56	1.49
Percent of beds in ICU	0.54	0.47	114.35	85.61	1.78
Control over new staff	0.11	−0.24	−0.55	0.69	0.64
Administrative influence in own area	−0.27	−0.03	−0.20	1.57	0.02
Multiple R = 0.86		R^2 = 0.75		Overall F at final step 2.56	
C. Quality: In-hospital Mortality					
Average yrs since residency	0.60	0.73	0.0013	0.0006	4.70*
Administrative influence in own area	0.54	0.55	0.0056	0.0026	4.62*
Ratio of direct care nurses to ADC	−0.25	−0.33	−0.0067	0.0045	2.24
Control over new staff	−0.28	−0.38	−0.0014	0.0010	1.89
Percent of beds in ICU	−0.32	0.46	0.17	0.13	1.82
No. of clerks on ward	−0.58	0.08	0.0006	0.0024	0.07
Multiple R = 0.85		R^2 = 0.72		Overall F at final step 3.04	
D. Costs: Expenditures per Patient Episode					
Percent of residents	0.71	−0.09	−152.59	1432.32	0.01
Control over new staff	−0.10	−0.02	−2.44	43.27	0.003
Administrative influence in own area	0.69	0.48	151.58	100.57	2.27
No. of different facilities	0.65	0.47	12.29	15.39	0.63
No. of clerks on wards	0.06	−0.21	−47.28	68.08	0.48
Total no. of staff	0.62	0.28	0.076	0.17	0.20
Multiple R = 0.85		R^2 = 0.73		Overall F at final step 3.58†	

*All measures of services and quality rates have been standardized to take into account patient mix of hospitals. Note that, since quality is measured by death rate, a negative correlation reflects a lower standardized death rate and thus better quality of care. *Abbreviations:* ICU = intensive care unit; ADC = average daily census.
†Significant at ≤0.05.

beds in the intensive care unit (ICU) were strongly associated with longer than expected service duration; control over new staff was strongly associated with shorter than expected service duration. Explicitness of nursing policies was also significantly associated with shorter than expected duration of services. Of those variables significantly associated with service duration, only proportion of beds in the ICU changed the direction of its association, its zero-order relation being negative and its partial relation becoming positive. The combined effect of these variables was strongly significant. And, in combination, these variables accounted for 98% of the variance in the average service duration.

Table 4 *B.* reports a multiple regression with the index of average-adjusted service intensity as the dependent variable. Unlike the previous equation predicting service duration, in the equation predicting average service intensity none of the individual predictor variables reached significance nor was the combination of variables significant. The strongest individual predictor was size of staff, which tended to be associated with a higher than expected level of service intensity. Proportion of beds in the ICU was the next strongest measure. Both of these measures assess hospital capacity, and the direction of their association is as predicted. Although none of the individual variables was significant, in combination the variables accounted for 75% of the variance in the average service intensity.

Table 4 *C.* reports the regression of the measure of quality—standardized mortality rate—on selected measures of hospital capacity and control. Only two of the variables were significantly associated with average mortality: average years of practice for surgeons and administrators' within-domain influence were positively associated with adjusted death rate. Two other measures—of labor intensity and control over new surgical staff—were negatively associated with death rate (that is, positively associated with better outcomes) but neither association was strong enough to be significant. The overall F at the final step measuring the significance of the combination of predictive measures did not reach significance. The combined variables accounted for 72% of the variance in average-adjusted mortality.

Table 4 *D.* reports results of the regression of average expenditures per patient episode on selected measures of hospital capacity and control. No single predictor variable attained significance, but in combination the variables were significant at the 0.05 level. The strongest single predictor variable was administrators' within-domain influence, a measure positively associated with higher costs, but this relation was not statistically significant. The combined variables accounted for 73% of the variance in expenditures per patient episode.

Two measures tend to stand out in Table 4 and in similar regression equations examined but not reported here. They are average years of practice for surgeons and administrators' within-domain influence. Each merits further brief examination.

Average years in practice since residency for surgeons is a measure based on data obtained from the study hospital or from AMA records. To a surprising degree, this measure tends to be positively associated with both average-adjusted service duration and mortality. We should recall that these two measures were themselves strongly associated (0.64). Moreover, this measure tended to be negatively associated with a large number of indicators that were themselves negatively associated with both mortality and length of stay. These measures include frequency of case discussions with pathologists (-0.71), control over new surgical staff (-0.13), proportion of beds devoted to ICU (-0.38), ratio of total staff to average daily census (-0.29), ratio of supervisors to direct care personnel (-0.50), number of clerks on wards (-0.53), and a number of other indicators of control and coordination developed but not included in this report.[10] These indicators of control and coordination were not themselves highly intercorrelated, but the consistency of their negative association with average years of surgeon practice is striking. The question was raised earlier about the proper interpretation of this indicator: these data suggest that a higher average number of years of practice for physicians was associated with more lax control and coordination arrangements.

As described in Appendix B, the indicator of administrators' within-domain influence is based on a question assessing the relative power of hospital administrators to influence a decision regarding contracting for a service such as a laundry. Like years of surgeon ex-

---

[10]However, note that two measures of physician staff control are notably absent from this list: control over tenured physicians and proportion of contract physicians. These two measures were positively associated with years of physician experience (0.25 and 0.15, respectively) and, as reported in Table 3, were positively associated with service duration and mortality. As previously noted, these associations were unexpected.

perience, administrative influence was positively associated with both average-adjusted service duration and quality, even when the effect of related variables was taken into account. And like years of surgeon experience, administrative influence was negatively associated with variables that were themselves negatively related to both mortality and length of stay. For administrators, these variables included most of the measures of coordination within the hospital: administrative influence was negatively associated with ratio of supervisors to direct care personnel (-0.41), number of clerks on the wards (-0.51), explicitness of nursing policies (-0.46), and ratio of total staff to average daily census (-0.38). As might be expected, given the pattern of relationships just described, administrative influence was positively associated with years of experience for surgeons, but only moderately so (0.24). Thus, both the measure of administrators' influence and average years of surgeons' experience appeared to be related to larger complexes of coordination and control measures that help to explain their observed association with differences in average service duration and quality of care.

Summary and Conclusions

It is not easy to summarize these results relating hospital characteristics to measures of services, outcomes, and costs. The small number of hospitals studied—only 17—severely limits the confidence to be placed in any generalizations relating hospital characteristics to these dependent variables. Nevertheless, the opportunity to study structure (hospital characteristics), process (service intensity and duration), outputs (patient care outcomes), and costs in a single study encouraged us to carry out this exploratory analysis.

The prediction that hospitals characterized by greater capacity would tend to provide more services than expected received some empirical support in our analysis. Zero-order correlations showed that hospitals with larger staffs, a higher proportion of residents, and more elaborate facilities exhibited higher levels of average service intensity and duration. When the effects of other variables were controlled in multiple regressions, partials for ICU beds, and resident and staff size, tended to be associated with longer than expected service duration; and ICU beds and staff size were slightly associated with a higher than expected service intensity. For the most part, indexes of staff qualifications were unrelated to services, with one important exception: the average number of years since residency for surgeons was positively associated with service duration but negatively associated with service intensity.

Measures of capacity to deliver services showed only a slight association with quality of care as measured by standardized mortality rates. Measures of labor intensity tended to be slightly associated with better outcomes as assessed by both zero-order and partial correlations. Again, measures of qualifications were not associated with quality of care, with the exception of average years since residency for surgeons; this indicator was negatively associated with higher quality of care.

Measures of service capacity were positively associated with costs of patient care in zero-order analyses: staff size, facilities, proportion of residents, and proportion of board-certified surgeons were all positively associated with higher costs per patient episode. The only measure of capacity negatively related to costs was an indicator of labor intensity. When examined in multiple regressions, however, none of these measures remained significantly associated with costs.

Turning to measures of coordination and control, we find that most of the measures of coordination were positively associated with better quality care, as predicted. When the effect of other variables was controlled, however, few of these measures exhibited partials large enough to be significant. Contrary to expectation, two of the measures of physician staff controls—control over tenured staff and proportion of contract physicians—tended to be associated with poorer quality care.

No predictions were developed relating coordination and control to measures of average service intensity and duration. In general, coordination measures were negatively related to duration but positively related to service intensity. The two measures of physician staff control discussed above showed just the opposite pattern.

Finally, administrators' within-domain influence was positively related to service duration and higher costs but negatively associated with quality of care.

The negative association between control over tenured physicians and between administrators' influence and quality of care was not only unexpected but is contrary to the results of our earlier study using these same measures (Flood and Scott, 1978). Even though the hospitals and the measures of these independent variables are the same in these two studies, discrepant results are quite possible given differences in the patient populations and outcome measures employed: briefly, the earlier study was based on a small subset of surgical patients treated during 1973 and 1974 and included measures of morbidity as well as mortality in the outcomes assessed. Nevertheless, we were surprised by the inconsistent results in these two similar studies.

Although the specific associations revealed in these analyses were not as clear and consistent as we would have preferred, the general research approach employed, which combines measures of organizational structure, processes, and outcomes into a single design and which attempts to adjust process and outcome measures for differences in the types of clients served, seems to us promising. Indeed, the low and/or inconsistent associations observed among these three types of measures indicate the dangers entailed in using one type of measure as a surrogate for the others—a practice all too common in health services research specifically and, more generally, in research on organizational effectiveness.

We recommend that analyses of the type explored here be carried out in a larger sample of hospitals. Increased sample size would greatly assist in sorting out the complexities of associations that seem to characterize the relations among the types of variables considered. Of course, improved measures of costs that take into account differences in patient mix are essential. Finally, we hope that others will explore the uses of patient abstract data as a potential source of information on that most elusive of all measures in service organizations—the outcome experienced by clients.

References

Blau, P. M., and Schoenherr, R. 1971. *The Structure of Organizations.* New York: Basic Books.

Brook, R. H. 1973. *Quality of Care Assessment: A Comparison of Five Methods of Peer Review.* DHEW Publication HRA 74-3100 (July). Washington, D.C.: Bureau of Health Services Research and Evaluation.

Child, J. 1974 and 1975. Managerial and Organizational Factors Associated with Company Performance: Parts I and II. *Journal of Management Studies* 11: 175–189; 12: 12–27.

Cohen, H. A. 1970. Hospital Cost Curves with Emphasis on Measuring Patient Care Output. In Klarman, H. E., ed., *Empirical Studies in Health Economics.* pp. 279–293. Baltimore, Md.: The Johns Hopkins University Press.

Commission on Professional and Hospital Activities. 1969. *Cholecystectomy Mortality: A Study from PAS and MAP.* Ann Arbor, Mich.: Commission on Professional and Hospital Activities.

Donabedian, A. 1966. Evaluating the Quality of Medical Care. *Milbank Memorial Fund Quarterly/Health and Society* 44 (Part 2, July): 166–206.

Flood, A. B. 1976. Professions and Organizational Performance: A Study of Medical Staff Organization and Quality of Care in Short Term Hospitals. Unpublished Ph.D. dissertation, Stanford University, Department of Sociology, Stanford, Calif.

————, and Scott, W. R. 1978. Professional Power and Professional Effectiveness: The Power of the Surgical Staff and the Quality of Surgical Care in Hospitals. *Journal of Health and Social Behavior* 19 (September): 240–254.

————, ————, Ewy, W. et al. 1977. Effectiveness in Professional Organizations: The Impact of Surgeons and Surgical Staff Organizations on the Quality of Care in Hospitals. Paper presented at the meetings of the American Sociological Association, Chicago, Ill., September, 1977.

————, ————, ———— et al. 1978. The Relationship Between Intensity of Medical Services and Outcomes for Hospitalized Patients. Paper presented at the meetings of the Pacific Sociological Association, Spokane, Wash., April, 1978. (Revised, December, 1978.)

Forrest, W. H., Jr., Brown, B. W., Jr., Scott, W. R. et al. 1977. *Studies of the Determinants of Service Intensity in the Medical Care Sector.* Report to the National Center for Health Services Research, DHEW, under contract HRA 230-75-0169 (September). Stanford, Calif.: Stanford Center for Health Care Research, Stanford University.

Fuchs, V. R. 1974. *Who Shall Live? Health, Economics, and Social Choice.* New York: Basic Books.

Georgopoulos, B. S., and Mann, F. C. 1962. *The Community General Hospital.* New York: Macmillan.

Goodman, P. S., and Pennings, J. M. 1977. *New Perspectives on Organizational Effectiveness.* San Francisco, Calif.: Jossey-Bass.

Goss, M. E. W. 1970. Organizational Goals and Quality of Medical Care: Evidence from Comparative Studies of Hospitals. *Journal of Health and Social Behavior* 11 (December): 255–268.

Kohl, S. G. 1955. *Perinatal Mortality in New York City.* Cambridge, Mass.: Harvard University Press.

Lipworth, L., Lee, J. A. H., and Morris, J. N. 1963. Case-Fatality in Teaching and Non-Teaching Hospitals, 1956–59. *Medical Care* 1 (April/June): 71–76.

Longest, B. B., Jr. 1974. Relationship Between Coordination, Efficiency, and Quality of Care in General Hospitals. *Hospital Administration* 19 (Fall): 65–86.

Morse, E. V., Gordon, G., and Moch, M. 1974. Hospital Costs and Quality of Care: An Organizational Perspective. *Milbank Memorial Fund Quarterly/Health and Society* 52 (Summer): 315–345.

Neuhauser, D. 1971. *The Relationship Between Administrative Activities and Hospital Performance.* Research Series 28. Chicago, Ill.: Center for Health Administration Studies.

Price, J. L. 1972. The Study of Organizational Effectiveness. *The Sociological Quarterly* 13 (Winter): 3–15.

Pugh, D. S., Hickson, D. J., Hinings, C. R. et al. 1968. Dimensions of Organization Structure. *Administrative Science Quarterly* 13 (June): 65–91.

———, ———, ——— et al. 1969. The Context of Organization Structures. *Administrative Science Quarterly* 14 (March): 91–113.

Roemer, M. I. 1959. Is Surgery Safer in Large Hospitals? *Hospital Management* 87 (January): 35–37ff.

———, and Friedman, J. W. 1971. *Doctors in Hospitals.* Baltimore, Md.: The Johns Hopkins University Press.

Rushing, W. 1974. Differences in Profit and Nonprofit Organizations: A Study of Effectiveness and Efficiency in General Short-Stay Hospitals. *Administrative Science Quarterly* 19 (December): 474–484.

Scott, W. R. 1977. Effectiveness of Organizational Effectiveness Studies. In Goodman, P. S., and Pennings, J. M., eds., *New Perspectives on Organizational Effectiveness* pp. 63–95. San Francisco, Calif.: Jossey-Bass.

Shortell, S. M., Becker, S. W., and Neuhauser, D. 1976. The Effects of Management Practices on Hospital Efficiency and Quality of Care. In Shortell, S. M., and Brown, M., eds., *Organizational Research in Hospitals.* Chicago, Ill.: Blue Cross Association, Inquiry Book.

Stanford Center for Health Care Research. 1974. *The Study of Institutional Differences in Postoperative Mortality: A Report to the National Academy of Sciences-National Research Council.* Springfield, Va.: National Technical Information Service.

Steers, R. M. 1977. *Organizational Effectiveness: A Behavioral View.* Pacific Palisades, Calif.: Goodyear.

Appendix A
Rationale and Procedures Used to Standardize Services and Outcomes for Patient Health Status

The rationale and procedures for standardization are essentially the same for service intensity, duration, and outcome. To simplify this discussion, we use services as the primary example.

The Rationale for Standardization

Our approach makes the important assumption that patients with a given initial health status (including the disease for which they are being treated and their general condition at the time of admission) have a "need" for services which is (can be viewed as) constant across all hospitals. To estimate what types and amounts of services are needed by what types of patients, an empirical regression procedure is employed based on the experience of all patients in the study, ignoring in what hospital they are treated. Having determined what each patient "needs" in the way of services, we can also determine what services the patient has actually received in the study hospital under the assumption that the types and amounts of services hospitals actually provide will vary greatly. It is the discrepancy between what services a patient needs and what services are actually received that is the datum of primary interest.

How best to assess the need for services is a difficult question, both theoretically and empirically. Clearly, one of the most important determinants of the amount and types of services needed is the nature of the disease and the general condition of the patient on admission. A second important determinant, whether the patient undergoes surgery, increases the likelihood of receiving specific amounts and types of services—for example, the need for blood. A third determinant, complications that arise during the hospitalization (intermediate outcomes), also increases the likelihood of requiring additional services. A fourth determinant, leaving the hospital before complete recovery, clearly implies some "need" not only for more days of care but for specific types of services as well. Death in hospital is, of course, the extreme example of incomplete recovery and immediately ends the "need" for services.

To assess the four types of factors affecting need for hospital services, we defined four basic sets of standardization variables, incorporating over 40 different measures:

1. *Admission Status.* This set of variables included the major diagnosis explaining admission to the hospital using 332 diagnostic groups; several indicators of the patient's physiological status such as additional diagnoses, admission test findings, and severity of the disease; and several demographic characteristics such as age, sex, and a height-weight index.

2. *Surgical vs Medical Treatment.* For surgical patients, the indicators included the number of (non-diagnostic) operations and the severity of the operations undergone.

3. *Complications.* This set of variables included in-hospital infection as well as other complications.

4. *Discharge Status.* This set of variables included death at discharge, transfer to another facility, or discharge with incomplete recovery.

For most of the analyses reported here involving service intensity and duration, all four sets of standardization variables were used. The only exception occurred when the relation between services and outcomes was assessed and then, of course, the variables measuring death in hospital were excluded as predictors of services.

These four factors affecting the need for services were used to estimate the impact of a patient's health status on the amounts and types of services needed. But before detailing the standardization procedure, let us turn briefly to two additional considerations incorporated into our approach: the unit of analysis in assessing intensity of services, and the assumption of the independence of sets of services.

During a hospitalization episode, a patient can receive varying amounts of several different types of services. Some authors point out that the *rate* of services consumed during a single hospitalization is not constant, but varies by day of stay—usually being a higher rate at the beginning of the stay. We chose not to focus on the rate at which a patient consumed services, in defining the intensity of services. Instead, we examined two different measures summarizing the total amount of services received during the entire stay. We called the total amount of a given specific service consumed the "intensity" of that service delivered to the patient. The total length of stay we called the "duration" of routine services. The duration of services reflects the total amount of routine nursing and hotel services consumed. (Note that intensive nursing care is treated as a specific service and variations in nurse/patient ratios are examined as a capacity measure.)

The second assumption incorporated into our approach is the independence of services consumed, for purposes of defining the "need" of the patient for each service. In defining the seven specific medical services, we took care to group interdependent services to the extent possible. Thus, categories of drugs were grouped together as one type of service; radiographic examinations for diagnostic purposes were grouped, and so on. In this manner, we have assumed that the seven types of services can be delivered independently of the other classes of services. For example, we assume that the number of drugs does not depend on blood use, etc. Therefore, the "need" for each service can be derived independently. The one major exception to this assumption was the belief that surgery (a class of service) is interdependent with the other services so that, for example, the need for intensive care, blood, and drugs does depend on whether the patient underwent surgery. We handled this interdependence by using surgery as one of the predictor sets in assessing the need for other services.

Standardization Procedure

The standardization procedure involves assessing the needs of a patient for a given service by comparing that patient with other similar patients. The first step in determining what patients are similar is to group patients into one of the 332 diagnostic categories on the basis of their final diagnosis explaining admission. Within each diagnostic group, the standardizing variables (age, additional diagnoses, operation, discharge status, etc.) are used to predict the amount of service needed by each patient. It is important to note two consequences of this procedure. The assumption of independence of need for each service (except surgery) is made only for services supplied to the same diagnostic category of patients. And the impact of each standardization variable for predicting the need for each service can vary across diagnostic groups. For example, age could be a very important predictor of intensive care for gallbladder patients, but not so for cardiac patients. The standardization procedure described below was then performed for each of the seven specific services reported here and for duration of services separately for each of the 332 diagnostic categories, or $8 \times 332 = 2656$ times. The final index of specific service intensity was based on the seven independently adjusted measures, combined to reflect their relative costliness as detailed in the main part of this paper and in footnote 3.

In the standardization procedure, data obtained from the PAS abstracts of all 603,000 patients are pooled into one of 332 groups by final diagnosis explaining admission. Through linear regression, an estimate is obtained of the impact of each of the predictor variables on the amount of medical services of a given type received by a patient. Each estimate of the impact of the predictor variable (i.e., the unstandardized coefficient) is multiplied by the actual value of each predictor variable (e.g., age, diagnosis, number of operations, and so on) observed for a given patient. The sum of these products for a given patient provides an estimate of the amount of the service "needed" by that patient. The estimate of what is needed is based on the average experience of similar patients in the "standard hospital"—which, in this case, is simply all hospitals combined. Having determined the amount of service needed by (predicted for) the patient, we also assess the amount of service actually received. The estimate of services needed is used as the baseline for a given patient against which we can observe whether more or fewer services were actually received than expected on the basis of the patient's health status.

In a similar manner, the likelihood of dying in the hospital is calculated for each patient based on the experience of all patients having similar characteristics in the study hospitals combined, and is compared with information on whether the patient actually did die. Discrepancies are measured and, as with services, can occur in either direction. The greatest disparities occur, of course, when a patient with a low likelihood of dying actually does die and when a patient with a high likelihood of dying is discharged alive instead.

Since our primary interest is in examining the relation between structural features of hospitals and service intensity, duration, and outcome, the final step is to aggregate the standardized measures of each of these variables for all patients in each study hospital. In this paper, only a composite measure of the intensity of the specific services is examined. The composite, which combines the adjusted measures to reflect their relative costliness, is also aggregated for all patients in the study hospitals. The measures reflect whether patients in each hospital received more or fewer services than expected, remained in the hospital a longer or shorter time than expected, and experienced a better or poorer outcome than expected in comparison with other patients with similar characteristics but treated in different hospitals.

Appendix B
Measures of Hospital Control

Influence Measures

To determine the relative influence of the administrator and the heads of the physician staff in affecting various types of decisions in the study hospitals, we asked informants in each hospital to rate, on a five-point scale, the amount of influence exercised by a given position on a specific, hypothetical decision. Responses were obtained by interview or questionnaire from the following types of informants: hospital administrators, chiefs of surgery, chiefs of anesthesia, directors of nursing, ward supervisors, head nurses, and ward nurses. Positions rated include the hospital administrators, chiefs of surgery, the director of nursing services, and physicians as a group. Ratings from all respondents in the same position were first averaged; then these position scores were themselves averaged. Respondents within hospitals exhibited a very high degree of consensus in their assessments of the influence exercised by the various positions on specified decisions.

After combining the data from all hospitals, we observed that the distribution of influence by position, as expected, varied greatly by type of issue. Based on these profiles as well as on the content of the decision items, we distinguished between the "within-domain" influence of a role group and its "encroachment" into the decision terrain of other role groups. The decision item used to assess the within-domain influence of the hospital administrator was "a decision to purchase contract services, e.g., laundry." The average rating given by the respondents in each hospital to the administrator provided the hospital's score on this indicator. The same decision item also served to assess the extent of encroachment by the physicians on the terrain of the hospital administrator: the greater the reported influence of physicians as a group on this item, the higher the encroachment. To assess the within-domain influence of the chief of surgery, responses to three decision items were combined: "a decision to add a clinical service, e.g., an intensive care unit"; "a decision to add an ear-nose-throat specialty room in the operating suite"; and "a decision to terminate a major department head, e.g., the operating-suite nursing director." As before, responses from all respondents were combined into a single score for each hospital.

Coordination Measures

The ratio of supervisory to direct care personnel measures the number of supervisory and managerial personnel to the staff engaged in patient care activities. The latter group does not include physicians but does include all personnel engaged in technical support activities, such as in the laboratories. Data are drawn from a questionnaire completed by each hospital administrator. The measure of the average number of ward clerks and secretaries—a measure of coordination activities at the ward level—is based on data supplied by head nurses for each ward.

To assess the extent to which coordination was effected through use of formal rules, nursing respondents from each hospital were asked to rate on a five-point scale the degree to which explicit general nursing policies had been developed. The specific items included were dress or attire on the wards; returning to work after an illness; and conditions for which nurses could be requested to work overtime. For each hospital, average ratings were obtained from the ward supervisors as a group, the head nurses as a group, and from non-rotating staff nurses working on the day shift as a group. The ratings were then combined into a grand mean for each hospital.

Control Within the Physician Staff

To assess the extent of control exercised by the physician staff over new staff members, several questions were asked of the chief of surgery. The questions sought information on: 1) the existence of separately defined probationary periods for different surgical specialties; 2) the presence of any waivers of probationary period (no waivers receiving a higher score); 3) the number of groups or positions that must review applications for staff privileges; and 4) the length of the usual probationary period. Reponses to these questions were standard-Z-scored, and then added together to provide a composite index.

A similar approach was used to assess the control exercised by the physician staff over its tenured members. The questions provided information on: 1) restrictions on the surgical privileges granted to general practitioners; 2) the use—not simply the existence—of written procedures to review the surgical privileges already granted; 3) the number of years for which privileges are granted (item reversed so that shorter periods received higher scores); and 4) the existence of explicit criteria defining who can serve as the first assistant to the surgeon. As before, all information was obtained through an interview with the chief of surgery; items were standard-scored before being combined into a composite index.

Roemer and Friedman (1971) have argued that the proportion of contract physicians on the medical staff is a good indicator of the extent to which the physician staff organization is tightly organized. Information for this measure is provided by the administrator for each hospital.

The larger project of which this study is a part was carried out under Contract HRA 230-75-0169 with the National Center for Health Services Research, Health Resources Administration, Department of Health, Education, and Welfare.

The Commission on Professional and Hospital Activities (CPHA) of Ann Arbor, Michigan, collaborated with the Center to provide data for this study. These data were supplied by CPHA only at the request and upon the authorization of the hospitals whose data were used. Any analysis, interpretation, or conclusion based on these data is solely that of the Center, and CPHA expressly disclaims any responsibility for any such analysis, interpretation, or conclusion.

Acknowledgments: We are indebted to all our colleagues at the Stanford Center for Health Care Research at Stanford University. We particularly acknowledge the help of William H. Forrest, Jr., director of the Center; Byron William Brown, Jr., who contributed statistical advice; and Betty Maxwell, coordinator and administrative assistant, who provided innumerable support services.

Address correspondence to: Prof. W. Richard Scott, Department of Sociology, Stanford University, Stanford, California 94305.

Prepaid Group Practice
and the
New "Demanding Patient"

ELIOT FREIDSON

Based on an extensive field study of the practitioners in a large, prepaid service contract group practice, this paper discusses how a prepaid service contract and closed-panel practice brings a new dimension into doctor-patient relations and how physicians respond to it. Unable to manage "unreasonable" demands for service by use of a fee-barrier or encouragement to "go elsewhere," as in traditional, solo, fee-for-service practice, they were particularly upset by a new type of "demanding patient" who claimed services on the basis of contractual rights and threatened appeal to higher bureaucratic authority. Modes of dealing with such patients are briefly discussed.

The future dimensions of medical practice in the United States are beginning to emerge now, both through the steady increase in prepaid insurance coverage for ambulatory care, and through the pressure on physicians to work together in organizations. But what will be the impact of those changes on the people involved, and on their relationships with each other? What will the doctor-patient relationship be like? There can be little doubt that prepaid medical care insurance plans will, by changing the economic relationship between doctor and patient, also change many ways in which they interact with each other. And there can also be little doubt that when physicians routinely work in organizations where they are cooperating rather than competing with colleagues, other elements of their relationships with patients and colleagues will change.

Obvious as it is that change will occur, we have rather little information relevant to anticipating its human consequences. We have fairly good estimates of the economic consequences of those changes in the organization of medical care, and we have hopeful evidence on how the medical quality of care might be affected, but between the input and output measures there is only a black box: we have little information on how the human beings in medical practice produce the results which are measured, on the quality of their experience in practice, and on the characteristic ways they try to manage their problems at work. Without knowing something about that, it is rather difficult to anticipate how doctor-patient relationships will change and what problems will be embedded in them.

This paper is an attempt to provide some information about how the participants in a medical care program which anticipated present-day trends responded to each other and to the economic and social structure of practice. The data upon which I shall draw come from an eighteen-month-long field study of the physicians who worked in a large, prepaid group practice. Most of the primary practitioners (internists and pediatricians) worked on a full-time basis in the medical group, and most of the consultants worked part-time, but all fifty-five of them were on salary, officially employees of the institution. Their medical group contracted with an insurance organization to provide virtually complete care to insured patients without imposing on them any out-of-pocket charges. In studying the physicians of the medical group, a very large amount of observational, documentary, and direct evidence was collected in the course of examining files, attending all staff meetings, listening to luncheon-table conversations, and carrying out a series of intensive interviews with all the physicians in the group. The research obtained a systematic and comprehensive view of how the group physicians worked and what their problems were. Because of a lack of space here, however, only a summary of findings bearing on a single issue is possible.

The Administrative Structure of the Group

To understand practice in the medical group, it is necessary to understand the framework in which it was carried out. The group did not have an elaborate administrative structure, since it lacked clear gradations of rank and authority and had rather few written, formal rules. It was not organized like a traditional bureaucratic organization. The few rules which were bureaucratically enforced all dealt in one way or another with the *terms* of work—with how and what the physician was to be paid, and the amount of time he was to work in return for that pay. Ultimately, the terms of work were less a function of the medical group administration than of the health insurance organization with which the medical group entered into a contract. The absolute income available for paying the doctors derived primarily from the insurance contract, which specified a given sum per year per insured person or family, plus additional sums by a complicated formula not important for present purposes. The administration of the medical group could decide how to divide up the contract income among the physicians but had to work within the absolute limits of that income.

By the same token, critical aspects of the *conditions* of work stemmed more from the terms of the service contract than from the choice and action of the group administration. The most important complaint of the physicians about the conditions of work in the medical group was of "overload"—having to provide more services in a given period of time than was considered appropriate. Such "overload" was a direct function of the prepaid service contract, which freed the subscriber from having to pay a separate fee for each service he wished, and encouraged many physicians to manage patient demands by increasing referrals and reappointments.

It was around these externally formulated contractual arrangements that we found the administration of the medical group establishing and enforcing the firmest bureaucratic rules, perhaps because it had no other choice than to do so in order to satisfy its contract to provide services. The prepaid service-contract arrangement could be conceived of as purely economic in character —simply a rational way of *paying* for health care, which did not influence health care itself. But it was much more than that, since it organized demand and supply, the processes by which health care takes place. In fact, it was closely connected with many of the problems of practice in the group. This is not to say that it created those problems in and of itself. Rather, it gave rise to new possibilities for problematic behavior on the part of both patient and physician and prevented the use by both of traditional solutions. To understand its relationship to the problems of practice in the medical group, to the way the physicians made sense of their experience, and to the ways they attempted to cope with it, let us first examine the way the physicians responded to the differences they perceived between prepaid service-contract group practice and private, fee-for-service solo practice.

The Meanings of Entrepreneurial and Contract Group Practice

All of the physicians interviewed, including those who had left the group and were solo practitioners at the time of being interviewed, had at one time or another worked on a salary in the medical group. Thus, they reported on circumstances in which they could not themselves charge the patient a fee for the services they rendered. Their income was independent of the services they gave, just as the cost to the patient was independent of the services he received. The patient demanded and the physician supplied services on the basis of a prepayment contract which established a right for the patient and an obligation for the physician. Furthermore, the group was organized on a closed-panel basis, so that in order to obtain services by the terms of his contract, without out-of-pocket cost, the patient had to seek service only from the physicians working at the medical group, and no others.

Virtually all of the physicians interviewed had also had occasion to work on the traditional basis of solo, fee-for-service "private" practice. In that mode of organizing work and the marketplace, the physician makes a living by attracting patients and providing them with services paid for by a fee for each service. The physician's income is directly related to the fee charged and the number of services provided. He has no contractual relationship with patients. He must attract them by a variety of devices—accessibility, reputation, specialty, referral relations with colleagues—and maintain a sufficiently steady stream of new or returning patients to assure a stable if not lucrative practice. In theory, the patient is free to leave him for another physician, and relations with colleagues offering the same services are at least nominally competitive.

How did the physicians interpret these different arrangements and what did they emphasize in their experience with each? In the interviews, the prepaid group physician was often represented as helpless and exploited, with words like "trapped," "slave," and "servitor" used to describe his position. Since the contract was for all "necessary" services, however, it was hardly accurate to say that the physicians had to provide every service the patient demanded. They could have refused. But at bottom it was not really the formal contract which was the issue. Rather, the physicians were responding to the absence of a mechanism to which they were accustomed, a mechanism which, by attesting to the value of the physician's services in the eyes of the patient, and by testing the strength of the patient's sense of need, precluded the necessity of actually refusing. The physicians were responding to the absence of the out-of-pocket fee which is a prerequisite for service in "private practice."

The fee was seen as a useful barrier between patient and doctor which forced the *patient* to discriminate between the trivial and the important before he sought care. The assumption was that if the patient had to pay a fee for each service, he would ask only for "necessary" services, or, if he were too irrational or ignorant to discriminate accurately, he would at the very least restrict his demands to those occasions when he was really greatly worried. The fee served as a mechanical barrier which freed the physician of the necessity of having to refuse service and of having to persuade the patient that his grounds for doing so were reasonable. Since a fee operates as a barrier in advance of any request for service, it reduces interaction between physician and patient. In the prepaid plan, the physicians were not prepared for the greater interaction which the absence of a fee encouraged.

In addition to the service contract, there was also the closed-panel organization of the medical group. The physicians themselves were aware that some patients often felt trapped, since, in order to receive the benefits of their contract, they had to use the services only of a physician employed by the medical group. If he wanted to be treated by a particular individual in the group, he might nonetheless have had to accept another because of the former's full panel or appointment schedule. And when patients were referred to consultants, they were supposed to be referred to a specialty, not to an individual specialist. Some of the physicians themselves found this situation unsatisfactory because they were not personally chosen by patients, but were seen by patients because they happened to have appointment time free or openings on their panel, not because of their individual reputation or attractiveness.

Finally, there was the issue of group practice itself, of the constitution of a cooperative collegium rather than, as in entrepreneurial practice, an aggregate of nominally competing practitioners. In the latter case, the physician may be "scared that somebody would . . . take his patient away," or that the patient may "walk out the door and you may never see him again." Nevertheless, if he can afford it, the physician in fee-for-service solo practice can choose to refuse to give the patient what he asks for, and can even discourage him from returning. But in the group practice, the physicians did not generally have the option of dropping a patient with whom they had difficulty. The reason was not to be found in any potential economic loss, as in entrepreneurial practice, but rather in the closed-panel practice within which colleagues were cooperating rather than competing. When physicians form a closed-panel group, they cannot simply act as individuals, "drop" a patient who is troublesome, and allow him to go to a colleague, for if each of the group dropped his own problem patients, while he would indeed get rid of the ones he had, he would get in return those his colleagues had dropped, as his colleagues would get his. And so the pressure was to "live" with such patients and try to manage them as best one could— something for which the physician with ideological roots in private practice was poorly prepared.

From the view which the physicians presented, it seemed that the medical group involved them in a situation in which traditional safety valves had been tied down and the pressure increased. The service contract was thought to increase patient demand for services, while at the same time it prevented the physician from coping with that demand by the traditional method of raising prices. The closed-panel arrangement restricted the patients' demands to those physicians working cooperatively in the medical group, so the physicians could not cope with the pressure by the traditional method of encouraging the troublesome patient to go elsewhere for service. Confrontation between patient and physician was increased, and both participants explored new methods for resolving them. Indeed, the insurance scheme itself provided the resources for some of those new methods of reducing the pressure on demand and supply.

Paradigmatic Problems and Solutions

The basic interpersonal paradigm of a problematic doctor-patient relationship may be seen as a conflict between perspectives and a struggle for control or a negotiation over the provision of services. From his perspective the patient believes he needs a particular service; from his, the physician does not believe every service the patient wishes is necessary or appropriate. The content of this conflict between perspectives is composed of conceptions of knowledge, or expertise, the physician asserting that he knows best and the patient insisting that he is his own arbiter of need.

The conflict, however, takes place in a social and economic marketplace which provides resources that may be used to reinforce the one or the other position. In the case of medicine in the United States, that marketplace has in the past been organized on a fee-for-service basis, practitioners being entrepreneurs competing with each other for the fees of prospective patients. The fee the patient is willing and able to pay, in conjunction with the physician's economic security, constitute elements which are of strategic importance to private practice. If the physician's practice is well enough established, he can refuse service he does not want to give or does not believe necessary to give, even though he loses a fee and possibly a patient. On the other hand, if he desires to gain the fee and reduce the chance of "losing" the patient, he may give the patient the service he requests even if he believes it to be unnecessary. Like a merchant, he is concerned with pleasing his patients by giving them what they want, suspending his own notions of what is necessary and good for them in favor of his gain in income should he desire such gain.

The patient, on the other hand, has his fee as a resource (if he is lucky), and the freedom to turn away from the practitioner who does not provide him with the service he wants and pay it instead to the physician who does. He may take his trade elsewhere, but before he does he may introduce pressure by implying that if he does not get what he wants he will find someone else. In essence, the patient can play "customer" to the physician's merchant.

In contrast to these marketplace roles, there are those more often ascribed to doctor and patient by sociologists—that of expert consultant and layman. The layman is defined as someone who has a problem or difficulty he wishes resolved, but who does not have the special knowledge and skill needed to do so. He seeks out someone who has the necessary knowledge and skill and cooperates with him so that his difficulty can be managed if not resolved. In dealing with the expert, the layman is supposed to suspend his own judgment and instead follow the advice of the expert, who is considered to have superior knowledge and better judgment. When there are differences of opinion of such character that the patient cannot bring himself to cooperate, the *generic* response of the expert is to attempt to gain the patient's cooperation by persuading him, on the basis of evidence which the expert produces, that it would be in his interest to cooperate and follow the recommended course. To *order* him to comply, or to gain compliance by some other form of coercion or pressure, is a contradiction of the essence of expertise and its "authority." Analytically, expertise gains its "authority" by its persuasive demonstration of special knowledge and skill relevant to particular problems requiring solution. It is the antithesis of the authority of office.

As a profession, however, medicine represents not only a full-time occupation possessed of expertise which participates in a marketplace where it sells its labor for a profit, but more particularly an occupation which has gained a specially protected position in the marketplace and a set of formal prerogatives which grant it some degree of official authority. For example, the mere possession of a legal license to practice allows the physician to officially certify death or disability, and to authorize pharmacists to dispense a variety of powerful and dangerous drugs. Here, albeit in rudimentary form, we find yet a third facet by which to characterize a third kind of doctor-patient relationship—that of the bureaucratic official and client. The latter seeks a given service from the former, who has exclusive control over access to services. The client seeks to establish his need and his right, while the official seeks to establish his eligibility before providing service or access to goods or services. In theory, both are bound by a set of rules which defines the rights and duties of the participants, and each makes reference to the rules in making and evaluating claims. In a rational-legal form of administration, both have a right of appeal to some higher authority who is empowered to mediate and resolve their differences.

In the predominant form of practice in present-day United States, the physician is more likely to be playing the role of merchant and expert than the role of official, though the latter is real enough and too important to be as ignored as it has been by sociologists and physicians alike. It is, after all, his status as an official which gives the physician a protected marketplace in which to be a merchant. Nonetheless, to be a true official virtually precludes being a merchant, so that only in special instances in the United States can we find medical practice which offers the possibility of taking the role of official on an everyday rather than an occasional basis.

The medical group we studied was just such a special instance, for it eliminated the fee and discouraged the profit motive, while setting up its physicians as official gatekeepers to services specified in a contract with patients, through an insurance agency with supervisory powers of its own. The contractual network specified the basic set of systematic rules, and established the official position of the physician. Under the rules, the physician served as an official gatekeeper to and authorizer of a whole array of services— not only his own, but also those of consultants who, even though "covered" in the contract, would not see a patient without an official referral, and those of laboratories, which do not provide "covered" tests without an official group physician's signature. In other reports of this study I show how the physicians were led to use their official powers to cope with problems of work, and how they exercised their role of expert. I also show how some railed against a situation which prevented them from using the more familiar techniques of the merchant to resolve their problems.

Here, however, I wish to point out that in the medical group the physician was not the only participant to whom a new role was made available. The situation, which left open the option of official and closed the option of merchant for physicians, also left open the option of bureaucratic client and closed the option of shopper or customer for patients. And when the patients acted as bureaucratic clients they posed different problems to the physician than they did when they acted as a customer, or as a patient: they asserted their rights in light of the rules of the contract. This untraditional possibility for patient behavior was one which upset the physicians a great deal and served as the focus for much of their dissatisfaction. Most of their problems of work stemmed ultimately from their relationships with patients and tended to be characterized in terms of the patient, so that it is important to understand the way the physicians saw their patients. Typically, work problems stemmed from patients who "make demands"; "the demanding patient" was seen to lie at the root of those difficulties.

Three Types of "Demanding Patients"

It is very easy to get the impression from this analysis that the work-lives of the group physicians were constantly fraught with pressure and conflict. Such an impression stems partially from the strategy of analysis I have chosen, a strategy which focuses on work problems rather than on the settled, everyday routines which stretch out on either side of occasional crises. Without remembering that most medical work is routine rather than crisis, one could not understand how physicians manage to get through their days. Indeed, the kinds of medical complaints and symptoms which are most often brought into the office were such that the daily routine posed a serious problem of boredom to the practitioners. Furthermore, most patients were not troublesome. As members of the stable blue- and white-collar classes, most knew the rules of the game, respected the physicians, and were more inclined than not to come in with medically acceptable (even if "trivial") complaints.

Nonetheless, the fact of routine, even boredom, would be difficult to discern in the physicians' own conversations. They did not talk to each other, or to the interviewers, about their routines; they talked about their crises. They did not talk about slow days, but about those when the work pressure was overwhelming. They rarely talked about "good" patients unless they received some unusual letter of thanks, card, or gift of which they were proud; they talked incessantly about troublesome or demanding patients. They almost never talked about routine diagnoses and their management, but talked often about the anomaly, the interesting case, or one of their "goofs." So the analytical strategy for reporting this study is not arbitrary, since it reflects the physicians' own preoccupations. It was by the problematic that they symbolized their work and it was in terms of the problematic that they evaluated their practice. Even though all agreed that "demanding patients" were statistically few in number, many who left the medical group ascribed their departure to their inability to bear even those few patients.

Most important for present purposes was the fact that, upon analysis of the physicians' discussion of "demanding patients," it was discovered that the most important type was a new one for them. They posed demands which the physicians were unaccustomed to dealing with, for the demands stemmed from the contractual framework of practice in the medical group and were generic to the role of the bureaucratic client rather than the customer or layman. Perhaps this was why they seemed so outrageous and insulting, for such demands treated the physicians as if they were officials rather than "free professionals." The distinction between that kind of demandingness and others was more often implicit than explicit in the physicians' talk when they were asked to characterize demanding patients. The tendency, however, was to distinguish one kind of demanding patient as dictatorial and another as essentially the opposite—eternally supplicant.

Of the two kinds of demanding patients, one would be familiar to the informed reader as the ambulatory practice version of the "crock" met in complaints by medical students and the house staff in the clinics of teaching hospitals. The crock was the person who played the respectful patient role, but presented complaints for which the physician had no antibiotic, vaccine, chemical agent, or technique for surgical repair. All the physician could provide for such complaints was what he considered "palliative" treatment rather than "cure." He neither learned anything interesting by seeing some biologically unusual condition nor felt he accomplished successful therapy. And he worried that he might overlook something "real."

Clearly, this kind of demanding patient was irritating because he had to be babied rather than treated instrumentally and because the doctor had to devote himself to "treating people [whom he considers to be] well, or have the same kind of anxieties we all have." Furthermore, he confronted the doctor with failure: he "can never be reassured. You know you are not getting anywhere with him and you just have to listen to him, the same chronic minor complaints and the same business." "I'm just not satisfied with my results, and the patient just keeps coming back, worse than ever."

In light of the distinctions I made earlier, it should be clear that this kind of demanding person was not playing either the role of bureaucratic client or that of customer. The role of the helpless layman was adopted, which did not contradict the role the physician wished to play. The problem was that the nature of the complaints was such that the medical worker could not play his role in a satisfying way—he could not really help, and his advice that there was no serious medical problem was refused.

The other kind of demanding patient was quite different, however, for he did not ceaselessly *beg* for help so much as *demand* services on the basis of his economic and contractual rights. Such rights do not, of course, exist in fee-for-service solo practice, but the analogue in such practice would be the demanding customer. Such a person is more likely to shop around from one physician to another rather than stick to one and demand his service. Given the structure of fee-for-service solo practice, we should expect in it rather less confrontation with demanding customers, though the physicians did tell stories about some who openly threatened to take their business elsewhere if they did not get what they wanted. Rare as such confrontation was, when it did occur, it was described with the same shock and outrage as was observed in the physicians' stories about demanding contract patients.

The "power of the contract" which one physician spoke of implied correctly that some patients, playing the role of bureaucratic client, threatened to and on occasion actually employed the device of an official complaint. They could complain either to the administration of the medical group or to an office established by the insuring organization to receive and investigate complaints. After all, if one has a contract, one also has the right to appeal decisions about its benefits. And naturally, the more familiar and effective with bureaucratic procedures the patients were, the more were they able to make trouble. The seventeen physicians who generalized about the social characteristic of demanding patients yielded in sum a caricature of the demanding patient as a female schoolteacher, well educated enough to be capable of articulate and critical questioning and letter writing, of high enough social status to be sensitive to slight and to expect satisfaction, and experienced with bureaucratic procedures. In the physicians' eyes, they were also neurotically motivated to be "demanding."

Also specially nurtured in the framework of the prepaid group practice—contrary to the ideal of bureaucracy but faithful to its reality—was the use by the bureaucratic client of "pull" or political influence to reinforce his demands and gain more than nominal contract benefits. Analogous to political influence in the free medical marketplace is the possession of wealth or prestige, making one a desirable customer who may refer his friends to the physician. Another form of "pull" lies in having connections with an especially influential and prestigious medical colleague. Both types of patients gain special handling in solo practice. In the medical group, however, "pull" was more related to influence in those segments of the community engaged in negotiating insurance contracts. There were occasional instances when a demanding patient was also an important member of a trade union, or had friends in high political places. Managing such patients was particularly difficult for the administration, since it was unable to protect its own staff in the face of such political influence.

Managing Demanding Patients in the Future

In this paper I have assumed that a prepaid service-contract medical group has important characteristics which will become more common in the future and which, therefore, allow us to make plausible and informed anticipations of the problems of medical practice in the future. On the basis of extensive interviews with physicians who worked in such a medical group, I suggested that a new kind of problem of management was posed to them by the social and economic structure of their practice. Ostensibly, the problem was the familiar and traditional one of the "demanding patient." Looking more closely at the usage of that phrase, however, led to the conclusion that there was more than one kind of "demanding patient." Indeed, on the basis of the physicians' discussions of their problems, I suggested that there were three types of demanding patients, each posing a different problem of management and a different challenge to medical self-esteem.

Virtually unmet in the medical group (but mentioned by the physicians) were those who acted like demanding customers by insisting on either obtaining the services they wished or of taking their business (and fees) elsewhere. Such a strategy is of course generic to entrepreneurial practice, and most effective with weakly established practitioners in a highly competitive medical market. The second type of demanding patient was the traditional "crock," what a spokesman for Kaiser-Permanente once called "the worried well." Such a patient persisted in seeking consultation for complaints which the physicians felt were trivial and essentially incurable. They were a more serious problem in the medical group than they were reported to be in fee-for-service solo practice because their demands could not be reduced by the imposition of a fee barrier or by suggesting that they go elsewhere for service. The third type of demanding patient was new and particularly disturbing to the physicians—the patient who demanded services which he felt he had a right to under the terms of his prepaid service contract and who had recourse to complaining about the deprivation of his rights to the bureaucratic system of appeal and review.

In the future, with prepaid group practice far more common, we should expect new problems in the doctor-patient relationship as that new kind of demanding patient is met with by more physicians. Insurance coverage in the future may be such as to maintain some kind of fee barrier (as in prepaid plans which now impose small charges for house calls), but the barrier will be less than that to which physicians were accustomed in fee-for-service practice and will be less effective in discouraging demandingness. In addition, since he will be working cooperatively with colleagues in group practice, the physician will be less able to simply "drop" his demanding patients. Unable to use money or evasion to cope with his relationship to problem patients, the physician will have to use other methods. What options are open to him?

Just as the structure of fee-for-service solo practice produces the possibility of using mechanical financial solutions, so does the structure of prepaid service-contract practice also produce the possibility of using mechanical solutions. The mechanical solutions observed in the medical group studied lay in providing all services covered by the contract which were not inconvenient to the practitioner—office visits, referrals, and laboratory tests. (The house call was not convenient, and was resisted strongly.) But whereas the former solutions were traditional and so regarded as "natural" and "reasonable," the use of the latter was regarded as "giving in," and treated with resentment and concern. Both are, analytically, equally mechanical, an equally passive reflex to the organization of the system of care.

The consequences of passive response to the new conditions by which patient demand will be structured are already clear. In the face of rising services and costs, strong administrative, financial, and peer-review pressures will force the physician to limit his "giving in" and restrict the supply of demanded services. But how exactly can the physician limit services, and what kind of inter-action will go on between him and his patient under such circum-stances? I cannot provide empirical evidence from my study be-cause in the medical group there was rather little organized pressure to limit services. The physicians could "give in" when they chose to. But the logic of my analysis would lead me to expect that when there is pressure to limit service to demanding patients in a structure like that of the medical group, the structure taken by itself provides the opportunity for doing so on the bureaucratic grounds of the official authority of the physician as a gatekeeper to benefits. He can simply refuse the patient, standing on the of-ficial position which the structure provides him.

But it need not be that way. While the prepaid service-contract group practice virtually precluded the adoption by physi-cian and patient of a merchant-customer relationship, and allowed the adoption of an official-client relationship which was precluded in private solo practice, it did not *force* the practitioners to manage their problems that way. Some chose to adopt the interactional strategy which is an inherent possibility in medical practice no matter what the historical framework in which it takes place—the strategy of the expert consultant who relies neither on his position in the marketplace nor on his official position in a bureaucratic system but on his knowledge and skill. Some physicians were persuaded that if they invested extra attention and energy in "educating" their patients and developing a relationship of trust they would ultimately have fewer "management" problems. To cope with suspicion on the part of the patient they initially pro-vided services on demand in order to show that they recognized the legitimacy of the patient's contractual rights, and that they were not motivated to withhold services from them. At the same time, however, they tried to explain to the demanding patient the grounds for their judgment that the services were medically un-necessary. They undertook, in other words, to persuade and demonstrate, and avoided mechanical solutions to the problem of demandingness. The social, moral, and technical quality of the medical care of the future will depend on whether medical practice will be organized in such a way as to encourage such a positive mode of responding to patient demands, or whether it will, like traditional practice, be merely a fiscally and technically functional structure which does not take cognizance of the human qualities of those it traps.

E. Freidson
Rm. 308, Sociology
19 University Place
New York University
New York, N.Y. 10003

Abridged version of a chapter of Eliot Freidson, *Doctoring Together* (Chicago: Aldine Publishing Company, forthcoming). Copyright © 1974 by Eliot Freidson. All rights reserved. The study reported here was partially supported by USPH grants RG-7882, GM-07882, CH-00025, CH-00414, and HS-00104.

Index

Accessibility, in health services system, 94, 95

Accountability
bureaucratization and, 51
of consumer representative, 22–25, 35
in licensure process, 240
of professional associations, 239

Accreditation, 233

Administration, hospital
and competition for physicians, 351
efficiency of, 50–51
and hospital stay length, 401
and hospital structure measurement, 393–394
influence of, 414–415
medical staff and, 339, 340
National Health Service, 375
and per patient expenditures, 404
power of, 192
and quality of care, 400–401, 404–405

Administration, program, 20. See also Health Services Agencies

Admissions, hospital. See also Hospital utilization
and costs, 347–348
prepaid group practices and, 264–265
rates, 105–106
societal norms and, 98

Advertising, 283

Advisory Committee, National Health Services, 376

Age
adult, and treatment decision, 321–323
and patient satisfaction, 172, 173, 180, 184–185
and physician-patient relationships, 214–215
and response to symptoms, 121
and utilization behavior, 131

Agencies, health care. See also Bureaucracy
consumer interaction with, 142
middle class and, 145–146
stigmatization, 136
working class and, 143–144

Agency capture, 20

Alienation
of lower class, agencies, and 143–144, 149

and utilization, 139–142

Ambulatory care
inpatient costs and, 76–79
physician direction of, 259–264
and professional authority, 211

American Hospital Association (AHA)
and creation of Blue Cross, 195
and physician participation in hospital management, 365

American Medical Association (AMA)
and alternative payment methods, 357
and hospital administration, 240–341, 366
and physician participation in hospital management, 365

Ancillary services. See also Physicians' assistants
in group practice, 296, 353
licensing of personnel, 235
management and, 297
in measurement of hospital structure, 393
method of payment and, 287–288
in National Health Service, 370–371, 375
office vs. hospital, 344
in office practice, 290
physicians and, 262, 286
and professional authority, 210, 218
transference of function to, 342
size of sector, 279
utilization, per patient day, 346, 347

Anencephaly, 328, 330

Attitudes. See also Ideology; Patient satisfaction; Values
concerning health and illness, 126
family, and critical illness treatment, 325, 326
and individual utilization, 101–102, 109
and patient satisfaction, 151–156
and professional authority, 226
traditional, 144
working class, 143–144

Autonomy
credentialing system and, 233
institutional licensure and, 243
professional licensing and, 234–237

Bed/population ratios, 94

436

437

438

inputs vs. health outcomes, 352
rights to, 88
Medical necessity
and admissions to hospital, 348
and appropriate use, 77–78
differential experience of symptoms
and, 121–122
and illness, perception of, 128
perception of, 118–128, 349
stress and, 122–126
Medicare
Analysis of Days of Care (MADOC),
265
dual billing and, 342–343
and increases in services to, 287
and monitoring of physician services,
250
and utilization review, 250
Medicare Act of 1965, 250, 251–252
Medicredit, 202
Mental damage, 311, 314, 316, 319–
321
Mental illness
changing norms of, 96
stigma of, 138
Middle class. *See* Social class
Minimum wage laws, 342
Minority groups. See Culture; Race;
Social class
Models of man, and policy, 1–13
Monopoly
demonopolization of knowledge, 211
health care providers, 202
and Hirschman analysis, 9, 10–11
on information, 50
physician services, 283–284
and professional authority, 209, 227
Mortality trends, 96
Myelomeningocele, 330–331

National Advisory Commission on
Health Manpower, 365
National health insurance
income and consumer use of, 66
and monitoring of physician services,
250
physician payment and, 297
and systemic model, 198
National Health Planning and Resources Development Act of 1974,
16, 45, 255
accountability in, 25
and conflicts, 49–51
and litigation, 41–45
planning, organization, and responsibilities under, 381, 382
and representation, 27, 30–31

National Health Service (NHS), British
and organization, 376–377
and district organization, 369–376
and Hirschman's model, 9
and implications for U. S., 381–383
machinery in practice, 378–383
and national organization, 377–378
and regional organization, 377
Need for care. *See* Medical necessity
Neurosurgery and financial burden of
illness, 324
questionnaires, 306–307, 310, 312
New York Health Insurance Plan.
(HIP), 287
NHS. *See* National Health Service,
British
Non-medical benefits, and professional
authority, 225
Non-profit motivation model, of medical organization, 194–197
Norms, 93. *See also* Values
and individual utilization, 102, 109,
110
of medical profession, USSR, 249
and societal determinants of utilization, 96
and stigmas, 133–139
Nurse practitioners, 243. *See also* Ancillary services
patient satisfaction with, 173
and professional authority, 210
Nurses
and duration of services, 403
in NHS, 375
transference of function of, 342

Occupational therapy, 238. *See also* Ancillary services
Office practice
ancillary services in, 290
costs of, vs. hospitalization, 289–290
vs. outpatient care, 77
Organization. *See also* Hospital
organization
in health services system, 94, 95
innovation in forms of, 150–151
and orientations towards clients, 143
Organizations, social control of, 191
idiosyncratic needs model of, 200–202
medical, 192–193
models of behavior and control of,
193–202
non-profit motivational models of,
194–197
sociological imagination and, 203–204
systemic model of, 197–200
Outpatient care. *See* Ambulatory care

Paraprofessionals. *See* Ancillary services
Participation, public, and accountability, 23, 25. *See also* Consumer representation
Parsons, R., 120, 304
Patient care
bureaucratization of, 211
physician participation in hospital management and, 367
Patients. *See also* Clients; Consumers; Consumer use; Critically ill patients; Doctor-patient relationship
expectations of, 254
medical error and, 270
and PSRO decisions, 255
Patients, demanding. *See also* Doctor-patient relationship
and future management, 429–432
and physician attitudes, 425
in prepaid group practice, 421–422
three types of, 426–429
Patient satisfaction. *See also* Doctor-patient relationship; Physician authority
and availability of medical services, 89
categories of, 171–174
continuity of care and, 183–184
and evaluations of care, 176–178
medical encounter characteristics and, 181–184
and patient characteristics, 176, 179–180
and patient encounter form, 176
and utilization behavior, 151–156
with waiting time, 172–173
Payment. *See* Physician payment
Peer review, and treatment decisions, 331. *See also* Professional Standards Review Organizations
Pediatricians
and brain death criterion, 328
and financial burden of illness, 324
patient satisfaction with, 172–173
questionnaires for, 306, 308–309, 315
treatment decisions of, 319, 326
Personnel. *See also* Ancillary services
and individual utilization, 102, 109, 110
middle class interaction with, 145
new categories of, 150
and per diem hospital costs, 341
physician participation in decisions, 365
population ratios, 94
and stigma, 136
Physician authority, 208
age and, 214–215
bureaucracy and, 217–219

education and, 215–217
future of, 225–229
history, culture, and ideology of, 220–225
individual characteristics of, 214–217
research findings on, 212–225
societal characteristics of, 217–225
technology and, 219–220
theoretical issues of, 208, 212
Physician payment
and hospital utilization, 350–351
and hospital cost containment, 357–360
and surgical utilization, 349
Physician payment, alternative methods of
and efficiency of physician practice, 295–296
and location decision, 291–293
and National Health Insurance, 297–298
physician pricing, income vs. utility maximization, 282–285
policy issues of, 285–287
and specialty choice, 293–295
three methods of, 280–282
and treatment setting, 288–291
and utilization of physician and non-physician services, 287–288
Physicians. *See also* Doctor-patient relationship; Hospital decision-making, physicians and; Specialists; Surgeons
and admission decisions, 347–349
and ancillary personnel use, 342, 344, 346, 347
dual billing and, 338
economic incentives and, 350–351
and euthanasia, 327
experience of, and hospital stay length, 401
financial risk, and hospitalization, 290
free hospital services to, 289
and group practice, 420–422
and hospital behavior models, 338–339
and hospital costs, 343
income vs. fees for, 343
and internal efficiency of practice, 295–297
and medical necessity, 78
in NHS, 374–375, 380, 381 (*see also* National Health Service, British)
and office care vs. outpatient care, 77
and readiness to initiate care, 129, 130
and resource decision, 339–340
response to utilization of, 77
role of, 423–425

440

vs. individual determinants, 90–92
and policy, 110, 111
social structure and, 101, 109, 110
trends and relationships in, 95–98
Sociological models
doctor/patient relationship, 423–424
of man, 4
Soviet Union
vs. Great Britain, socialized medicine
in, 212–213
physician visits in, 249
Soviet Union, professional authority in,
213, 228
age of patient and, 215
education and, 215–217
history, culture, and ideology in, 222–
225
technology and, 219–220
Specialists
capitation and, 295
and referral rates, 253–264
third party payments and, 294
Specialization
choice of, payment methods in, 293–
295
technology and, 356
of treatment centers, 346
Staff, physician, 415–416
Staffing, hospital, 403
State. *See also* Government
and licensing boards, 240
and professional autonomy, 233–234
Status. *See also* Social class
alienation and, 140
chronic illness and, 125
stigma and labeling process, 133–139
Stay length. *See also* Hospital utilization
as measurement of service duration,
389–390
organizational capacity and, 398–401
physician and, 265
predictors of, 401
Stigma, and utilization behavior, 133–
139
Stress, and illness, 122–126
Strikes, physicians and, 381
Supply, physician
and medical utilization, 284–285
restricting, and competition, 283
Surgeons
fee-for-service systems and, 293
third party payments and, 294
treatment decisions, 306–309, 310,
312, 317, 319
Surgery
comparative rates for selected operations, 271

GHI vs. HIP plan, 349
per patient day, 345
surgeon supply and, 284–285
unnecessary, 269–270, 294
in U. S. vs. Great Britain, 288, 350
Sweden, utilization in, 61, 65
Symptoms
and decision to seek care, 129–130
differential experience of, 121–122
vs. measure of perceived illness, 103
recognition of, 119–121
stress and, 122–124
Systemic model, of medical organization, 197–200

Tastes
as determinant of care use, 59, 66–68
and level of care, 78–80
Technology, 93
and growth in ancillary service use,
346
and health planning, 47–51
and health services system, 96
and hospital utilization, 355
and professional authority, 220–221,
227
specialization and, 356
Terminal illness, 316, 318
Testing, diagnostic, hospitalization for,
344
Third-party payment plans
and accessibility, 95
and hospital care costs to consumer,
337–338
and special vs. primary care physicians, 294
societal norms and, 97–98
Trustees, hospital, 340

United States
National Health Services model and,
381–383
surgery and radiology utilization in,
350–351
surgical rates in, 271
User charges
and consumer use, 70–74
with indemnity insurance, 79
Utilization, of services, 99–108. *See also*
Consumer use, economic aspects of;
Hospital utilization; Physicians, and
health services use; Price and consumer use
alienation and, 139–142
characteristics of, 90–92
consumer-agency interactions, 142–
157

443